Socialism Mediated

Socialism Mediated

The Making of Soviet Culture in Central Asia

CLAIRE ROOSIEN

OXFORD
UNIVERSITY PRESS

OXFORD
UNIVERSITY PRESS

Great Clarendon Street, Oxford, OX2 6DP,
United Kingdom

Oxford University Press is a department of the University of Oxford.
It furthers the University's objective of excellence in research, scholarship,
and education by publishing worldwide. Oxford is a registered trade mark of
Oxford University Press in the UK and in certain other countries.

Published in the United States of America by Oxford University Press
198 Madison Avenue, New York, NY 10016, United States of America

British Library Cataloguing in Publication Data
Data available

Library of Congress Control Number: 2025950272

ISBN 9780198971184

DOI: 10.1093/9780198971153.001.0001

Printed and bound by
CPI Group (UK) Ltd., Croydon, CR0 4YY

The manufacturer's authorized representative in the EU for product safety is
Oxford University Press España S.A. of Parque Empresarial San Fernando de Henares,
Avenida de Castilla, 2 – 28830 Madrid (www.oup.es/en or product.safety@oup.com).
OUP España S.A. also acts as importer into Spain of products made by the manufacturer.

FSC
www.fsc.org
MIX
Paper | Supporting
responsible forestry
FSC® C013604

For Robert Bird

Contents

Figures, Tables, and Charts

Figures

Tables

Charts

Note on Transliteration

This book uses sources in three languages, three scripts, and even more script variants, since the scripts used for Uzbek and Tajik have changed multiple times over the course of the twentieth and twenty-first centuries. Any transliteration system will be imperfect under these circumstances. In order to avoid confusion, I have transliterated all Uzbek-language materials published in Arabic script, Cyrillic, or in other versions of Latin script, into the version of Latin script that has been used in Uzbekistan since 1995. Particularly in the case of workers' correspondent reports, this has the unfortunate effect of flattening vernacular dialectal variation. Readers with an interest in historical linguistics and dialectology are encouraged to refer to the original materials. The only exceptions to this transliteration principle are the names of familiar toponyms with an accepted English-language transliteration: hence Uzbekistan, not O'zbekiston; and Samarkand, Bukhara, and Andijan, not Samarqand, Buxoro, and Andijon. In order to avoid confusion, I use *boi* instead of *boy* when referring to the class category.

My Uzbek-language transliteration system thus diverges from the Library of Congress system for transliterating Uzbek, which presumes a Cyrillic-script source text and would introduce inconsistency based arbitrarily on the year of publication. I have, however, used the LOC system for Russian and Tajik, with the exception that I follow the Arabic-script transliteration norms for Sadriddin Ayni, while dropping the `ayn for simplicity's sake, and I use the accepted romanization of widely familiar names even when they do not follow LOC norms: Gorky, Krupskaya.

Many individuals published or were discussed in multiple languages as well as multiple scripts. For consistency's sake, in the text I use the transliteration appropriate to the language the individual used most in public: hence Qahhor and not Kakhkhar, Ayni and not Ayniy. To facilitate ease of finding, in the notes and bibliography I have transliterated from the script in which the text being referenced was published. Readers interested in, say, the writings of Abdulla Qahhor, should look under both Kakhkhar and Qahhor in the bibliography; the titles of Russophone materials on Tojixon Shodieva give her name as “Tadzhikhan Shadieva.” In the 1930s, Oydin published using her pen name (Oydin), but in most library catalogs, and therefore in the bibliography here, her name is given as Oydin Sobirova, using the surname derived from the first name of her father.

All translations are mine unless otherwise noted.

Acknowledgments

Gratitude comes with a debt of responsibility. Many people have shaped me and my work in this book, and by thanking them, I acknowledge my gratitude for their help while absolving them of responsibility for its flaws.

The first phase of my research on this project was funded with the generous support of the Beinecke Scholarship, a Hanna Holborn Gray Advanced Fellowship, and an Arnaldo Momigliano Dissertation Research Travel Grant. In a moment when the US federal funding that has historically provided so much support to the study of Central Asia and the Soviet Union is under attack, it is with bittersweet gratitude that I acknowledge the support of FLAS and Fulbright-Hays DDRA fellowships. Later phases of this research were supported by the A. Whitney Griswold Faculty Research Fund Award, and the Frederick W. Hilles Publication Fund of Yale University supported some of the production costs for the book.

Portions of an early version of Chapter 1 appeared in "'Not Just Tea Drinking': The Red Teahouse and the Soviet State Public in Interwar Uzbekistan," *Kritika: Explorations in Russian and Eurasian History*, 22, no. 3 (2021): 479–510, and portions of Chapter 2 were previously published in "'I Dress in Silk and Velvet': Women, Textiles and the Textile-Text in 1930s Uzbekistan," *Central Asian Survey*, 41, no. 1 (2022): 1–21. I am grateful for permission to republish them.

Without my friends, hosts, and colleagues in Uzbekistan, this project would have been impossible. I am especially grateful for the expert input, logistical support, and warm hospitality of Shahnoza Madaeva, Nodira Mustafoyeva, Saodat Nazarova, Bahrom Irzayev, Shokir Pidaev, Sayyora Ismailova, Svetlana Matyoqubova, Dilorom Karomat, Feruz Narmanov, and Nodira Jalolova. The staff at the National Archives, National Library of Uzbekistan, Alisher Navoiy Literature Museum, and Institute for the Study of the Arts (San'atshunoslik) in Tashkent provided essential support. I am also grateful to the Higher School of Economics, Liudmila Novikova, Sergei Abashin, and Samuel Hirst for supporting my early research in Moscow and St. Petersburg, and I thank the staff at RGASPI and RGALI for their assistance. I will never forget my earliest teachers from Samarkand, especially my language teachers: Sanobar Haydarova, Fotima Fayzullayeva, and Liliia Arkadievna.

The Departments of History and Near Eastern Languages and Civilizations (now Middle Eastern Studies) at the University of Chicago provided fertile ground for cultivating my research at early stages. Holly Shissler's creative, enthusiastic support for my work cultivated the project at its root. She opened my eyes to the interconnectedness of the Turkic world and the ferment of the interwar, and her kindness made her a true friend as well as a mentor. Faith Hillis's unassuming brilliance continues to inspire me. She taught me how to be a historian, but also showed me what it meant to be a good human being in academia. Frank Lewis, taken from us far too soon, taught me much about Persian and the Persianate, and his gentle erudition and hospitality will always be a model for me. Although not technically based at the University of Chicago, Christina Kiaer brought early shape to my work on this project and has been an encouraging presence ever since. I am also grateful for the support of Leora Auslander, Eleanor Gilburd, Na'ama Rokem, Kağan Arık, Saeed Yousef, John Woods, Leah Feldman, Lina Steiner, C. Ryan Perkins, Bill Nickell, and William Mazzarella. Flora Roberts, Kara Peruccio, Misha Appeltova, Abigail Bratcher, August Samie, Roy Kimmey, Michael Bechtel, Ahona Panda, Katie Tucker, Maryam Sabbaghi, Ilana Miller, Madeleine Elfenbein, Annie Greene, and Zachary King were both interlocutors and friends. The members of the Student Parent Group and GSU—especially Devin and Marcos Gouvêa, Amanda Valdez, Abhishek Bhattacharya, Jorge Lefevre, Joey Cross, Andrew Yale, Basil Salem, and Irami Osei-Frimpong—were a lifeline.

My pandemic year in the History Department at Providence College might have been entirely miserable if not for the generosity of colleagues and co-teachers, especially Colin King, Jennifer Illuzzi, Alex Orquiza, Alyssa Lopez, Anthony Jensen, Bruce Graver, Terry McGoldrick, Colin Jaundrill, and Ted Andrews. I learned much of importance for this book from them, and a part of me will always regret leaving them so soon.

My colleagues at Yale have been instrumental in shaping the trajectory of my research. Edyta Bojanowska, Marijeta Bozovic, Molly Brunson, Jinyi Chu, Nari Shelekpayev, John MacKay, Sergei Antonov, Egor Lazarev, Ernest Mitchell, David Engerman, Doug Rogers, Erika Valdivieso, Nana Osei-Quarshie, Hannah Shepherd, Serena Bassi, Mukaddes Muhetaer, Ayesha Ramachandran, Isaac Nakhimovsky, Jonathan Wyrtzen, Leslie Gross-Wyrtzen, Cajetan Iheka, Allison Harris, Nurfadzilah Yahayah, Shawkat Toorawa, Denise Ho, and AZ Zayaruznaya have given generously as colleagues and friends. Nathan Low provided invaluable advice on political theory. I am especially grateful for the crew that came with me to Yale from Chicago:

Jane Mikkelson, Sonam Kachru, and Sam Hodgkin. Christina Andriotis, Carly Koebel, Cheryl Morrison, and Sam Meade have made all the logistics possible with skill and warmth. Umid Usmanov helped track down some key sources. We lost Katerina Clark not long after I got to Yale, but I continue to find her fingerprints on my work.

At every stage, this project took shape with the generative feedback of many colleagues. The Midwest Russian History Workshop was where I presented the very first iterations of this project; I am eternally grateful to Chuck Steinwedel, for driving me and a baby all the way to Indiana to get feedback on my very first draft of my very first chapter. The participants of the History and Literature Workshop organized by the American University of Central Asia provided formative commentary on multiple portions of the book. I am especially grateful to James Pickett, Azhar Dyussekenova, Christopher Baker, Naomi Caffee, Donohon Abdugafurova, Gabriel McGuire, Kristen Fort, and Emily Laskin. Marianne Kamp read the entire manuscript at multiple stages and gave essential feedback at every juncture. Adeeb Khalid, Bruce Grant, Ali İğmen, and Kevin Platt also gave incisive comments on the entire manuscript, without which the book would be much weaker. Erin Hutchinson, Zukhra Kasimova, Nergis Ertürk, Alexander Herbert, Jeff Sahadeo, and Anna Whittington were also helpful interlocutors at critical junctures along the way. My editors at Oxford University Press, Tom Stottor, Imogene Haslam, and Zara Cannon-Mohammed have helped usher the book through to completion. Audra Wolfe and Anne Amienne helped organize and shape the manuscript, and Charlotte Kasza brought coherence to the book at the last.

None of this would have been possible without the many people who cared for my children so I could work: Bronwyn Koehl, Mara Farcasanu, Trish Ryan, Sophia Zaferes, Basia Tracz, Arcadia Davies, Sayonte Baldwin, Chloe Richards, Susan Papademetris, and the teachers at Kids International, Edith B. Jackson, and Worthington Hooker School. For their moral support, I thank Fr. Elijah Mueller, Rebecca Luft, Fr. Stephen Voytovich, and Cindy Voytovich.

To my family, I owe a debt of gratitude that goes beyond what words can express. My children, Iva, Danny, and Isaac, have been a source of inspiration and a grounding force. I will always miss Sofia and count her as my fourth, though she is no longer with us. My parents, Kathy and Andy; my siblings, Emma, Maggie, and Joseph; and my in-laws, Terri, Kevin, Nikki, Dustin, Trevor, Paige, Celeste, and Ben, along with the many wonderful people they have brought into my life, have enriched my thinking in more ways than I can yet apprehend. As I worked on this book, Mark has been my constant conversation partner, cheerleader, proofreader, developmental editor, travel companion, and so much more. Without him this book could never have come to be.

The first kernel of this book emerged in conversation with Robert Bird. We met when I was eighteen years old: he believed in me before I believed in myself. He shaped my thinking, my writing, my teaching, my being-in-the-world in ways that I am just beginning to appreciate. When he died of cancer in 2020, at the age of fifty, it ended a conversation I felt was only just beginning. I miss him always. Although I'm sure he would make many line-edits and conceptual reconfigurations of this book, I dedicate it to him, in all its imperfection.

Preface

When the USSR established itself in southern Central Asia, in many ways it continued a Russian colonial enterprise that had begun at least five decades before. The Soviet Socialist Republics of Uzbekistan, Turkmenistan, Kyrgyzstan, Tajikistan, and Kazakhstan largely coincided with the borders of the Russian Empire that had occupied, settled, and massacred its way to hegemony across the decades leading up to the revolution of 1917. Seated in the former colonial capitals, European overseers in the Soviet Union reported back to Moscow about "native" morale and local "backwardness." For years after 1917, indigenous fighters in Central Asia's mountain and forests took up arms to struggle against the foreign dominion of their godless exploiters. In response, the Soviet authorities imprisoned, executed, or exiled those who dared resist them.

For many Central Asians, the continuities between the Soviet and imperial orders were unmistakable. And yet, the Soviet state insisted on its *discontinuity* with the past legacies of empire. If the empire of old had ruled on behalf of a capitalist ruling class, the Soviet government claimed to represent Central Asia's "masses": the factory workers and farmers, hired hands and hardworking women they saw as their natural allies. Never mind that the societies of Central Asia were predominantly Muslim and largely agrarian—a far cry from the industrial European cities where the Soviet ideas had been forged. The new Soviet overseers believed their ideas of revolution, internationalism, and solidarity held universal validity, whether in the steppes and oases of Central Asia or the fields and forests of Russia.

Central Asians had their own ideas about what made a just and prosperous society. Some Central Asians believed the Soviet project was fundamentally at odds with their vision of human thriving, and sacrificed their lives to resist it. Others joined the Soviet endeavor, inevitably staging an encounter between the world they envisioned and the world their European Soviet comrades imagined. By mediating between the two, these Central Asians conjured a new rendition of public life in the early decades of the Soviet experiment. In a context that was arguably more neo- than anti-colonial, their work legitimized the Soviet state as—ostensibly—ruling on behalf of, rather than in opposition to Central Asia's "masses." But in articulating their own visions of what a Soviet public would look like in Central Asia, they often pointed toward the tensions and contradictions in that project. This book captures that fraught effort through scenes of cultural encounter in the nascent Soviet Socialist Republic of Uzbekistan. Along the way, I suggest that the story of Uzbekistan's culture can tell us a great deal about the Soviet experience elsewhere, with its chaotic, brutal, and often self-contradictory efforts to make new social worlds from old.

The story of this encounter emerges through sites of mediation: the social spaces that Central Asians inhabited and the cultural forms they used. But it is perhaps best encapsulated through attending to one of the personalities who came to stand in for the Soviet encounter in Central Asia.

Consider Tojixon Shodieva (1905–81), among the most famous in the pantheon of Soviet Central Asia's heroes of socialist labor. She entered the public view with a spectacular scene of unveiling at the Sixth Congress of the Komsomol, held in Moscow in 1924—or so the story goes as related by Fannina Halle in her book *Women in the Soviet East*. An enthusiastic German observer of Soviet women's affairs, Halle was not personally present at this scene of Shodieva's unveiling, and relates the entire story in quotation marks without attributing a source.[1] With its spectacular reveals and potent visual language, unveiling was perfectly suited to the new cinematic era. It is entirely appropriate, then, that Halle tells the story as if mediated through a camera lens, in a series of vividly drawn shots and reverse shots.

Shot: we first see Shodieva from her audience's perspective. She appears seated in a "prominent place near the chairman and several guests of honor," wearing a Central Asian veil, a "red silk *paranja* and a black horsehair *chachvan*." Members of the Communist Youth League (Komsomol)—a women's delegation from a textile factory in Krasnokholm, Orenburg Oblast; a young man from the Don Basin—deluge Shodieva with notes demanding that she remove her veil. Lenin's widow Nadezhda Krupskaia, seated near Shodieva, personally relays the demands of the crowd that Shodieva remove "that instrument of the oppression of women."[2] After receiving the request from Krupskaia herself, Shodieva hesitates.

Reverse shot: peering out through her veil, Shodieva sees "through the black lattice-work how the whole hall came nearer to her, as if it made up one great unit." But in that moment of hesitation, Shodieva looks out once more, and sees, in the front row, "a group of her own countryfolk."

Shot: Shodieva's fellow Central Asians "did not take their eyes off her." Then, "the Uzbek woman tore off her *chachvan* and her *paranja* and hung both on the banner at the edge of the platform. The film operators and photographers straightway placed their apparatus."

The "film operators and photographers" make explicit what should by now be clear: Shodieva's unveiling was a media event as much as it was a personal transformation. It was a cinematic spectacle that made her visible: not only to her audience at the Komsomol Congress, but also to the mass media, and thereby to Uzbek, all-Soviet, and global publics. Halle belonged to that global public herself: she never met Shodieva, learning of Shodieva largely from her "biographer" Valeriia Gerasimova, whose articles about Shodieva circulated widely in the Soviet press through the 1960s.[3] Beginning in the late 1920s, photographs of Shodieva's unveiled face circulated throughout the Soviet Union and the world in newspapers and newsreels, posters and press releases; the story of her unveiling and activism was told in poems, stories, and films in multiple languages (Figure 00.1). Shodieva was the paragon of Soviet socialism's claim to represent Central Asia's masses. But by 1938, the Soviet secret police had swept Shodieva away to a hard labor camp along with much of the Uzbek Communist Party leadership. Her image, once so ubiquitous, vanished suddenly from public view. Now designated an enemy of the people, in the gulag she may well have become a fellow-prisoner with some of the very people she once denounced in her role as collective farm administrator.

Our sources on the life and times of Tojixon Shodieva are many but strikingly inconclusive. Should we call her a victim of totalitarianism or colonialism? Or, perhaps, a perpetrator? A Stakhanovite labor hero?[4] A courageous woman's organizer?[5] An Uzbek national exemplar? A type of Soviet celebrity? Tojixon has been described in all these ways—but only because each of these personas represent a facet of the emergent media persona of "Tojixon," distinguishable from a historical figure, "Shodieva." As a model for mobilization, Tojixon needed to represent her public: cultural directives were quite clear that Central Asian women needed to be able to see themselves in her and follow her example in the cotton fields that would "free" the Soviet Union of its dependence on Western capitalist cotton. Yet the very qualities that made her exemplary also rendered her inaccessible. The mediated representations of Tojixon reveal anxieties about whether that mobilizational project was in fact feasible, or whether Tojixon would always remain an unattainable vision to her Central Asian public. Moreover, in the eyes of some European observers, Tojixon represented not a model for emulation but a racialized icon of Eastern femininity, making her the object of oversight rather than an object for imitation. To her publics, Tojixon was always seductively close and impossibly distant.

As valuable as it is to understand who Shodieva was as a historical figure, we learn a great deal from Tojixon as an object and agent of mediation. Tojixon's mediatized persona reflected core tensions in the Soviet project: between voluntary participation and manipulation, between the disciplining Party vanguard and the purportedly undisciplined masses. Beginning with Tojixon, we see that the project of socialist construction in Central Asia was always already

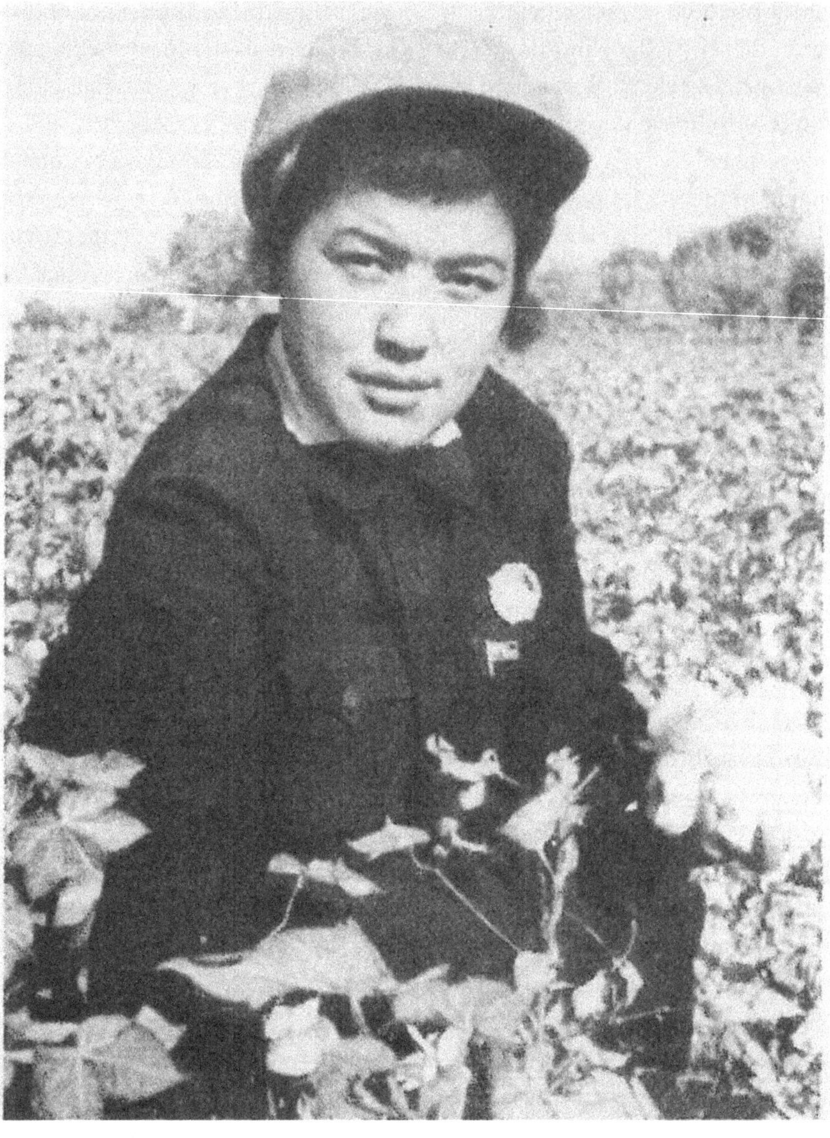

Figure 00.1 Portrait of Tojixon Shodieva, plate from Fannina W. Halle, Women in the Soviet East (E.P. Dutton & co., inc, 1938).

a project of mediation—across cultural difference, aesthetic forms, social divides, and geographical distance. The pages that follow trace how Central Asians mediated socialism, with all the tensions, conflicts, and contradictions inherent to that project. By the end of our journey, I hope, we will have the tools to better understand not just Tojixon Shodieva, but also the many others like her who mediated, and were mediated by, socialism in Central Asia.

Socialism Mediated: The Making of Soviet Culture in Central Asia. Claire Roosien, Oxford University Press.
 DOI: 10.1093/9780198971153.003.0001

Introduction

In mid-April 1929, *Pravda Vostoka* (*Truth of the East*), the official Russian-language newspaper of the Communist Party's Central Asian Bureau, published a photograph showing activists storming the minaret of a brick mosque in Tashkent's old city (Figure 0.1).[1] The Bolsheviks had just intensified their campaign against Islamic institutions—closing religious schools, confiscating pious endowments, burning women's veils—and the mosque had just been closed. In the picture, five young male activists looked eagerly up from the base of the minaret, while two others leaned out of its windows.[2] Some of the activists waved (presumably) red flags from the minaret—one flag on the right, and one on the left. The caption claimed that these young men, members of a poor peasants' group, were in the process of converting the now-defunct mosque into a club for the Komsomol, the Communist Youth League. "In place of a mosque, a club," the caption summarized triumphantly.

The editors responsible for publishing the photograph evidently printed it to celebrate the "victories" of socialism in Central Asia. But within days, they came under attack from propaganda official and future film magnate, Boris Shumiatskii, who claimed that the image gave precisely the wrong impression. "This photograph documents for the viewer," he complained, "that the closure of the mosque is being carried out not by masses of the population, but only by Komsomol members; that even the Komsomol members do not appear as a mass, but merely in a group of seven; and that the closed mosque is not being handed over to the population, but merely as a club for the Komsomol cell."[3] Shumiatskii feared that in looking at *Pravda Vostoka*, Central Asian audiences would fail to imagine themselves as participants in a shared Soviet project. Instead, they would passively observe the activists' youthful zealotry; or, worse from his perspective, they would identify those zealots as the front for an illegitimate claim of popular sovereignty—in this case, a claim made by a Russian-language newspaper on behalf of a largely Muslim population that mostly spoke not Russian, but Persian and Turkic.

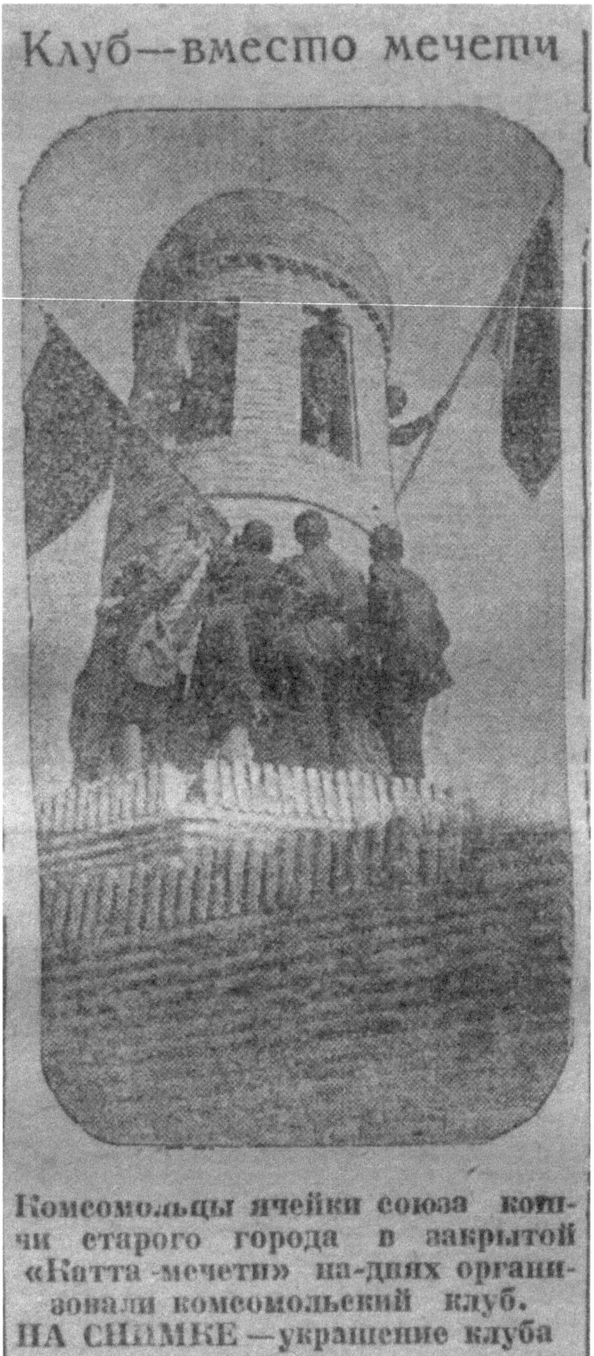
Клуб—вместо мечети

Комсомольцы ячейки союза кошчи старого города в закрытой «Катта-мечети» на-днях организовали комсомольский клуб.
НА СНИМКЕ—украшение клуба

Figure 0.1 Young activists raising flags over a former mosque, "Vmesto mecheti—klub." *Pravda Vostoka*, April 15, 1929, 5.

For some viewers from Central Asia, the photograph must have confirmed that the Bolsheviks governed on behalf of Europeans, over and against the Muslims of Central Asia. In so many ways, the photograph undermined the very justification for Soviet sovereignty in the region: Central Asia's people.

This ephemeral episode illustrates a much broader dynamic in the crisis of legitimacy that faced the Soviet state when it consolidated its power in Central Asia. Tenuously integrated into the Russian Empire and closely linked to the Middle East, the steppes, fields, and cities that became the republics of Central Asia were a far cry from the societies where Marxism-Leninism was forged. To establish a foothold in what became the republics of Uzbekistan, Tajikistan, Turkmenistan, and Kyrgyzstan, the Soviet state depended on mediation by a narrow segment of the population, mostly comprised of a small cohort of Central Asian urban elites who made common cause with European Bolsheviks—Russians, Ukrainians, Germans, and Ashkenazi Jews, much like the colonial administrators who had governed before. Eventually, as agricultural collectivization and cottonization extended the Soviet reach further into the countryside, young rural activists joined the struggle; but the ranks of Party activists always represented a small proportion of the region's broader population.[4] Despite their initially narrow social base, Soviet authorities represented themselves as acting for the benefit of Central Asia's "masses"—a representation that became increasingly urgent as the Communist Party enacted ever more aggressive policies of social engineering beginning in the late 1920s, from agricultural collectivization, to women's unveiling, and ultimately, the mass political violence of the Great Terror.[5]

As the hand of the state became heavier, the Party's claim to represent the people of Central Asia became more difficult to maintain. When the Bolsheviks emerged victorious in the Russian Revolution of 1917, they had professed they would undo the dark legacies of Russian imperialism. In a statement in 1917, Lenin and Stalin offered the Muslims of the Soviet Union the right of self-determination, urging them to voluntarily make common cause with the Bolsheviks on behalf of the toiling masses of the Muslim world.[6] According to Lenin and Stalin, the Soviet Party-state was supposed to govern on behalf of the formerly colonized peoples of Central Asia, not to reproduce the colonial hierarchies of the Russian Empire that it inherited. But the Bolsheviks encountered stiff resistance from a range of historically Muslim Central Asian communities, and the Communist Party struggled to back up its claim that it governed in the name of the people of Central Asia. Even though the Party-state emphasized the Soviet Union as a benevolent alternative to the rapacious empires of the capitalist world, many of its practices were all too familiar: European settlement, indigenous dispossession, cultural erasure, forced labor, and economic and environmental extraction.[7] For the Party-state to maintain legitimacy as a government rooted in popular sovereignty rather than imperial fiat, it needed to show that the Central Asian people were on its side and that socialism was on the side of the Central Asian people. More importantly, it needed to mobilize Central Asian people as voluntary participants in the Soviet project—or at least to plausibly represent them as so mobilized.

This book is about how Soviet culture bridged this gap in the newly formed republic of Uzbekistan. Culture legitimized the Soviet state as representing the people of Central Asia rather than re-subjugating them. An army of local mediators made Soviet culture in Uzbekistan—writers, composers, activists, organizers, intellectuals, and performers. In the eyes of the European Bolsheviks, their lived experience and cultural knowhow equipped them to enculturate Soviet dogmas, and the identities they assumed as non-European, "proletarian" men and women made them indispensable representatives to Central Asians and to the outside world. Over the early Soviet years in Central Asia, they built a new culture. When they wrote in Uzbek or Tajik, they helped to codify novel literary languages, drawing from but significantly altering the long legacies of literary production in the region. They tapped into historic traditions of folk song and classical poetry, but they combined them with new mediums like the novel and the cinema. They identified the social institutions they thought held the most potential for building socialism, and helped to reform them: in their words, to make them "Red." Their cultural creativity, their organizational experience, and their social networks made the Soviet Union Central Asian and made Central Asia Soviet.[8] At the same time, their work often brought the inherent contradictions and injustices in the Soviet project to the fore. Too often, these mediators have been trivialized, either as useful idiots for the Moscow-centered state, or as essentialized spokespeople for their nation, their religious background, or their regional position. In this book, I argue that we might understand them best as mediators, not easily reducible to trite binaries: victims versus perpetrators, heroes versus villains. It is in the process of mediation that the core tensions in the Soviet Union's project of anti-colonial neo-imperialism come to the fore.

Mediators for the Age of Mass Society

The mediators at the heart of this book harked from the non-European and predominantly Muslim population of Central Asia. By using the term "mediator," I intend to highlight the creative and interpretive role that these

Central Asian cultural producers embodied. I draw on Bruno Latour's distinction between "intermediaries" and "mediators." For Latour, "intermediaries" convey meaning without altering it: they are passive conduits.[9] Mediators play a more active role: they "transform, translate, distort, and modify the meaning or the elements they are supposed to carry." The actors in this book are mediators in this sense. Although the Party-state needed local allies to legitimate their claim to popular sovereignty, in practice, those mediators did more than rubber-stamp Moscow's projects and propaganda. Instead, they interpreted, appropriated, re-formed, and re-mediated socialist culture. Indeed, they *made* socialist culture in Central Asia. In this book, consequently, cultural production comprises an archive not only of top-down messaging and its appropriation, but also of the tensions and conflicts inherent in the project of building Soviet culture.

Nearly all the mediators I discuss belonged to the Party or its junior wing, the Communist Youth League (Komsomol). Most mediators crafted an autobiographical narrative about some sort of "proletarian" origins, but that rhetoric masked a wide range of social, educational, and economic backgrounds. Some harked from renowned intellectual milieux. The Bukharan intellectual Sadriddin Ayni (1878–1954) was educated in the best Islamic colleges, or *madrasas* of Bukhara, while the Tashkent-based woman writer Oydin (1906–53) had the distinction of being brought up in classical Persianate learning before the revolution. Before becoming a devout Communist, Soviet Uzbek singer Muhiddin Qori-Yoqubov (1896–1957) earned renown as a Qur'an reciter. Others came from more humble origins: the novelist Husayn Shams (1903–42) learned to read on the job as a typographer, while collective farm celebrity Tojixon Shodieva rose through the ranks of the Communist Party after escaping an abusive marriage, and popular singer To'xtasin Jalilov (1895–1966) began life as the son of a wagon-driver. Many other mediators in this book are unnamed or known only by the initials they used to sign their reports to Soviet newspapers. Despite their anonymity, these schoolgirls, collective farm activists, and factory workers comprised a crucial cohort, interpreting socialism for their own communities and attempting to make sense of the new ideology for themselves and their world.

While some were literate in the former prestige languages of high Persian and Arabic as well as the Turkic and Persian vernaculars, the new generation of mediators worked exclusively in newly codified vernacular languages. These included the languages of the newly formed national republics—Uzbek, Tajik, Kyrgyz, Kazakh, and Turkmen—as well as non-titular national languages like Uyghur and Judeo-Tajik. Vernacular languages were boosted by a reform in 1928–29 that replaced the Arabic script, in which most Central

Asians had previously written, with several versions of Latin script.[10] Mediators envisioned Latinization as a strategy to make literacy accessible to the vast majority of Central Asians: they perceived Arabic script as difficult to learn, lacking vowels and associated with a high register of vocabulary.[11] In contrast, Latin script was largely phonetic and ostensibly better suited for Turkic languages.[12] Government statistics for Russian imperial and early Soviet Central Asia are notoriously unreliable, but without question, literacy rates ballooned during the late 1920s and the 1930s, as the Party-state initiated aggressive campaigns for mass literacy in the newly implemented Latin script. The script reform also cut many Central Asians off from the long Islamic textual traditions of Transoxania. Moldering in inaccessible archives and hidden in secret family collections, the Arabic and Persian manuscripts that had once comprised the core of Islamic education in the region all but disappeared from view, as quietly influential as they may have continued to be.[13] From now on, mediators would cite the Collected Works of Marx more than collections of *hadith*.

Mediators were also overwhelmingly young. With few exceptions, they were in their teens, twenties, or at most their thirties. Their youth was no accident: in the late 1920s, a purge of so-called "bourgeois nationalists" swept the Soviet national republics, sidelining much of the older generation of intellectuals, including Central Asia's modernizing Jadids.[14] Some of the elders were executed and others imprisoned, while still others simply retreated to "safer" pursuits like translating the Russian classics into Uzbek. In their stead, an energetic but highly inexperienced cohort emerged. Young mediators must have feared the dark fate that befell so many of their mentors, but nevertheless, they continued to draw on what they had learned from them in Jadid schools and cultural circles. They were undoubtedly aware of the critiques some elders had made of the Soviet order—that it turned Central Asia into a repository of raw materials for its neo-colonial economy, that it repressed their shared Turkicness in favor of a deracinated national project—but in their public work, they rejected those critiques out of hand.[15]

In the climate of fear that reigned after the terror of the late 1920s, the safest option was to lie low, stay anonymous, and keep away from the roving and repressive eye of the state. Instead, these young people devoted their energies to imagining and building a new world on behalf of the Party. Young men seized mosques against the protests of their elders; young women performed on Soviet stages despite a spate of femicides against such performers; aspiring poets published experimental free verse in official journals. Quite a few perished violently. Some died in clashes with the anti-Soviet resistance, but the Party wiped out many more through repression, imprisonment, and summary execution. Others survived, often by the skin of their teeth, and built long careers as cultural leaders in Soviet Uzbekistan.

These individuals can be called "mediators" in two main ways. First, they mediated between the Soviet state and Central Asia's "masses," interpreting and communicating state policies through cultural institutions and media. Mediators were embedded in rapidly entrenching hierarchies: they received top-down directives for culture and propaganda workers, including literal lists of slogans they were called upon to promulgate. Many mediators enjoyed special privileges as a reward for their creative and organizational labor, and as I demonstrate in Chapters 1 and 2, they came to comprise a new cultural elite in Central Asia, supplanting and subsuming the pre-revolutionary elites that had once dominated cultural production. But as they brought their own intellectual and personal commitments to bear on their work, and as they confronted regional sociocultural realities, mediators inadvertently pointed out the inconsistencies in the Soviet project of popular sovereignty. In their role as employees or activists for the Party, mediators legitimized Soviet power on behalf of the masses by virtue of their identity as Central Asians, workers, or women. But by inviting their participation, the Party-state made space for mediators not only to parrot but to create. As they imagined the shape socialism would take in their political, historical, cultural setting, they amplified unexpected resonances and unpredictable dissonances in the Soviet project for legitimation through the masses.

Second, in addition to mediators' position between Moscow and Central Asia, they "mediated" by working through the mass media. When the Bolsheviks consolidated their hold over Central Asia in the late 1920s, they created a media infrastructure that was completely unprecedented in the region. Newspapers had existed in Central Asia before the Revolution, but they were largely the province of a rarefied circle of modernizing intellectuals. By the late 1920s, new Soviet infrastructure distributed newspapers and journals much more widely than before. Print runs ballooned as the new publications promoted collectivization and cotton production. The Uzbek-language daily newspaper, *Red Uzbekistan*, reported a daily print run of 25,000 in 1930, which increased to 44,927 by May 1932.[16] The number of books printed in the Uzbek language in Uzbekistan increased from 1909 in 1928 to 8738 in 1933.[17] In 1928, there were twenty-five newspapers in any language in Uzbekistan; by 1933, there were forty-nine newspapers in the Uzbek language alone.[18] Newspapers increased in frequency as well: a 1929 resolution, for example, called for several major newspapers to publish three or four times per week, rather than one or two.[19] Railroads made it possible to disseminate print media much more broadly and regularly than before.

Broadcast media was almost unheard of in Central Asia before the Revolution, but by the late 1920s, radio and even film technologies began to proliferate; the number of film projectors (*kinoustanovki*) in Uzbekistan nearly quadrupled, reaching 469 in 1932 from 121 in 1928.[20] Mediators were the vanguard of an unprecedented form of mass society in Central Asia.

Sources on mediators are both plentiful and compromised. This book is based on work in rare book collections and archives in three countries. Official state and Party archives, including the Russian State Archive of Social-Political History (RGASPI) and the Komsomol Archive (RGASPI-M) maintained under its auspices; the Russian State Archive of Literature and the Arts (RGALI); and the National State Archive of Uzbekistan (O'zMDA) offer critical material on the institutions in which mediators worked. Their stenographic records, meeting protocols, planning documents, statistical accounts, and official reports reveal the inner workings and the driving logic of Party-sponsored cultural work. By and large, the documents held in these archives were produced as official accounts of the work of institutions sponsored by the Party-state, with all the biases to be expected in such accounts: they tend to overemphasize the "victories" and exaggerate the challenges mediators faced, as bureaucrats benefited from showing visible results and looked better when juxtaposed with "delinquent" enemies. Furthermore, the vast majority of documents in these archives are in Russian. I supplement these sources with lesser-known archives focused on cultural work, including the Alisher Navoiy State Literature Museum archive (ANLM), which contains the personal papers of over 160 writers from Uzbekistan; and the Archive for the Study of the Arts (O'zRFASI) under the auspices of the Republic of Uzbekistan Academy of Sciences. One of the richest sources for this book, however, is the vast body of published material—newspapers, journals, books, and other ephemera—that mediators consumed and produced. These materials are often as difficult to find, access, and read as archival materials, produced as they were in multiple different scripts and subjected to repeated rounds of censorship, suppression, and republication. Read attentively and critically, however, published materials present a unique archive of cultural conversations as they took shape in languages other than Russian.[21]

Difference and the Soviet Public

The interwar period was a global age of self-determination. In the liberal west, the Wilsonian doctrine called for national self-determination as a fundamental principle for the post-World War I order. By replacing the Old World empires with newly founded nation-states, the doctrine remade the maps of Europe, the Middle East, and beyond. Globally, state sovereignty came to be decisively linked to the people—the nation, or, in the Soviet case, both the nation and the proletariat. The Soviet Union's ideological stance only amplified the urgency of legitimation through self-determination. Indeed, early Soviet ideology insisted that the state existed only as a temporary stopgap. The Bolsheviks had long promoted a vision that mass participation and Party control would one day converge. According to this vision, once the proletariat had smashed bourgeois domination, the state and its trappings would wither away and a classless, communist society would prevail. In the coming communist order, the state would be supplanted by a society so just, enlightened, and democratic that the state's coercive force would no longer be necessary and the sovereign people would reign supreme.[22] The "masses," defined in terms of both the all-Soviet proletariat and the nations that comprised it, became central to legitimizing the Soviet state.

In addition to its legitimizing role, mobilizing the masses had significant implications for agricultural and industrial production.[23] This became especially salient with the advent of collectivization and the Five-Year Plans that demanded unprecedented, if not impossible production levels in all industries. As the Soviet Union fought to escape economic dependence on the capitalist world, it turned to the fertile, sunny lands of southern Central Asia to grow cotton—a cash crop that promised to facilitate Soviet autarky. If Ukraine has been called the "bread-basket" of the Soviet Union, then Uzbekistan might be called its wardrobe.[24] Uzbekistan was a major producer of cotton, and the lynchpin of Stalin's ambition to achieve cotton autarky. Collectivization in Uzbekistan entailed sowing cotton on land that had previously been used for food production—a hard sell for farmers who were rightly suspicious of the ability of the central state to provide their families with the food they needed to survive. In the Soviet "cotton belt," stretching across the most populous regions of Uzbekistan, Kyrgyzstan, Turkmenistan, and Tajikistan, the Party-state mobilized to produce unprecedented amounts of raw cotton that would power textile mills in the industrial regions of central Russia and Eastern Europe.[25] In the context of this economic program, the state could no longer rely exclusively on the thin ranks of urban elites to prop itself up in the region. The Party needed all hands on deck, from peasants and youth to workers and women. By the late 1920s, then, in Soviet Central Asia the bulk of official culture and propaganda work existed primarily to mobilize the masses for feats of production. Official culture revolved around cotton production and the catalogue of agricultural processes surrounding it: sowing, irrigation, cultivation, harvest.

Although the Party-state under Stalin became increasingly authoritarian, it never relinquished its distant aspiration for a stateless society. This produced an ideological double-bind. The Soviet state maintained legitimacy only insofar as it convincingly claimed that it governed on behalf of the proletarian masses. In order for socialism to come into fruition anywhere in the Soviet Union the proletarian masses needed to appear alongside the state as active participants in its mobilizing mission. But as time passed, the disjuncture broadened between actually existing Central Asians—who acquiesced to state policy sometimes through persuasion, but often also through a cocktail of coercion, cooptation, and violence—and the Party-state that claimed to govern on their behalf. The gulf between the Party and Central Asia's masses threatened to delegitimize the entire Soviet project.

Bridging this gap were Uzbekistan's mediators, who took it upon themselves to *imagine*, *address*, *organize*, and ultimately, *mobilize* a public: a collective organized around mass institutions (the club, the Red Teahouse) and imagined through the mass media (the newspaper, the radio, the film). To convey the concept of "public-ness" in a less clunky locution, I employ the term "publicity." My usage should not be confused with the more conversational use of the term "publicity," in the sense of marketing or advertising.

My study traces the making of a Soviet public during the tumultuous early years of Soviet rule in Central Asia: the 1920s and 1930s. In so doing, this book aims to deprovincialize Central Asia by demonstrating how it participated in global processes while also showing the distinctive features of Soviet mass publicity in the imperial periphery. The book homes in on the Soviet project to accommodate *difference* in a public that was, fundamentally, universalizing. That is to say, it chases down the contradictions in a project of public-making that on the one hand celebrated difference—indeed, created new categories of difference—and subordinated those categories of difference to a universalizing project. Readers will notice that thus far, I have spoken intermittently of Central Asia rather than Uzbekistan. As a case study I focus on the Soviet Socialist Republic of Uzbekistan, but rather than taking the Uzbek nation as a starting point, I emphasize the contingency of the national borders of Central Asia. Many of the patterns I identify in Uzbekistan can be observed in other Central Asian republics as well, and many of the individuals I discuss identified with non-titular nations within the republic of Uzbekistan. The book examines the making of Soviet culture in Uzbekistan, but it presumes that *Uzbek* was just as contingent a category as *Soviet*, and most of my conclusions can be applied elsewhere in Central Asia's "cotton belt."

Soviet publicity was, in aspiration, universal. Bolshevik ideologues understood the revolution as a global phenomenon, bringing together workers of the world across their differences: gender, race, ethnicity, nationality, and geography. Paradoxically, however, the Soviet government began its efforts at mass publicity by reinforcing and even creating new categories of difference. From 1918, when the first nationally defined republics emerged in the Caucasus and Eastern Europe, national identity was among the most important of these categories. The process of creating new nationally defined Soviet republics expanded to Central Asia in 1924, creating the Union Republics of Uzbekistan and Turkmenistan and an Autonomous Republic of Tajikistan under the auspices of the Uzbek Republic.[26] This concluded a process of carving the Soviet Union into nationally defined administrative units, populated by categories such as "Uzbek" and "Tajik" that imperial ethnographers and local elites formulated collectively.[27]

Nation, Empire, and the Soviet Public

The nation was far from a foregone conclusion as the organizing principle for Central Asia's people. During the fifty years before the 1917 Revolution, the territory that came to comprise the national republics of Central Asia was organized not in a national, but a traditionally imperial administrative structure. Tashkent was the Russian administrative capital for much of southern Central Asia, which comprised the Russian Governor-Generalship of Turkestan. The Russian Empire also governed through protectorates: the Emirate of Bukhara, the Khivan Khanate, and until 1876, the Khanate of Khoqand, most of whose territory eventually ended up in the Soviet republic of Uzbekistan.[28] The Bukharan emir and the Khivan and Khoqandi khans are examples of a broader phenomenon. The Governor-Generalship of Turkestan had a Russian bureaucracy, but also left local institutions, including courts, religious institutions, markets, and guilds largely intact.[29] Although the Russian imperial administration sometimes spoke in terms of a civilizing mission, in practice efforts to convert or "civilize" Central Asians were few and far between.[30] Russians, including tsarist administrators, settler peasants, and industrial or railway workers, comprised a tiny minority of the population of modern-day Uzbekistan, and were concentrated in a few urban regions. Even in Tashkent, there was little mixing of Central Asians with their European colonial administrators: Tashkent, like Samarkand, was divided into a native "Old City" and a European quarter.[31]

For the mostly Muslim population of Central Asia, sedentary cultural life was polycentric, focused in cities like Tashkent, Samarkand, Bukhara, Shahrisabz, and the Ferghana Valley. Samarkand and Bukhara in particular were historic cultural hubs and home to world-renowned *madrasas*, or Islamic colleges, which drew students from throughout the Islamic world.[32] These cities, like most of the region, were ethnically diverse. The most significant groups of the population included Sarts, or sedentary Turkic-speakers; Tajiks, or sedentary Persian-speakers; and Qazaqs, or Turkic-speaking nomads.[33] Most people spoke multiple languages for different purposes. Persian and Arabic were prestige languages, used for high culture—poetry, religion—while state bureaucracy operated largely in Persian and Chagatay Turkish, which differed in turn from the vernacular Persian and Turkic that was spoken on street and steppe. The highly contingent modern idea that a people corresponded to a single ethnically defined nation, a single national language, and a bounded territory was new to Soviet Central Asia.

It was also unexpected that the Bolsheviks recognized the nation as a meaningful social category at all. At the time the Soviet Union was founded, many Communists believed that nationalism had no place in their movement, and vehemently rejected all national projects as ideological constructions that were inherently bourgeois. Lenin and Stalin made the highly controversial choice not only to *recognize* nationhood, but to enshrine it as the primary organizing principle for their federative administrative structure.[34] Both Lenin and Stalin conceded that the nation would eventually vanish in the coming communist order, but for the time being, it was necessary to allow local nationalisms time to develop. This was particularly true of the most "backward," most oppressed nations, such as those of Central Asia. This ideological concession would permit the new Soviet state to overcome the legacies of Russian empire, which early Soviet historiography and Lenin himself described as a "prisonhouse of nations."[35] Central Asian intellectuals eagerly adopted the national project as their own. Although the idea of the nation was relatively marginal in Central Asia, even before the revolution a small but significant group of the Muslim intelligentsia believed that the nation was a necessary component in the passage to modernity and participated eagerly in the early Soviet nationalizing project.[36] They defined the borders of Uzbekistan and Tajikistan, and they did the intellectual work to create "Uzbek" music, literature, and culture as a category of their own, separate from other regional cultures.

The efforts of these nationalizing elites dramatically transformed how Central Asians identified themselves. If you asked a rural Turkestani cotton farmer to introduce himself in 1906, he might have told you he was a Muslim or shared his village or family name. By 1939, in contrast, the Soviet census asked all Central Asians to identify with one of sixty-two recognized Soviet nationalities, and most could respond. To make matters more complicated, no Soviet republic was populated exclusively by its titular nationality. The creation of Uzbekistan minoritized large numbers of Tajiks, Qazaqs, Turkmens, and Kyrgyz people who found themselves stranded in the titular republic of another nation; there were also considerable populations whose nationality corresponded to no Soviet republic, such as Uyghurs and Persian-speaking Jews.[37]

Making Soviet culture in Uzbekistan entailed making nations, and in turn, attaching cultural and linguistic practices to those newfound national categories. Mediators wrote "Uzbek" poetry, composed "Uzbek" songs, drafted the "Uzbek" national novel, and wore "Uzbek" national textiles. At the same time, many cultural practices fit awkwardly within a national frame. The teahouse, for example, belonged to all the sedentary people of Eurasia; and it belonged to none of them in particular. *Atlas* silk fabric was at once an Uzbek national textile and the shared patrimony of the Kyrgyz, Tajik, and Uzbek nations. Indeed, in some cities such as Samarkand, vast proportions of the population had shifted on paper from "Tajik" to "Uzbek" in the course of less than ten years, as the result of coercion, falsification, or both in the 1926 census.[38] While these national categories were not without precedent in the region, and although the nation looms large in my study, I consequently resist the temptation to back-project "Uzbekness" in a moment when Uzbekness, Tajikness, etc. were under construction. Instead, I lean into moments of supranational and subnational identification. For the purposes of this book, I take the nation not as a given, but as a contingent project. More importantly, Soviet publicity subordinated nationality to its agenda to build a public that transcended national difference even as it subsumed it.

The Soviet federative structure explicitly disavowed empire and imperialism, but many features of its political organization were continuous with the Russian imperial order. Although the national republics had considerable autonomy in some spheres and at certain moments, ultimately, in the early Soviet years, all major decisions were funneled through the Party top brass in Moscow, including the ability to appoint republican leadership. The Soviet Union gave empire a distinctive form, but it should still be understood as a type of empire. We might draw on Ronald Suny and Valerie Kivelson's fourfold definition of an empire as "exhibiting some or all of the following four characteristics": empires comprise a "collection of disparate lands and peoples"; they are "based on inequitable, hierarchical relations of power" between metropole and periphery; and their "form of rule is exercised through difference rather than through integration or assimilation."[39] In this respect, the Soviet rhetoric about multinationality might be viewed prismatically: from one angle, it amplifies the ideals of socialist internationalism, with its stated emphasis on inclusion and equality; from another perspective, it reinscribes imperial diversity for the new age of popular sovereignty and Westphalian nationalism. Mediators participated in what Leah Feldman has termed a *translatio imperii* between tsarist empire and Soviet empire by another name.[40]

Gender and the Soviet Public

The nation was not the only category of difference that the Soviet Party-state created and cultivated. In the Central Asian context, gender intersected with empire and nation, as women's "emancipation" became a major focus of Soviet policy in the 1920s and 1930s. In the process of litigating gender relations in Central Asia, the Bolsheviks instigated an upheaval in the categories of masculinity and femininity.[41] The place of women in society had been debated in Central Asia long before the Bolshevik revolution, but in 1927, the Women's Division of the Communist Party instigated an aggressive campaign for women's "emancipation," calling it the *hujum*, or "attack" on women's oppression. The campaign initiated a broad swath of policy efforts: it expanded women's education, liberalized divorce law, and encouraged women to pursue work outside the home, but its most visible effect was unveiling. In grand public spectacles like Tojixon's cinematic unveiling, Central Asian women tore off the black *paranji* and *chachvon* that they had once worn and cast them into roaring bonfires. Unveiling represented not only a sartorial choice, but also a rejection of a broader system of women's seclusion, in which veiling both covered women and allowed them to venture into public without being seen by the prying eyes of non-kin men. Joined by Russian Women's Division activists, some Central Asian women eagerly participated in the Hujum, seeing in it an opportunity to advance women's affairs that they held near and dear.[42]

Authorities rolled back the most aggressive Hujum measures in response to local backlash, and in reality many Central Asian women continued veiling until as late as the 1950s. Still, the rhetoric of women's emancipation endured. Women's "emancipation" served the broader Soviet agenda for collectivization and cotton and silk production. If half the adult population was not "free" to work outside the home, how would the Five-Year Plan ever be fulfilled? The rhetoric about the Hujum intersected with transnational colonial discourses about helpless colonized women in need of "rescue" by their colonizers. At the same time, particularly on the part of Central Asian activists, it resonated with programs for women's modernization elsewhere in the Middle East: both Turkey and Iran launched aggressive campaigns for unveiling within a decade of Central Asia's own campaign.[43]

Although official Soviet discourse generally upheld a rigid gender binary, in Central Asia, the Hujum forced mediators to reinscribe the boundaries of masculinity and femininity. Official Soviet narratives represented the Party as a benevolent parent, undermining men's perceived traditional roles as providers and protectors of their families. Newly "emancipated" women cut their hair short, socialized in mixed company, and took on leadership roles that had historically been held by men. Some activist women even spurned marriage and childbearing—a dramatic break with rigid societal expectations that women marry young and bear sons as quickly as possible. To many Central Asians, Soviet women appeared less feminine than their veiled and secluded counterparts. Soviet men, in turn, struggled to envision a mode of masculinity that would be compatible with Soviet public life. The Hujum inaugurated a moment of gender-bending, as cultural intermediaries struggled to imagine new ways of masculinity and femininity-in-public.

Class and the Soviet Public

Soviet publicity aspired to *integrate* Central Asia's population along lines of nationality and gender. Although it created new forms of national identification, and instigated a radical campaign for women's "emancipation," ultimately Soviet publicity was supposed to subsume and integrate national and gender difference rather than reifying it. Class operated quite differently. When it came to class, Soviet publicity emphasized exclusion rather than integration. During the collectivization drive of the First Five-Year Plan, the Unionwide Party agenda called for the "liquidation of the *kulaks* [roughly, 'wealthy peasants'] as a class," utilizing class categories specific to the Russian Empire after the Great Reforms.[44]

The process of defining class in Central Asia, as elsewhere in the Soviet Union, was highly contingent and often emerged less from "objective" economic markers than from happenstance and personal connections. Social and economic hierarchies did exist in Central Asia, but they did not map neatly onto the categories of state economic policy. There were strong incentives to identify with the state-provided categories, however: benefits accrued to some class markers, while repression followed others. This system motivated Soviet people to craft "proletarian" or "peasant" class identities even when their bona fides were weak.[45] Although all prior Marxist theory had understood class status to have objective material roots, paradoxically, in the Soviet system class in a material or sociological sense mattered less than class ascription—how successfully a person cultivated a bureaucratic identity and performative self-presentation as a "proletarian" or "peasant."

Things were further complicated in Central Asia, since the categories of proletarian, peasant, and *kulak*, formulated as they were in the aftermath of Russian serfdom and urban industrialization, rested uncomfortably on Central Asia's agrarian society. Central Asia had never practiced serfdom in the same way as central Russia, so to an even greater extent than elsewhere, identifying *kulaks* (Uzb. *quloq* or *mushtumzo'r*) in Central Asia was a contingent process depending on the affinities of local activists. Uzbek rural activists spoke primarily of "making *quloqs*" rather than merely eliminating them, implying the category was more constructed than apprehended objectively.[46] Other class categories were applied, all equally contingent—*boi* (the wealthy), the bourgeoisie; while Islamic clerics came to be rhetorically linked to the ruling classes regardless of their material situation. If Soviet publicity was inclusive along lines of class and gender, then, it was exclusionary along class lines, and being designated as a *quloq*, *boi*, or other class enemy could mean expropriation, exile, or even death. In this way, class thus became an imagined category of Soviet publicity, just as much as gender and the nation.

Organizing the Public

This book examines the role of local mediators in shaping a shared space of state-sponsored discourse, which I term a "state public sphere." By using this language, I interrogate the relationship between state and society in the context of Soviet empire. For the last thirty-five years, the absence of a Habermasian public sphere—that is, an intermediary category between society and the state that facilitated rational-critical deliberation on policy, organized around a nexus of voluntary social institutions (coffeehouses) and the print media (newspapers)—has loomed large over the study of Soviet culture and society.[47] Jürgen Habermas's *The Structural Transformation of the Public*

Sphere was translated into English in 1989, triggering a deluge of scholarship across the humanities and social sciences. Some readers developed trenchant critiques of the liberal-normative public sphere in terms of race and gender, pointing out that the ideal-normative Habermasian sphere excluded women, nonwhite people, and non-propertied men, and arguing that a stark separation between state and civil society may not actually be desirable.[48] Furthermore, the eighteenth-century public sphere was not as autonomous of the state as Habermas implied, dominated as it was in France and Germany by the "service elite."[49] Nevertheless, the vision of a field of political discourse that would be autonomous of the state proved tantalizing for the post-Cold War generation of Sovietologists. In the historiography of the Russian Empire and Soviet Union, a vast scholarly debate emerged surrounding the relative strength of Russia's civil society or public sphere, and the presence or absence of a precedent for the institutions of liberal democracy in Russia and its empires.[50] A sizable body of scholarship has considered the Russophone category of *obshchestvennost'* as a possible analogue for the public sphere as theorized by Habermas, while others have rejected the analogy altogether, especially when it comes to the Soviet period.[51] It speaks to both the kinship and mismatch between the categories that Russophone scholars have vacillated between a cognate with the English, *publichnost'*, and the Russian term *obshchestvennost'*, with the former serving generally as a normative category and the latter a descriptive one.[52]

The translators of Habermas could not have foreseen the collapse of the Soviet Union, but the booming popularity of Habermas in the early years after the Soviet collapse is no accident. Habermas framed his theory of the public sphere in nostalgic terms for a long-lost eighteenth century that never really existed, but his readers adapted that historical model and attempted to apply it to any number of contexts, setting up the autonomous public sphere as an implicit model for democratization in an era of US hegemony.[53] As Francis Fukuyama proclaimed the "end of history" and the reign of a new liberal order, the Soviet Union and its satellites seemed to be consigned to the dustbin of history. Their future seemed to hinge on their ability to construct a civil society and public sphere on the Habermasian model, or rather, on the model of Habermas's Anglophone readers in the 1990s.

It never made sense to conceive of the world in binary terms, as divided between the settled liberal public spheres of Euro-America and the illiberal authoritarianisms of Eastern Europe, Russia, and Eurasia. But as Soviet successor states in both Russia and Central Asia turn to new forms of authoritarianism, the specter of the liberal public sphere has continued to haunt the scholarship on Soviet and post-Soviet politics and culture as well as the popular discourse about it, usually setting up the liberal-normative public sphere as an unattained or unattainable goal.[54] From the vantage point of 2025, as I finish this introduction, the familiar dichotomy between illiberal Eurasia and the liberal west seems increasingly quaint.

To be sure, I concur with the scholarly consensus that the ideal-normative public sphere has little analytical purchase for the Soviet period, and especially for the period of Stalin's rule. After all, during the 1920s and 1930s the Soviet state consolidated its grip over cultural production and banned all forms of associational life outside the bounds of the Party-state. Independent publications ceased to exist, replaced by newspapers and journals that were funded, distributed, and censored by various wings of the Party-state. Organized state violence exceeded what had previously been imaginable, stamping out all remaining self-organized cultural, intellectual, and political life. In Uzbekistan, a series of major purges—erupting most violently in 1929 and again in 1937–38—largely eradicated the prerevolutionary intelligentsia and along with it many of Central Asia's truest believers in the Bolshevik cause. Over the course of the 1920s and 1930s, secret police shot many of Uzbekistan's best and brightest, burying their bodies in unmarked graves; others languished in prison camps for decades, leaving their families disgraced and destitute. The Habermasian ideal of a deliberative public sphere functioning autonomously from the state has no application here, if anywhere.

My purpose in using the term, then, is not to belabor the tired debate about whether the Soviet Union ever had or might have had anything like a Habermasian public sphere. Instead, I aim to understand cultural production as an interface between state and society by historicizing the specific shape that mediators gave Central Asia's public. The Russian imperial and Soviet cases should not be dismissed as aberrations from liberalism, but rather as variations on a transnational phenomenon that took shape differently in different conditions.[55] Rather than taking the liberal norm as a benchmark against which all public cultures should be evaluated, I suggest that Soviet publicity bears a "family resemblance" to other kinds of publicity, both liberal and nonliberal.[56]

In focusing on the Central Asian periphery of the Soviet Union, I also bring a long-neglected dimension to the debate about Russian imperial and Soviet publics, which has until recently focused almost entirely on the metropolitan center. In so doing, I emphasize the multinational character of the Soviet public, which took shape atop the ashes of a transnational Islamicate sphere. The language mediators used for state publicity is instructive here.

In the 1920s and 1930s, Uzbek-speakers in Central Asia adopted the term *jamoatchilik* as a counterpart for *obshchestvennost'*, but that term in turn tapped into longstanding associations with Islamic communal forms and trans-imperial self-organization.[57] *Jamoatchilik* derives from the Arabic *djamāʿa*, a term that had long designated both the worldwide community of Muslims (similar to its corollary, the *umma*), and the face-to-face congregation of believers assembled in prayer.[58] By the early twentieth century, some Central Asian intellectuals began using *djamāʿa* and its derivatives to refer to what Adeeb Khalid describes as a type of public sphere, although it differed from the Habermasian paradigm in its dependency on the colonial state and lack of a coherent bourgeois class affiliation.[59] Called "Jadids" from the Arabic, Persian, and Turkic word for "new" (*jadid*), in honor of their commitment to new educational methods, these intellectuals gathered in political and intellectual societies and published their works through the mass-circulation media—especially newspapers. Indeed, Jadids often represented themselves visually as men wearing European-style suits and waving newspapers in the face of their detractors. The Jadids' interest in the mass-circulation press cultivated a new kind of transnational, transimperial intellectual community. Jadids read newspapers and journals published in Baku, Istanbul, Orenburg, and Ufa; they imagined themselves as part of a shared community of progressively minded (*taraqqiyparvar*) Muslims and modern Turkic people.[60] The newspaper-toting Jadids also built public institutions, facilitating self-organized circles and societies and establishing the first modern theaters in Central Asia.

The Jadids overlaid their practices of public life on a diverse range of longer-standing venues for collective engagement. At the *madrasas* of Central Asia's towns, erudite scholars expounded their interpretations of Islamic law, while at Sufi *khanaqas*, or lodges, spiritual guides with cross-regional ties led their followers on the path to spiritual enlightenment—and, often, political power.[61] Groups of men or women (*gap* or *gashtak*) would agree to gather regularly for tea, music, and conversation, rotating the venue from house to house and offering one another mutual aid. In the markets and teahouses of Central Asia's villages, people met daily for entertainment and to catch up on the day's news. While the Soviet public profoundly reshaped Central Asia's society, it could never fully replace or eliminate everything that came before.

The Soviet public sphere thus created a space which on the one hand legitimated Soviet rule and facilitated mass mobilization; on the other hand, it initiated cultural and social dynamics that the state could neither predict nor control. Because it is predicated on mass participation, the public is always unpredictable, always containing energies and attachments that the state can never fully contain, no matter how hard it may try. Alexei Yurchak described the poets, writers, and musicians who sought sinecures in Soviet boiler-rooms as an example of the way that apparently non-state cultural production was nevertheless imbricated with the Soviet state, while Kyrill Kunakhovich argues that official spaces like theaters became "Communism's public sphere," serving as key venues for oppositional discourse in Cold War-era Poland and East Germany.[62] In both cases, state publicity facilitated self-organization: sometimes in support of state policy, occasionally in opposition to it, but more often in ways that cannot be reduced to flat binaries of collaboration and resistance, official society and civil society. The state public sphere was a space of mass participation, and that participation was inherently unstable. Cultural mediators attempted to mobilize the masses on behalf of a Soviet project, but also recognized (and sometimes feared) the potential of culture to move the masses in other directions.

Cultural mediators worked to build a state public sphere in two main ways: by organizing and by imagining it. State-sponsored "mass institutions" served as venues not only for imbibing propaganda, but also for organizing the masses around state discourses and state projects. Central public institutions in the Soviet Union included workers' clubs, women's clubs, cultural circles, the Soviet Writers', Composers', and Artists' Unions, and most of all for Central Asia, thousands of Red Teahouses. By organizing the Soviet public, these "mass institutions" sought to render Central Asians readily *addressable* by the mass media. These organizational efforts are the subject of Chapters 1 and 2. Chapter 1 examines the premiere institution of the Soviet public sphere in Central Asia, the Red Teahouse. European administrators and Central Asian administrators alike believed the Red Teahouse would help them both to recognize and to integrate Central Asians' cultural difference in an official cultural institution. But the harmonious overlap between Central Asian social practices and Soviet state publicity never materialized. I show that cultural intermediaries used teahouses both to create a public and to police its boundaries—generating a new elite that marginalized ordinary Central Asians as much as it mobilized them. In Chapter 2, I turn to the Soviet Writers' Union of Uzbekistan, formed in 1932 with the stated goal of mobilizing Central Asia's "masses" both as readers and as writers. In fact, the Writers' Union completely reoriented literary and cultural life around a narrow group of insiders based in Tashkent and defined by informal social networks. Paradoxically, Soviet publicity facilitated a "shadow public sphere" that existed only thanks to state patronage but also outside of its control. By the late 1930s, these dynamics informed the logic of Terror.

Imagining the Public

This book's initial chapters focus on the organizational work of the state public: the state-run institutions that structured the Soviet public sphere. But the rest of this book proceeds from a second presumption: that a public is imaginary, and that institutions only organize a public insofar as they help to *imagine* that public.[63]

In the Soviet Union, some categories had profound administrative significance. Whether one was designated as a *kulak* or a peasant, the member of a titular or a non-titular nation, could have life-or-death consequences. But at the same time as it constructed and reified new social categories through bureaucracy, the Soviet Party-state embarked on a massive project of mass publicity: not just to designate the masses *on paper* as "proletarians" or "Uzbeks" or Soviet people, but also to cultivate a sense of belonging to those collective categories through address. It is in this sense that "women," "Uzbeks," and *dehqons* (farmers), became categories of mass publicity as well as categories of bureaucratic administration. Furthermore, as Soviet publicity expanded beyond discourse into such embodied media such as material culture, dance, and popular song, it functioned on an affective as well as an intellectual level. This process took shape dialectically, as cultural intermediaries created their publics through address, and audiences (at least in aspiration) responded by imagining themselves—and feeling themselves—as belonging to that public. When a novelist addressed a "proletarian" public in novel form, he helped his readers to begin understanding themselves as proletarians. When a Red Teahouse patron heard a section of that novel read aloud, he could begin to imagine himself as one among many Central Asian "proletarians," most of whom he would never meet. When an Uzbek Stakhanovite wore a factory-woven *atlas* silk dress, she remembered her position as part of a broader political society extending beyond her family or her village. At least, such were the ambitions of Soviet mediators.

The making of the Soviet public in Uzbekistan coincided with two major developments in Soviet culture. First, in the mid-1930s Socialist Realism came into its own as the sole mode for Soviet cultural production. The consolidation of Socialist Realism coincided with the codification of national cultures in the non-Russian republics and autonomous regions of the USSR. Although the two developments were basically contemporaneous, Socialist Realism has usually been studied independently of national cultures, while studies of national cultures have historically sidestepped the ways that

Socialist Realism both amplified imperial histories and catalyzed national cultural construction.[64] At its origins, though, Socialist Realism was always already national. At the First Congress of the Soviet Writers' Union, held in Moscow in 1934, Socialist Realism was promulgated as the sole mode of Soviet cultural production. At that same congress, gigantic banners bearing Stalin's famous slogan adorned both the outside and the inside of the meeting hall: "Proletarian in content, national in form—such is the all-human culture toward which socialism is proceeding." Over the ensuing years, a revised version of the slogan, "national in form, socialist in content," became a rallying cry for an entire generation of Soviet national writers in the Socialist Realist mode.

Like many slogans, this one had a pleasant ring but left much to creative interpretation. First, what constituted "form" and how was it possible to separate "form" from content? My reading of "national form" takes its inspiration from the vast tradition of media studies that took shape in postwar Europe and North America.[65] The field is too heterogeneous to summarize in depth, but its core assumption is shared: that the process of mediation fundamentally shapes the meanings we make and the worlds we inhabit; or, to borrow Stalin's terms but not his assumptions, that form and content cannot, in fact, be so cleanly separated. In the Central Asian context, it became clear very quickly that form could not hold content as a glass held water. To the Central Asian musicians who rejected the *shashmaqam* classical music suite because of its religious and courtly associations, that musical "form" carried with it a great deal of thoroughly un-socialist content. The novel was almost unheard-of in prerevolutionary Central Asia, but it quickly became the premiere form of socialist literature for every national republic, including Uzbekistan. In this case, *language* became the primary signifier of national "form," while the generic and stylistic features that most contemporary literary theorists would consider "formal" came from a decisively extra-national origin—from the Russian, and before that, from the western European literary tradition. And yet, in practice, cultural producers used the slogan about "national form" to justify all kinds of creative approaches to enculturating socialist ideology. The Red Teahouse was a "national form" when it came to social life; artisanal woodcarving evoked "national form" when it came to architecture, even in an opera house; and the aria that was performed in that opera house comprised "national form" if it drew on a Persianate epic, was performed in a "national" language, or used folk ornamentation in its melodic line. Dangers abounded: emphasize the "national" or the wrong form of nation-ness too much and you could be condemned as a bourgeois nationalist.

Such was the fate of the Jadids. "National form" meant everything, and it meant nothing in particular.

The definition of "proletarian content" was still more complicated. Marx averred that capitalism took shape historically in the specific conditions of modern Europe; without the conditions of modern industrial capitalism, the proletarian revolution could not take place. Even Russia, with its mostly agrarian society and its limited industrial development, was the last place many Marxists anticipated a revolution would occur. When the Bolsheviks took over in Moscow and St. Petersburg, they shocked the world—communists most of all. If Russia was "backward" with respect to capitalist development from the perspective of Marxism-Leninism, Central Asia was all the more so. Without subscribing to the linear notions of progress and the Orientalist assumptions underpinning some traditional Marxist accounts, we might readily acknowledge the difficulties inherent in imagining "proletarianness" in Central Asia. To make Soviet culture, Central Asia's intermediaries had to forge a recognizably national "form," while simultaneously inventing a "proletarian" culture for an economic situation that differed fundamentally from that of the factory cities of Europe and Russia.

Although working under severe institutional constraints and in an environment of real precarity, mediators in the 1930s used Socialist Realism as a kind of laboratory: both for imagining socialism in Central Asia and for reckoning with the legacies of the past. In the Socialist Realist novel, writers produced new imaginaries of the nation and forged new categories of masculinity and femininity. Socialist Realism also went beyond the mediums usually associated with "high" culture: Sheila Fitzpatrick posits a "discourse of Socialist Realism," encompassing all areas of social communication, not just artistic and literary arenas. Against the everyday privations of life in the Soviet Union, Socialist Realism focused on a future-in-the-making as one of joyful labor, social equality, material plenty, and warm comradely relationships.[66]

Many attempts at Socialist Realism fell flat, as by the late 1930s, they were either denounced as insubordinate or condemned as aesthetically unsuccessful. We could see these novels, songs, and poems as aesthetic accomplishments. But beyond value judgment, I read them as embattled experiments in Soviet public-making. They grapple with the contradictions between the ostensible Soviet commitment to decolonize Central Asia and the persistence of imperial hierarchies; they struggle to imagine a Soviet Central Asian masculinity and a fully integrated femininity. When I emphasize that Central Asia's mediators worked within a Socialist Realist mode, then, I do not mean to suggest that they were hapless dupes or craven shills for an oppressive

Soviet agenda. Instead, they saw themselves as participants in a shared project of public-making. Mediators believed their creative work had the potential to shape the world they and their children would inhabit. In Socialist Realism, they strove to imagine a more just order in a world they knew was in fact quite unjust.

But the imaginative work of Socialist Realist cultural production went beyond merely *representing* the public. Its imaginaries of the public extended to its unprecedented efforts to address the "masses" as those "masses" learned to read for the first time. It *conjured* a public, to the extent that in conjunction with mass literacy programs and the organizational work of mass publicity, Socialist Realism made it possible for Central Asia's "masses" to imagine themselves as part of a shared public for the first time in a new way. If Chapters 1–2 emphasize the organizational work of making a Soviet public, then Chapters 3–5 turn to aesthetic media as modes to imagine, address, and ultimately, mobilize Central Asia's public. I have selected these examples among many other possible media—the theater of the period, in particular, remains understudied—but they serve as case studies of the intersection between media and state publicity.[67] In Chapter 3, I consider the three first Socialist Realist novels to be written in Uzbek, arguing that the novels can be read as artifacts of the tortured process of public-formation, much as official autobiographies have been read as archives of Soviet subjectivity. Still, despite official insistence to the contrary, novels remained an elite form, largely inaccessible to the average collective farmer. Accordingly, Chapter 5 addresses luxury textiles and the body of texts surrounding them, arguing that in response to the tension between women's "respectability" and their participation in the state public, luxury textiles came to play an outsize role in imagining women's roles in the official public sphere. It connects gender with the history of Socialist Realism through close readings of Uzbekistan's women's magazine, *Yangi Yo'l* (*New Way*), by setting up a distinction between a "Hujum aesthetic" of the late 1920s and a Socialist Realist mode beginning from approximately 1930. Chapter 4 turns to popular song as part of a broader discourse about setting socialist "tempos" for cotton production. The chapter examines how Uzbekistan's cultural intermediaries remade musical form and the social settings for musical performance in an effort to make music a medium of mass publicity, all the while working with musical forms that bore pre-Soviet and often un-Soviet associations. Both chapters demonstrate that women's participation constituted a major fault line in the project of Soviet publicity. In the conclusion, as a case study of Soviet publicity, I look at Tojixon Shodieva, the biggest celebrity from Soviet Uzbekistan, whose persona brings together all the phenomena discussed in the book's earlier chapters. Drawing on theories of celebrity from a range of modern mass societies, I argue that Shodieva's persona elucidates much about the dynamics of Soviet publicity more broadly: particularly, about the intersections of race, gender, nationality, and class ascription in producing a Soviet public—and the subterranean fault lines beneath the Soviet project for an ostensibly "universal" mass publicity.

Socialism Mediated: The Making of Soviet Culture in Central Asia. Claire Roosien, Oxford University Press.
 DOI: 10.1093/9780198971153.003.0002

1
Tea

Introduction

In April 1928, at the Third Convention of Uzbekistan's Communist Youth League, a young activist named Shcherbakov registered a serious concern about the Red Teahouse. Red Teahouses were the foremost institution for Marxist-Leninist instruction in Uzbekistan. But Shcherbakov complained that the patrons of some Red Teahouses were not studying the books that had been sent to them for political education. Instead, the books had been hung from the ceiling with ropes—dusty, torn, and unread.[1] Some Komsomol activists attracted teahouse patrons by sponsoring other entertainments: donkey races, musical performances. But if the primary function of the Red Teahouses was to promote socialist construction and spread Soviet culture to the masses, Shcherbakov believed they had failed.

Teahouses were immensely popular in Central Asia well before the Bolsheviks came to power and far beyond the Soviet realm. For centuries, travelers had remarked that in the absence of a culture of public alcohol consumption, caffeine ruled the day: teahouses were the most visible social spaces in the town squares and city centers of Eurasia.[2] At tea- and coffeehouses, men chatted and napped, recited poetry and enjoyed music, shared music and discussed matters of communal interest. It made sense, then, that beginning in the 1920s, the Soviet state sought to take advantage of the teahouse's popularity—and to curb its seditious potential—by making it "Red." From the Bolshevik perspective, the teahouse was perhaps the most ideologically palatable option for appropriation among the menu of Central Asian institutional forms. Markets, for example, were highly visible communal spaces in Central Asian towns, but their primary function was trade—unlike teahouses, which often adjoined markets, but whose commercial purpose was subordinated to the social one. Religious institutions, such as mosques and Sufi lodges, were obviously intolerable to Bolshevik activists. In contrast, not only were teahouses popular: they were popular among the right kind of people, rural peasants and urban "workers." Furthermore, as the reference book claimed, teahouses were already the locus of a type of public.

In other words: teahouses were *already* popular, and they were already places for associational life; why not put them in service of the state? Over the course of the first two Five-Year Plans, the Red Teahouse became the preeminent institution of the Soviet public in Uzbekistan, and indeed, in all of sedentary Central Asia.[3] Drawn to the teahouse because of its familiarity, Central Asia's masses would come for the tea and stay for the socialism. What could go wrong?

As it turned out, a lot went wrong: Shcherbakov was not alone in his concerns. As Red Teahouses proliferated throughout Uzbekistan in the late 1920s, so did anxieties about the teahouse public. These anxieties originated with European bureaucrats, but Central Asian Party activists quickly adopted them. In reams of archival and newspaper reports throughout the 1930s, horrified local correspondents complained of Red Teahouse users that they saw as behaving in an un-socialist way. Their reports revealed a fundamental contradiction in the project for Soviet publicity: in patronizing the teahouse, activists feared, the Party was underwriting practices that were fundamentally un-Soviet and also impossible to control—perhaps, even, a counterrevolutionary counterpublic.

Red Teahouses were such a major focus of Party activism that, unsurprisingly, they sometimes became lightning rods for popular disaffection with Soviet policy. Archival reports from the Soviet secret police describe several instances in which Red Teahouses were attacked by crowds of angry men. In August 1929, for example, seven men from the Ferghana Valley area of Vorukh were arrested for destroying a Red Teahouse after a Communist Party secretary, Saidov, requisitioned a beloved local shrine as an agricultural produce processing point.[4] For these men, the teahouse represented not a legitimate local institution, but the institutional face of Soviet power. On another occasion, the activist, poet, and musician Hamza (discussed further in Chapter 4) was murdered by a mob after trying to shut down another shrine in the Ferghana Valley; the crowd then went on to destroy a Red Teahouse.[5] In the grand scheme of things, however, such occasions of outright resistance were rare. From the perspective of the state, the Red Teahouse was problematic not because it was widely reviled, but to the contrary, because it was popular in all the wrong ways. Recognizing this problem, in 1925 an administrator for village work under the auspices of Uzbekistan's Commissariat of Enlightenment wrote a letter to all his subordinates in Central Asia. According to the letter, the teahouse model had failed. Instead of cultivating the masses, Red Teahouses had become almost indistinguishable from ordinary, "black" teahouses. The letter called for an overhaul of the teahouse system. In order to facilitate this, the writer proposed that Red Teahouses be renamed "Houses of Cultural Improvement" (Rus. *doma kul'turnogo vospitaniia*).[6] For the institution to become properly Soviet, in other words, it needed to be stripped of its identity as a local institution.

The proposed name change never took place, and 1925 was a profoundly different moment from the years of the First and Second Five-Year Plans, when the Red Teahouse reached its social-institutional apogee. But the anxiety about nomenclature revealed an enduring problem with Red Teahouse. By adopting the teahouse as the prototypical mass institution in sedentary Central Asia, the Bolsheviks hoped to attract Central Asian villagers and workers to the Soviet cause, demonstrating that Sovietness was compatible with "national form." But for the people of Central Asia, teahouses came with a host of associations, practices, and attitudes, some of which Party activists saw as incompatible with socialism. To local newspaper correspondents, normal social life at the teahouse was bourgeois, backward, even counter-revolutionary. In sponsoring the Red Teahouse, then, Bolsheviks created the conditions for pre-existing social practices to persist under the auspices of the state public—some of which were then pathologized as anti-Soviet.

This chapter zeroes in on how local activists attempted to mobilize "national form" by making the teahouse "red." I argue that we might understand the teahouse as an institution of an emergent public sphere in Central Asia. After the Bolsheviks incorporated the teahouse into their system of mediated mass publicity, it was subsumed by the state public sphere. Yet when the Central Asian population failed to comport with Soviet norms for "cultured" behavior, they inspired doubt about whether *all* the masses should be permitted to participate in the Soviet public. Likewise, tensions surfaced within the project for a proletarian public sphere, particularly along gender lines. As activists attempted to fulfill their directive to imagine, address, and mobilize a Party public at the teahouse, they often instead created civilizational hierarchies that fundamentally undermined the universal vision of proletarian publicity.[7]

Trans-Eurasian Teahouse Culture

In 1934, *Komsomol of the East* (*Komsomolets Vostoka*) published a print of a Central Asian teahouse by European graphic designer Semën Mal't (Figure 1.1).[8] While tea is present in the image, it appears as an afterthought: the teapot rests inconspicuously in the bottom right. Although two men hold tea

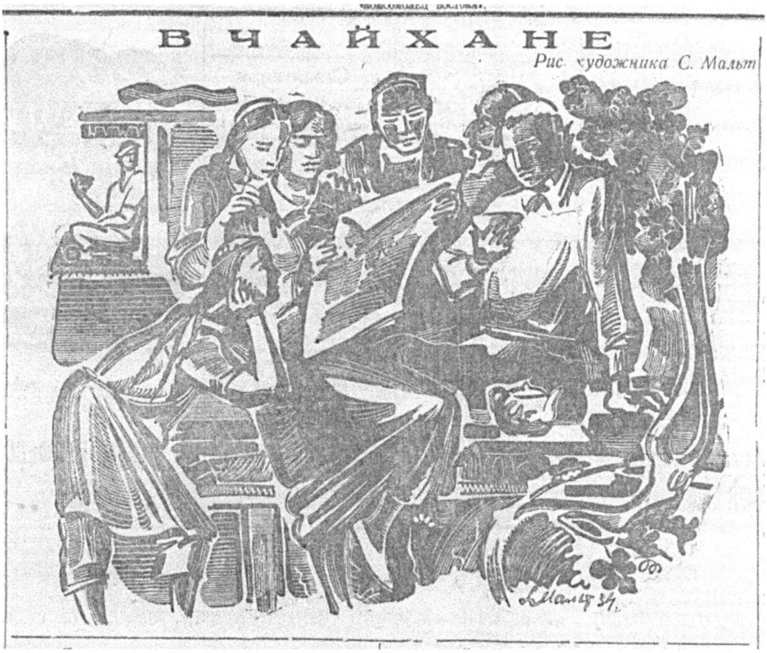

Figure 1.1 "At the Teahouse," engraving by Semen Mal't, *Komsomolets Vostoka*, June 26, 1934, 4.

bowls, their sight lines, like those of all the people in the image, are directed toward a different focal point—a newspaper, prominently placed in the center and jutting into the foreground, as if inviting the viewer to take a look at the headlines. The bodies of the seven figures curve around the newspaper, creating a rounded frame; even the grapevine on the right side leans in, as if to peek over the tea-drinker's shoulder. Remarkably, three of the figures are women: two girls wearing skull caps, braids, and Central Asian dresses peer at the newspaper; and another woman, wearing a European-style collared dress, holds the newspaper in her hands. Perhaps she is reading it aloud for the benefit of her less-literate comrades.

The image is entitled, quite simply, "At the Teahouse." But the women and the newspaper make it clear: this is no ordinary, "black" teahouse, but a Red one, organized not around a circle of conversing men, nor around a teapot or opium pipe, but instead around the primary medium of Soviet propaganda: the newspaper. In Mal't's representation, the teahouse brings together men and women, young and old, all as participants in a Soviet system of mass publicity. Mal't's engraving of a teahouse represents, in visual form, the Bolsheviks' vision for how the Red Teahouse would function in Central Asia:

as an institution through which Central Asians would be integrated in a mixed-gender, multinational, proletarian public, mobilizing around the Soviet mass media.

For many Central Asian viewers, this image of the teahouse would have been unfamiliar, and not because teahouses themselves were unfamiliar. Outsiders visiting Central Asia before the Revolution almost universally commented on the visibility of teahouses in Central Asian towns.[9] When Danish traveler Ole Olufsen visited the Emirate of Bukhara in the early twentieth century, for example, he represented the emirate's towns as an inhospitable landscape of blank walls, with houses that "look as if they had shot up from the earth like mole-hills." The sole exception was the market, and particularly its teahouses:

> If one does not enter the bazaar where there is life and bargaining in the shops or passes by to the ponds where the men come together to drink, wash themselves, gossip and smoke hookah on the stone-steps which lead down to the water or take tea in the tea-houses round the pond, one may very well drive through a whole town without seeing anything but clay-walls.[10]

Like most European travelogues on Central Asia, Olufsen's account was suffused with Orientalist tropes. The East was hidden and hostile; this was a society whose inhabitants, nearly indistinguishable from animal life, obscured themselves from the European gaze in a landscape that Olufsen described less as built environment than geological landscape. Teahouses, in contrast, offered themselves up to foreign observers as a rare example of "Oriental" public life outside of religious institutions. To quote the famed Hungarian travel writer and linguist, Ármin Vámbéry:

> To study that part of their lives which is before the public eye, we must first pay a visit to the tea-booths, which are the resorts of all classes. The Bokhariot, and the remark applies indeed universally to all Central Asiatics, çan never pass by a second or third tea-booth without entering, unless his affairs are very urgent indeed.[11]

Much like Olufsen, Vámbéry expressed a strange frustration when Central Asia proved inaccessible to his probing gaze: his discussion of teahouse culture was immediately preceded by a deprecatory discussion of women's veiling in Central Asia. Famed Russian photographer Prokudin-Gorskii, likewise, produced very few images of sedentary Central Asian women, and all of them were heavily veiled. In contrast, his photographs of teahouses bared masculine sociability to the imperial gaze (Plate 1).

For a nineteenth-century European, the teahouse was both the most visible and the most accessible social institution in sedentary Central Asia. While European travelogues reify their authors' presuppositions about somnolescent, decadent Oriental "leisure," they also comprise some of the most accessible sources on social life in prerevolutionary Central Asian teahouses. In contrast to local sources, in which genre norms tended to preclude extended discussions of everyday life and teahouses were considered too mundane to describe in detail, foreign travelers are among the most plentiful sources on teahouse life in prerevolutionary Central Asia. These foreign accounts demonstrate both the popularity of the teahouse and its perceived incompatibility with European modernity.

What happened at the teahouse? Imagine a Central Asian townsman visiting his local teahouse in the early fall. He walks to his local market, located at the town center, where the teahouses rub shoulders with shops.[12] The weather is hot and dry, and the townsman looks forward to sitting near a pleasant body of water—a man-made pool, an irrigation ditch—which humidifies the air and attracts birds, twittering and splashing in the background. Greeting his companions, the townsman seats himself on a wooden platform, or *supa*, furnished with comfortable mats and cushions, and situated under an awning or shade tree.[13] This teahouse is a well-appointed one: in addition to the basic provisions, hot water and tea bowls, the enterprising teahouse manager has arranged for bread and fresh fruit to be made available for his patrons.[14] The men at the teahouse might pass around a water-pipe, or *chilim*, from which they smoke tobacco, hemp, or opium.[15]

When one visits a teahouse, one comes to stay. Our townsman's teahouse is one of several at the market; the teahouse owners jockey for customers by hiring musicians to perform.[16] Because teahouses are spaces exclusively for men, women do not generally perform there. Instead, among the most popular musical entertainments are the adolescent boy dancers, or *bachas*, who sing, play, and serve patrons at the teahouse. *Bachas* often cross-dress and sometimes perform sexual services—to the scandal both of European observers and of Islamic modernizers.[17] Games and gambling also attract many patrons. Our townsman prefers chess, but there are many options: dice, dominoes, or European-style cards. Cockfighting and pheasant fighting are also common diversions.[18] At many teahouses, a man can even get a shave or a haircut if he feels the need to spruce up.

While teahouses provide various goods and services, their most important function is social. At a minimum, a teahouse might offer a samovar and a place to talk.[19] The European observers who pass through Central Asian towns tend to trivialize teahouse conversation as mere "gossip." Ella Christie says teahouse patrons "sit cross-legged…while gossiping to their hearts' content."[20] At another teahouse, Eugene Schuyler observes "a group of natives…discussing the latest local gossip, or the rumours from the Khivan expedition."[21] Ármin Vámbéry comments condescendingly that "the Bokhariot can…chatter away hours and hours, amidst his fellow tea-drinkers; for the meaningless conversations that are maintained weary him as little as the cup after cup of tea which he swallows."[22] For these European observers, teahouse talk is evidence of Oriental indolence, lacking in broader social or political significance.

Contrary to the presuppositions of many European travelers, not everyone saw teahouse talk as trivial. Despite dismissing teahouse talk as "meaningless," for example, Vámbéry noted that the Emir of Bukhara at the time of his travel, Muzaffar al-Din, "enforce[d] with severity the laws respecting religion and morals," referring specifically, upon leaving Bukhara, to the "drivers and peasants [outside Bukhara] discussing political subjects before the teashops, the prohibitions not being enforced as in Bokhara."[23] Vámbéry evidently believed that teahouse talk represented a political threat to the authoritarian Bukharan Emir. Many of the later Bukhara Emirs attempted to burnish their authority through adopting an image as defenders of Islam, including clamping down on teahouse behaviors they perceived as immoral, such as intoxication and gambling.[24] With respect to public discourse and teahouse sociability, this entailed what Vambery termed "espionage," state surveillance oriented toward the enforcement of moral prohibitions. While it is somewhat less well documented, researchers and practitioners have claimed that the last Bukharan Emir banned music at teahouses, presumably justifying himself through his interpretation of Islamic law.[25] But it is also quite plausible that in some cases, religion merely served as a pretext for broader anxieties about the teahouse's potential for sedition.

The political significance of the teahouse and of teahouse talk comes into focus when we recognize the teahouses of Russian colonial Central Asia as one case of a broader, trans-Eurasian institution. Indeed, Central Asia's teahouses came to exist thanks to the dissemination of tea culture from China, where it had millennia-long roots.[26] In west Asia, the coffeehouse was the dominant institution beginning in the early modern period, thanks to the spread of coffee from the Arabian peninsula through the Ottoman Empire and into Iran; in Iran, coffee came to be replaced by tea during the course of the nineteenth century.[27] And yet, regardless of the caffeinated beverage of choice, tea- and coffeehouse culture was remarkably continuous across Eurasia, from Izmir to Chengdu. Often situated at markets and crossroads, teahouses served not only locals; they also offered travelers a place to rest and refresh themselves. Olufsen pointed out, for example, that teahouses were "frequented by newly arrived caravan people."[28] At night, they served as a kind of inn for travelers. Muhammad Badi', a seventeenth-century Samarkandi intellectual and state functionary, traveled through Iran, stopping along the way at urban coffeehouses to collect the biographies of notable Persian poets. For Badi', the coffeehouses—along with Sufi shrines and madrasas—served as an informal network in a broader Persianate cultural sphere that spanned empires.[29] Teahouses often provided rooms to host travelers. In this sense, tea- and coffeehouses—particularly those located in important trade towns—should be understood not merely as a national, imperial, or local institution, but as transnational, transimperial, and trans-Eurasian.

Beginning in the early modern period, teahouses facilitated a kind of public sphere across Eurasia, although not identical to the bourgeois public sphere Habermas postulated.[30] Perhaps because of their status as nodes of cross-border exchange, modern tea- and coffeehouses shared many features, whether in Anatolia, Transoxiana, or China. Everywhere, tea- and coffeehouses were places of masculine sociability and leisure. Although sometimes segregated by social status, on the whole they drew patrons from across the social spectrum, including wealthy landowners, noble elites, or successful businessmen alongside peasants and day laborers.[31] There was striking continuity of entertainment across tea- and coffeehouses in Eurasia: Chinese and Turkish teahouses, like Central Asian ones, often attracted patrons through entertainment, such as bird fights and musical performance; in the Ottoman Empire, as in Central Asia, backgammon was a popular teahouse game. Likewise, tea- and coffeehouse culture was highly gendered nearly everywhere: whether in Chengdu, Samarkand, or Shiraz, "respectable" women did not visit teahouses.[32]

It is also notable that many of the European visitors observing the Central Asian teahouse compared it to European social institutions of the bourgeois public sphere. Scottish traveler Ella Christie, who visited Russian Turkestan during the 1910s, described visiting teahouses "which serve as a form of club to the natives."[33] Likewise with Russian observers: the Turkestan volume of the 1913 *Full Geographical Description of our Fatherland* claimed that "teahouses play the role of a restaurant or a club." These travelers saw in the teahouse an expression of a social practice that extended well beyond Europe, and indeed, did not originate in Europe. By the time of the Constitutional

Revolution in Iran, coffeehouses had become hotbeds of political discourse: "In many of the *Qahwa-khánas* (coffeehouses) professional readers are engaged, who, instead of reciting the legendary tales of the *Sháh-náma*, now regale their clients with political news."[34] Likewise, in the Russian imperial Caucasus, Azeri writer Memmedquluzade read aloud from his politically tendentious satirical journal *Molla Nesreddin* at local teahouses.[35] In Republican Turkey and Republican China, reforming elites often focused their efforts on tea- and coffeehouses both because they were popular social institutions and because, in the eyes of reformers, they were dens of backward behavior.[36]

Eurasian tea- and coffeehouses did not develop the same kind of public life that took shape in eighteenth-century Europe, and until the twentieth century, they did not facilitate the circulation of the periodical press or the forms of autonomous political organization that characterized Habermas's imagined bourgeois coffeehouses. Still, they should be understood as a Eurasian analogue—perhaps even a Eurasian *origin*—for the European coffeehouses that Habermas claimed as the incubator for the modern European public sphere.[37] They should thereby be placed in comparative perspective, not as a direct counterpart to the Habermasian coffeehouse, but as a social institution with a shared genealogy, representing an alternative form of social self-organization. Teahouses were not an aberration from modernity, but a component of it. It is therefore unsurprising that, when the Bolsheviks gained a foothold in the region, they turned to the teahouse as an institution from which to begin building a Soviet public in Central Asia.

Soviet Orientalists and the "Teahouse Text"

Mal't, the maker of the teahouse engraving, belonged to a circle of European artists and graphic designers at work in Central Asia during the early Soviet years, and he was far from alone in producing visual representations of teahouses. Unlike Mal't, though, other European artists continued prerevolutionary travelers' tradition of representing teahouses—whether "Red" or black—as sites of Oriental leisure. In 1924, Mal't's colleague, modernist painter Vadim Volkov produced his famed canvas, "The Pomegranate Teahouse" (*Granatovaia chaikhana*). The canvas is dominated by bright red: red turbans, red robes, red pomegranates, and even a red fruit motif on the teapot. But this is not the red of the communist international: it is a red representing, in Volkov's understanding of Sufi color symbolism, a mystical intuition (*irfon*).[38] The six male figures in the teahouses are rendered as six fractured triangles, with the men's downturned faces at the apex of each shape; the top three play stringed instruments, while the bottom figures are engaged, apparently, in mystical contemplation, harking to the "piala of Allah and the smoke of the kalyan."[39] As critic Natalia Apchinskaia suggests, the composition recalls Andrei Rublev's "Trinity," invoking both Orthodox and Islamic antecedents for the path of enlightenment. For Volkov, the teahouse was a place of spiritual enlightenment, not of political consciousness-raising. When Velimir Khlebnikov traveled to Central Asia, it is not for no reason that he set up shop in a teahouse, making himself out to be a kind of "Russian dervish." Khlebnikov's experiments with oriental mysticism found their ideal site in the teahouse.

Volkov and Khlebnikov were among many early Soviet intellectuals to see in the teahouse an "Oriental" spiritual vitality and aesthetic immediacy that they felt European societies had lost. According to his *Salyr-giul': Impressions of Uzbekistan,* Sigizmund Krzhizhanovskii's first impression upon arriving in Central Asia was of a Red Teahouse:

> It's two a.m. I return to the upper square. It is surrounded by murky lights behind transom windows. I walk up to one of them, hoisting my rucksack. The sign reads, "Kisil Caj-xana" [Red teahouse].
>
> Under the sign, behind the glass, or more precisely, in the display case, is an exhibit of mannequins: the teahouse patrons. The patrons are made not of wax and paper, but of flesh and blood. But they are arranged in mannequin-like immobility on the levels of the platform inside the teahouse...Behind the pillars of the canopy, under the soft light of a lamp, bundled up in its yellow glow, lie the specimens of the teahouse...a colorful heap of bodies and turbans, sunken into the black and red ornaments on the pillows. The murky patterns of the rugs laid out under a tangle of dreams, entwined with visions and sighs, all purchased for copper *tiyin*—all of this seems like some sort of orchestrated féerie, a tableau vivant, intended for a full theater of thousands. For me, the only person seeing it now, it is even a little awkward.[40]

Like Volkov, Krzhizhanovskii represented the Red Teahouse not as a modern newspaper room, but as a museum of oriental leisure. Enshrouded in the play of ornament and light, the teahouse patrons become a living exhibit. They are not candidates for mobilization: to the contrary, they are aesthetic objects, better suited for display than for action. Later in his impressions, Krzhizhanovskii stresses the teahouse as an ideal spot for beating the Central

Asian heat: "The best antidote to the heat is doing nothing (*nichegonedelan'e*) in the teahouse." The teahouse is a site for midday rest, obviously incompatible with socialist time-discipline. Krzhizhanovskii mentions the propaganda posters and advertisements at one teahouse: "a tractor, plowing furrows in a field... Chlorodont toothpaste on a toothbrush—a portrait of Lenin—an advertisement for Gutalin shoe polish—a poster reading 'Down with the veil!' "—but this enumeration serves only to accentuate that these items are out of place. In the teahouse ruminations that ensue, Krzhizhanovskii composes a series of fantastical fables, inspired by "oriental" folktales like the *Arabian Nights*. Unlike for the Bolshevik bureaucrats, for these modernists, the teahouse—even the Red Teahouse—represented a spectacle of oriental languor, not of Soviet modernity.

We might thus describe a two-pronged "teahouse text" in Central Asia. On the one hand, for some Party bureaucrats, the teahouse's popularity among the common folk made it ideal for adaptation as "Red"; on the other, to many European observers, it represented an appealingly un-modern space of Oriental leisure. While Volkov, Krzhizhanovskii, and Khlebnikov were soon marginalized from official Soviet culture, their Orientalist view of the teahouse's incompatibility with modernity persisted. Indeed, as Red Teahouses proliferated, so did an official discourse that represented the teahouse public as fundamentally undisciplined, even disloyal. The perception of Oriental leisure that so appealed to Krzhizhanovskii offended Soviet authorities and underpinned the pejorative discourse around "black" as opposed to Red teahouses.

The Red Teahouse and the State Public

While we have many photographs of Red Teahouses, some of which feature newspapers, very few of them—if any—show a gender-integrated teahouse clientele. Mal't's vision of the teahouse—significantly, a woodcut and not a photograph—is one that rarely, if ever, existed in reality. Still, it is a visual expression of the ideal-normative view of what the teahouse was to be under Party tutelage. And as the teahouse ascended in Soviet Uzbekistan, it formed a nascent public around it, as imperfectly as that public may have incarnated the Soviet ideal.

As Mal't's highly idealized engraving suggests, the Red Teahouse served not only to mobilize the masses, but to *represent* them as an already-mobilized public. The Red Teahouse's status as a *national* institution was essential to this project. When they adopted the teahouse form, Soviet administrators made it clear that they did so in an explicit effort to make the Soviet state public identifiably "national." In a 1923 letter defending the Red Teahouse as a propaganda institution as opposed to a commercial one, an agitprop officer called teahouses "a unique type of the cultural apparatus, adapted to local conditions."[41] As one Russian-language article about Red Teahouses affirmed, Central Asian farmers had been accustomed to spending time at teahouses "since time immemorial" (*ispokon vekov*).[42] A 1927 handbook for Red Teahouse activists echoed this language: the "specific conditions of Central Asia" made the Red Teahouse "one of the most basic instruments for making workers of the primary local nationalities participate in enlightenment work and the political life of the country."[43] A 1927 reference book about Central Asia made the goal explicit:

> Chaikhanas (teahouses) play a very significant role in the life of the sedentary population of Central Asia. Teahouses exist in every *kishlak* [village], and they are a peculiar type of club, where public opinion (*obshchestvennoe mnenie*) takes shape. It is clear, then, how significant it would be to organize a broad network of red teahouses with cultural-enlightenment goals.[44]

When Soviet administrators decided to adapt the teahouse as a state-sponsored facility, the Red Teahouse joined the ranks of a number of Soviet institutions, most of which also existed outside of Central Asia. These included women's clubs, workers' clubs, peasants' houses (*doma dekhkanina/doma krestianina*), and Houses of Culture.[45] In the earliest years, Red Teahouses focused on literacy programs and other "enlightenment" projects—hygiene instruction, agronomical training. Very quickly, however, the teahouse became the preeminent institution for mass mobilization in Central Asia. The land reform initiatives of 1925–26 took place in part at Red Teahouses. In the late 1920s, when the drive for collectivization began, Red Teahouses became central institutions for organizing and building support for collective farms and cottonization. By the mid-1930s, Red Teahouses became a major vehicle for promoting "culturedness." In each case, however, the teahouse facilitated both a sense of Soviet belonging and of local acculturation. As Table 1.1 shows, teahouses were by far the most numerous institution of mass publicity in Uzbekistan, eclipsing the number of collective farm clubs, the second most common institution, by a factor of nearly 20.

Red Teahouses, as opposed to black ones, were supposed to help Central Asians imagine themselves as belonging to national, proletarian, and

Table 1.1 "Club-type" institutions in the Uzbekistan SSR as of Jan. 1, 1934

	Total number	Number of paid employees	At these institutions				
			Permanent libraries	Radio receivers (with loudspeakers)	Radio receivers (without loudspeakers)	Permanent film projectors	Mobile film projectors
Red Teahouses	3324	3061	4	1225	94	2	12
Village/ kolkhoz clubs	177	210	51	82	7	18	21
National minority clubs	23	46	13	9	1	2	1
Women and girls' clubs	56	104	29	33	1	2	1
Children and youth clubs	24	44	7	11	1	5	0
Educational workers' clubs	23	50	14	11	1	5	2
Industrial cooperative clubs	4	13	4	3	0	1	0
Farmers' (Collective Farmers') Houses	9	18	3	4	0	0	0
Sanitary education houses	2	2	0	0	0	0	0
Other	46	75	25	28	0	5	6
TOTAL	3688	3623	150	1406	104	40	43

Notes: This table includes a rubric for Houses of Culture, but does not record their numbers.

These figures are in O'zMDA, F. 94, op. 5, d. 1257

gender-inclusive publics. Their ownership and management were the foremost factor in progressing those agendas. In the 1920s, most Red Teahouses were privately managed but tax-exempt because of their important role in Party work. By the time their numbers reached their peak in the 1930s, however, the vast majority of Red Teahouses were managed and funded by Party-state establishments: collective farm, workshop (*artel'*), city, village, or neighborhood budgets.[46] This "Red" funding promoted "red" activities. From the very beginning, teahouses modeled "modern," rational ways of everyday life. Chairs and tables replaced the more traditional cushions and rugs on the floor or a seating platform. A tea service was assumed but rarely discussed.

Teahouses began in the early 1920s as venues for mass "enlightenment," akin to village reading rooms elsewhere in the Soviet Union. Early Red Teahouse administrators placed great emphasis on "reference" (*spravochnaia*) work.[47] Farmers could ask a Party member about how land reform would affect them, consult an agronomist about why tractors were useful, or learn about how to take advantage of the latest legislative changes. For particularly difficult questions, the consultants were supposed to keep a notebook to jot down queries for future research.[48] It also appears that teahouses served as hubs for the administration of land reform, including serving as the space to interview local residents about the amount of land they held in preparation for redistribution.[49]

Throughout the 1920s and 1930s the teahouse system prioritized organizing Central Asians around the mass media, especially the periodical press. Even if they offered no other amenities, teahouse managers subscribed to the latest publications: the Party daily *Red Uzbekistan (Qizil O'zbekiston)*, the Komsomol newspaper *Young Leninist* (*Yosh Leninchi*), and the peasant-facing newspaper *Poor Farmer* (*Kambag'al Dehqon*).[50] The first priority in programming was to read newspapers aloud for the benefit of illiterate patrons. For the convenience of semi-literate patrons, teahouse managers were called upon to mark the most important articles and phrases with a red pencil.[51] Although the newspaper was the fundamental form of media at the teahouses, it was not the only one. Teahouse radio receivers increased in number during the course of the 1930s, although radio programming in Uzbek still consisted primarily of live readings from the newspaper.[52] Film projectors were far less widespread, but in the countryside, Red Teahouses constituted the primary venue for film screenings. Visual media, such as diagrams and posters that drew on the latest newspaper headlines, served to organize public opinion (*jamoat fikri*) at the teahouse.[53] In locales where there were insufficient resources for a full Red Teahouse, activists could open a "Red Corner," which could feature some Party literature, a poster or two, a wall newspaper, and some banners with slogans. In places where there was a Red Teahouse that served only men, "women's Red Corners" filled the gap, albeit unequally.

A reformed sense of temporality underpinned the Red Teahouse public: the Soviet public depended on newspapers arriving regularly and on time. Drawing on Walter Benjamin, Benedict Anderson argues that the nation comes to exist thanks to a changing conception of temporality. Anderson argues that sacral time presupposes a simultaneity of past and future—as when, for example, the Paschal liturgy purports to instantiate, rather than merely reenacting, an ever-existing moment of resurrection; or as when Muslims sacrifice a lamb for Eid al-Adha, participating in Abraham's sacrifice of the divinely provided lamb in the place of his own son. In contrast, in the modern world a new conception of time came to dominate, time became not sacral and simultaneous, but "homogeneous and empty."[54] In this new sense of time, the "clock and the calendar" mark the passing of time, and "temporal coincidence" rather than "prefiguring and fulfillment" are the dominant modes of experiencing time.

For Anderson, the medium of the newspaper makes it possible for readers to imagine *simultaneity* as they had not before. In a single issue of *Red Uzbekistan* newspaper, for example, a teahouse patron outside Bukhara might read of a zealous cotton-sowing brigade outside Namangan, a literary reading at a Tashkent club, and a tax-evading "black" teahouse owner in Stalin raion.[55] These events are unconnected except for their simultaneity on a date in, say, April 1931. By reading the newspaper, the teahouse patron begins to imagine himself as invested in these events, coming to belong to a public that comprises the Namangan brigadier, the Tashkent poet, and the frustrated correspondent in Stalin raion. Anderson calls this sense of temporal coincidence the "meanwhile," and identifies it as a distinctive feature of print culture after the eighteenth century. In this world of mobilization for mass production, the new temporality was constantly inflected by cotton. In the early spring, the cotton planting campaign dominated programming, while in the fall, cotton picking dominated the schedule. Agitprop officials had always demanded the timely circulation of newspapers, but in the context of ever-updated Plans and a production schedule that changed from week to week, demands for timely press distribution became ever more urgent.[56]

It would be possible to continue enumerating such examples endlessly, but the point should be clear: the Red Teahouse, like all other mass institutions, was intended to be a venue for promoting the Party line. As American traveler Anna Louise Strong asked about the Red Teahouse with more than a hint of Orientalism: "Is it possible that the East may lose its leisure, and drink its tea with one lump or two of propaganda?"[57] Indeed, by the late 1920s, Red Teahouses became not only a source for agronomical knowhow and generic "enlightenment," but a major venue for agitation and propaganda, that is, for conveying Party ideology and promoting collectivization. In Red Teahouses, activists held meetings agitating for villagers to enlist in collective farms, while newspapers, posters, and pamphlets popularized the latest slogans. Soviet archives and publications are studded with the lists of such slogans for propagandists working in Red Teahouses and other mass institutions.[58] In the 1930s state propaganda undertook an overarching, all-encompassing campaign to get Uzbeks to the cotton field. For example, one 1930 bulletin for cultural propaganda workers called on Red Teahouses "to help cotton growers learn the political life of the republic and the village (Uzb. *kishlak*)." "Political life" was shorthand for "the slogans of the Party (the cotton campaign, collectivization, work with poor people, and so forth)."[59] At teahouses, the author continued, cotton growers might meet textile producers and compare notes. While enlightenment-related projects like literacy and sanitation remained important, from now on, "production propaganda" became a major priority.

But more than passively receiving propaganda messages from Moscow, Red Teahouses also trained patrons to participate actively in reproducing and interpreting official state discourse. Teahouse visitors joined in discussions of the newspaper stories they heard, or wrote their own articles for wall newspapers.[60] Party administrators urged literate patrons to report on their local teahouse's activities by contributing to newspapers as a peasant correspondent. Teahouses sponsored circles for village or workers' correspondents, as well as for political education, literature, art, music, physical culture, or military preparedness. Cultural and educational circles served two goals: on the one hand, they served to inculcate socialist values and convey state agendas; on the other hand they attracted new participants by providing access to enjoyable activities and cultural amenities. Indeed, despite the constant emphasis on political education (Rus. *politprosvet*) and sloganeering, by the mid-1930s, by far the most common circles at Red Teahouses and clubs were general education (i.e., literacy) and musical (choral and instrumental) circles. Political reading groups and anti-religious clubs seem to have been far less common.[61] The aspiration was that, by attracting participants through enjoyable activities, Red Teahouses they would elicit active participation among young newcomers, not just the small existing cadres of Party activists.

In the context of collectivization and cottonization, the peasantry became the main focus of Party organization, and the number of Red Teahouses increased dramatically. In the mid-1920s, the number of Red Teahouses and the number of clubs had been comparable, but their numbers rapidly diverged during the first two Five-Year Plans, with the number of clubs remaining relatively flat when compared to the ballooning number of Red Teahouses. I have traced this rapid transformation in Table 1.2.

The vast increase in the number of Red Teahouses after the start of the First Five-Year Plan is a trend that can largely be explained by the rapid growth of their number in the countryside. While Red Teahouses continued to operate in cities, urban teahouses also came to focus their efforts on the countryside, prioritizing the cotton production agenda in their programming.[62] Successful urban institutions also often sent delegations to help rural ones get on their feet, a practice known as *shefstvo*.[63]

Shefstvo only went so far, however, and in this period of rapid growth, Red Teahouses began to depend on local, rural cadres. For the most part, the people who organized Red Teahouses are nameless and faceless; it would be very difficult to reconstruct the biography of any individual teahouse manager. However, it is possible to create something of a composite portrait of them based on passing references in the press. Many teahouse directors came by the work unwillingly, under pressure from the agitprop division, the Machine-Tractor Station (MTS), or some other such hierarchy. Still, some teahouse

Table 1.2 Growth in numbers of women's clubs, kolkhoz/village clubs, and Red Teahouses over time

Year[1]	Women's Clubs	Kolkhoz/ Village Clubs	Red Teahouses
1925	16	107	160
1926	32	130	177
1931		128	942
1932		109	1481
1933		217	2647
1934	56	177	3324
1935		141	2825
1936	28	222	2993
1937	29	429	3107

[1] These figures are compiled from O'zMDA, F. 94, op. 1, d. 65, l. 93; O'zMDA, F. 94, op. 5, d. 1219, l. 23; O'zMDA, F. 94, op. 5, d. 1914, ll. 35, 36; and O'zMDA F. 94, op. 5, d. 1257. 1925-26 figures for women's clubs come from Babadzhanova M. "Razvitie seti kul'turno-prosvetitel'nykh uchrezhdenii v kishlakakh Uzbekistana (1925-27 gg.)," From *Sbornik rabot aspirantov TashGU: Istoriia KPSS. Istoriia.* Ed. Iu. I. Ibragimov and V. P. Kharin (Tashkent: V. I. Lenin nomidagi Toshkent davlat universiteti, 1964), 152-156. The category of clubs changes over time: the 1925-26 statistics enumerate the total number of clubs; in the 1930s, the terminology shifts from "village" (sel'skie) to "collective farm" clubs, and in these statistics, urban clubs are excluded. The total number of clubs in the 1930s was thus probably a couple hundred more than reported in the official statistics.

managers took their work seriously. Most of these activist teahouse managers came to teahouse work from a variety of other state-sponsored organizations such as the Komsomol. For example, scholar Khushbekov notes that village teachers were the most consistent organizers of Red Teahouse activity.[64]

Komsomol members—who often overlapped significantly with village teachers—were particularly active in organizing Red Teahouses. It was not uncommon for administrators to call on the Komsomol to whip delinquent teahouses into shape. One report noted that in the town of Ko'lli Qo'rg'on, a group of "important men" (Uzb. *kattalar*) managed the teahouse, but were only interested in tea-selling, rather than the work of public organizing. The article called upon the local Komsomol to take over from those men, who were probably local elites of an older generation, accustomed to "black" teahouses.[65] In Naryn (Kyrgyzstan), according to the traveling editorial team of *Young Leninist*, the Red Teahouse had fallen into such disarray that the local trade union handed it over to the Komsomol's supervision. The local Komsomol cell agreed to take over with support from the newspaper staff, and even decided to rename the teahouse "Young Leninist," after the newspaper.[66] *Young Leninist* frequently called upon local Komsomol members to exert their influence over ineffective teahouse managers.[67] In summer 1932, claiming the Komsomol had not sufficiently addressed the problems at Red Teahouses, *Young Leninist* inaugurated a month-long Komsomol inspection of Red Teahouses around the Republic of Uzbekistan, aiming to align their work with the "production principle."[68] This approach proved effective in some cases. For example, in G'ijduvon, where more than a third of teahouse managers were illiterate, *Young Leninist* reported that the best-functioning teahouses were managed either by trained Komsomol members, or by sincere nonparty youth.[69]

Newspapers often showcased "exemplary" teahouses as inspiration for activists.[70] To give an example: a local correspondent, one Y. Hamdamov, wrote to *Yosh Leninchi* in 1935 to applaud his local teahouse, which operated under the direction of a certain Hasanov.[71] Hamdamov applauded the "expertise and beauty" with which the teahouse had been decorated. Its walls were adorned with posters, slogans, and pictures, while busts of Lenin, Stalin, and Uzbek Party and Party-state leaders Yo'ldosh Oxunboboyev and Fayzulla Xo'jayev rested on its tables. Those tables also enabled teahouse patrons to spread out and read the many newspapers and journals that were available there. The teahouse manager ensured the radio played frequently, and the teahouse was equipped with electric lights. The teahouse facilitated a chess club, and was equipped with dedicated corners for voluntary societies like military preparedness organization OSOAVIAKHIM and Red Cross analogue MOPR. Of course, there was always plenty of tea for thirsty visitors. An exemplary Red Teahouse that was commended in 1937 offered all of the amenities mentioned above, as well as two billiard tables, a monthly wall newspaper, musical instruments, and weekly performances from a local theater troupe.[72] All exemplary Red Teahouses facilitated newspaper read-aloud sessions for semi-literate patrons, and they were frequently commended for facilitating film screenings.

From the focus on enlightenment in the early 1920s, to the emphasis on mass mobilization of the late 1920s, by the mid-1930s, the activities of teahouses expanded to include a greater emphasis on "culturedness," part of a broader turn in Soviet culture toward what Vera Dunham has termed "middle-class values."[73] Scholars of Soviet history have shown that a discourse of "culturedness" took shape in the mid-1930s, officially sanctioning norms of cultural consumption and everyday life, many of which had once been considered "bourgeois"—wearing makeup, attending the opera, dressing fashionably. In Central Asia, the discourse of culturedness was deeply Eurocentric. To be "cultured" in Central Asia required one not only to bathe regularly and brush one's teeth, but also to dress in "European" clothes, to listen to and perform harmonized music, and to sit on a table and chairs rather than on the floor. Being cultured, in other words, was to become more European. At the same time, local activists saw "culturedness" as compatible with certain components of "national" identity. "Cultured" teahouse patrons might sit on chairs, but drink from tea bowls (fastidiously washed), rather than cups with handles. They might wear a skullcap, but not a turban; a headscarf, but not a *paranja*. They speak, read, and write in Uzbek, but also study Russian. Perhaps they play a stringed instrument like the *rubob*, but not in a solo improvisational tradition; instead, they join a folk orchestra sponsored by the Red Teahouse.

Before, teahouses were considered exemplary as long as they held read-aloud sessions, hosted consultations, and sponsored a few circles; now, their purview expanded to serving the entertainment needs of hard-working collective farmers, and keeping them comfortable. In addition to the usual newspapers and books, a 1937 charter for Red Teahouses called for supplies including a portable gramophone, billiard tables, chess sets and other table games, maps and a globe, a wall clock, and even barber equipment.[74] The priorities for teahouse managers still included political education, but also encouraged "cultured leisure."[75] The packed evening schedule—illuminated by electric lights—was to include discussions of world affairs, but also theatrical performances, musical interludes, and group games.[76] Strikingly, this charter barely mentioned tea. In their supplies, activities, and priorities, teahouses were converging with clubs throughout the Soviet Union.[77] In this sense, the colonial valences of the Soviet discourse of "culturedness" were clear.

In other ways, however, the growing discourse of "cultured leisure" facilitated a return to older modes of public life. Teahouses in Central Asia had always offered entertainment to attract clients, including dance, theater, and musical performances. Now, the Communist Party was emphasizing music just as much as it emphasized reading Lenin's works.[78] And these were no mere piano recitals. One workers' correspondence praised a teahouse for having a *dutor*, *chang*, and *nay*, traditional Central Asian string and woodwind instruments that travelers had reported seeing at teahouses already in the nineteenth century.[79]

With the new expectations came tighter control over teahouse administration. Since 1930, teahouses had been answerable to raion "cultural bases" (Rus. *kul'tbazy*), not all of which effectively fulfilled their mandate to supervise local Red Teahouses.[80] In 1935, as part of a broader effort to consolidate efforts, the *kul'tbazy* were renamed Houses of Culture. Now, their main job, according to a report from the Commissariat of Enlightenment, was to serve "the cultural needs of Stakhanovites" by increasing programming and improving staff.[81] Exemplary Houses of Culture would sponsor Saturday work days (Rus. *subbotniki*) and cotton-picking competitions, as well as a wide variety of educational and leisure clubs. The Andijon House of Culture, for example, facilitated aeronautics, sewing and knitting, drama, music, and Russian language clubs. Additionally, Houses of Culture served as both model and mentor for the "lowest-level" (Rus. *nizovoi*) mass institutions, the Red Teahouses.[82] Accordingly, in late 1936, the Commissariat of Enlightenment began issuing forms that all Red Teahouses were required to get signed at the House of Culture, confirming that they were indeed functioning as Red (rather than Black) Teahouses, and that they were being appropriately supervised.[83] As successful as the Red Teahouse model may have been, administrators still fretted that it was not doing enough to facilitate a "Red" public sphere.

The "Red" and the "Black"

The "redness" of the teahouse meant little to a large proportion of teahouse visitors. For mediators like activists and correspondents, on the other hand, the teahouse's main role was to induct their fellow Central Asians into a Soviet public that stretched beyond the local and the face-to-face: to help Central Asians imagine themselves as Uzbeks, as proletarians, and as Soviet people. On the part of Central Asia's new elites, the discourse about teahouse life thus contained an implicit anxiety that the Central Asian population was not "ready" for Soviet public life.[84] The popularity that legitimized the Red Teahouse as authentically national also made it less perfectly Soviet. For local activists, the Red Teahouse's failure to effectively mobilize the masses did not signal its illegitimacy or its inefficacy as an institution. To the contrary: the Red Teahouse was a perfectly legitimate institution, but saboteurs had undermined it. Workers' correspondents adduced these normal uses of the teahouse as proof of sabotage, or at least of undisciplined engagement. Because of their "backwardness," their lack of cultivation, these men were unready to participate in the state public. According to this logic, they deserved to be repressed. The narrative about disorderly teahouse patrons served to justify excluding and repressing them, even in a state that claimed to govern on behalf of the public.

Uzbek-language newspaper reports about Red Teahouses proportionately increased with their growing number throughout Uzbekistan. Since Red Teahouses usually operated under the leadership of youth activists, such reports appeared most commonly in *Yosh Leninchi* (Uzb. *Young Leninist*), the official organ of the Komsomol. Teahouse reports often appeared on the back page of the newspaper, frequently in batches of two or three per day. These correspondences fell into two main categories: first, and least frequent, commendations of exemplary teahouses; second, harsh critiques of poorly run teahouses and their managers, exhorting them to do better. It is difficult to ascertain with certainty the provenance of any individual article. Often no longer than a paragraph, the articles are often unsigned or signed with initials only, and even when an author's name appears, the individual is so historically obscure as to be unidentifiable. However, most such missives evidently came from village or worker correspondents (*rabdekhkor/ rabsel'kor*), amateur journalist-activists who contributed to regional newspapers.[85] In the village of Chinos, for example, one article reported that forty Komsomol members had taken up the mantle of workers' correspondents, forming an active circle of self-taught writers. Desiring further training, the group of aspiring correspondents wrote to the journal *Muxbirlar Yo'ldoshi* (*Correspondents' Companion*) in an attempt to drum up further support for their endeavors.[86] Stylistic inconsistencies and non-standard dialectal variants indicate that many of the authors of these articles did not come from highly educated backgrounds. Most correspondents likely belonged to the cadres of local youth activists. Many correspondents were students of one kind or another; village teachers, who comprised the primary social base of the Party in the Central Asian countryside, were another major source of village correspondents.[87] Village correspondent reports evince intense social conflict in the Central Asian countryside, often culminating around invasive policies like women's unveiling, collectivization, and anti-religious activism. Correspondents saw newspaper reports as a key tool to effect the changes they desired in their communities: their notes could result in serious disciplinary action against the people correspondents critiqued.

Teahouse correspondents' reports describe the on-the-ground realities of Red Teahouse life, often in greater detail than can be found elsewhere. Still, they should be read critically—not merely as *descriptive* sources, but as *normative* ones. Newspaper reports were often the first foray in campaigns to purge or punish the correspondents' opponents, often referring to the offending individuals by name. Indeed, as has been well documented elsewhere, newspapers were a key venue for denunciations during the Terror. In writing their reports, teahouse correspondents drew on widely circulating political scripts that linked drunkenness with counter-revolution, or excoriated profiteering ex-merchants. These scripts, in turn, derived from the Party education that correspondents received and the clear political imperatives of the workers' correspondence genre. Workers' correspondents felt that they stood to benefit from participating in Party agendas. By writing for the newspaper, correspondents consolidated their status as "Red," as loyal supporters of Soviet power. As Abashin notes, "public letters and secret anonymous notes," including correspondents' notes in newspapers, were an "instrument of power in the hands of teachers...they became a pseudo-public space of self-expression, in which Soviet people learned to speak a Soviet language and play the role of a Soviet citizen."[88] As Botakoz Kassymbekova has argued with respect to early Soviet Tajikistan, the workers' correspondent's movement was a "*process of disciplining*" that served as "an experiment both for constructing 'masses' and constructing 'the state.'"[89] Worker correspondents tended to stress the negative, because exposing "wreckers" and delinquents helped burnish their own self-image as diligent Soviet people and the state as responsible for maintaining law and order.

A cartoon published in satirical journal *Mushtum* (Uzb. *The Fist*) exhibits the layered power dynamics inherent in the worker correspondents' reports (Plate 2). In the cartoon, a portly patrician (Uzb. *to'ra*) seizes a worker correspondent by the throat, wagging a finger at a wall newspaper that contains a prominent image of that very scene. The patrician shouts, "Why did you put my picture in the wall newspaper, saying that I have been attacking correspondents? That's a lie! It's never happened, and never could happen!" The correspondent replies, "Don't you see? It's happening right now." The cartoon represents the worker correspondent as a victim: the patrician's large physique dominates the correspondent's angular frame. *The Fist* published the cartoon to critique a power differential that supposedly favored anti-Soviet elites like the patrician. Indeed, there is much evidence that worker and peasant correspondents, like other village activists, often experienced violent attacks.[90] *Muxbirlar Yo'ldoshi* (*Correspondents' Companion*), the official Uzbek journal for correspondents, even published images of correspondents who had been murdered.[91] But the image's self-referentiality undermines a straightforward reading of correspondents as victims. To the contrary: the wall newspaper looms large behind both figures, challenging the patrician's epistemic authority even while his physical dominance temporarily persists. The cartoon thus implies that in the new Soviet order, power lies not in brute force, but in mass publicity. In 1931 in Uzbekistan, a newspaper denunciation could be more dangerous than the fist—or, more precisely, a newspaper denunciation carried the full force of the state's monopoly on violence.[92] In emphasizing the patrician's violence, the cartoon occludes the Soviet state's own violence: in real life, that wall newspaper cartoon could justify expelling the so-called patrician from the Party, relieving him of his official duties, imprisoning him, or executing him. The satirical journal's title, *Mushtum* (*The Fist*), drove this point home.

We can read worker correspondent reports as a rare and untapped source on everyday life in early Soviet Central Asia. But they must also be recognized as a discursive project, drawing the parameters of the Party public and strictly policing its boundaries. They not only relate what happened at the Red Teahouse, but they also lay out norms for the Party public in Uzbekistan. Specifically, they counterpose an ideal-normative "Red" public sphere to what were understood as the "black" or "dark" masses, whose incontinent presence justified ongoing state intervention and violence. In this respect, the rhetoric around the Red teahouse tapped into longstanding categories of "blackness" in Central Asian society. As Donohon Abdugafurova has shown, "blackness" has a long history as a social category in Central Asia—"uneducated, ordinary, and poor people who are not from Sayyid or Kwaja [sic] (i.e., noble or high-status) lineages," but also as an ethical category.[93] "Blackness" represented social inferiority with relation to high-status individuals like the "white-boned" aristocracy.[94] In their representation of the Red Teahouse, mediators appropriated this component pre-Soviet discourse for ostensibly revolutionary ends. Instead of "black" as opposed to "white-boned," the Soviet system generated a discursive opposition between the "black" and the "Red," which in turn created a new Central Asian elite backed by the state's monopoly on violence.[95]

In making this effort, they tapped into a variety of representational traditions about the teahouse. On the one hand, they drew on ethnographers who identified the teahouse as a popular social institution: a "kind of club." On the other, as they began to appropriate the teahouse model, they constantly echoed European outsiders' Orientalist representations that saw teahouse "leisure" as incompatible with modernity. It is not for no reason that these anxieties about the public also appeared in the medium of the mass-circulation newspaper. If, as Benedict Anderson famously argued, the newspaper created new forms of "imagined communities," the worker correspondents' reports served as a device for imagining an identifiably national and fully Soviet public. If the teahouse was the crux of the Soviet effort to mobilize a state public around the mass media, teahouse reports delineated the parameters of that public.

Correspondents' reports should thus be taken not primarily as an accurate description of what transpired at the Red Teahouse, but as a discursive tool that distinguished the "Red" public from the "black" counterpublic. What forms of bad behavior did correspondents find at the teahouse? To answer this question, we might begin by returning to the 1925 administrator who hoped to rename the Red Teahouses. He felt that the population was using them, not as a locus of enlightenment, but as a space for vulgar commercialism. There were concrete material reasons for this state of affairs. Until the attempt to make them "red," teahouses had always been profit-making institutions. The fact that Red Teahouses were tax-exempt compounded this issue. In 1923, the question of profit generated an extended correspondence between educational officials (under the auspices of Turkpolitprosvet, the Central Asian administration for political education in the early 1920s) and the People's Commissar for Finances. The educators argued that it was unfair to exempt the Russian Peasants' Houses and Village Reading Rooms (*izby-chital'ni*) from taxation while not doing the same for Uzbekistan's Farmers' Houses and Red Teahouses. They continued that although Red Teahouses appeared to be commercial institutions, in reality they performed essential educational and propaganda functions. The Finance Commissar's office countered with an affected concern for "black" teahouse owners, arguing that exempting Red Teahouses would put all other teahouses out of business.[96] In passing—and probably revealing its true motives—the Finance Commissar's office also noted that exempting Red Teahouses from taxes would reduce state revenues.

Ultimately, Red Teahouses received at least some tax exemptions.[97] But teahouse correspondents consistently claimed that the tax exemptions and state subsidies granted to Red Teahouse workers encouraged the schemes of profiteering NEPmen and saboteurs. By creating a financial incentive, tax exemptions invited any teahouse owner, regardless of his Communist commitment, to register as "Red." By the late 1920s, many Red Teahouses were not privately run, but were instead expected to generate revenue for a sponsoring organization, such as a collective farm.[98] They were also supposed to attract clientele with their low prices—and therefore, to garner participation in Soviet culture and propaganda work.[99] In reality, correspondents complained, local teahouse operators were more profiteer than propagandist. As they claimed, some teahouses were run by men who were known to have been merchants before the Bolshevik ascendancy.[100] Other correspondents claimed that the unscrupulous took advantage of their position by pocketing the profits.[101] In one case, a Red Teahouse owner went beyond selling hot tea and became a wholesale broker of dry tea leaves.[102] Another bought bread from a nearby bakery and sold it at a profit at the teahouse he managed.[103] In the town of G'ijduvon, the head of the Red Teahouse under the sponsorship of the municipal police had even turned half of it into a for-profit barbershop.[104] In some instances, patrons reportedly had to pay just as much for tea at Red Teahouses as at black ones.[105] Many teahouses had purportedly made commercial work their primary focus, but one teahouse correspondent spoke for all activists when he insisted in his headline that a Red Teahouse's job was "Not Just Tea-Drinking."[106]

For correspondents, profiteering was just the tip of the iceberg. With Red Teahouses mushrooming in the largely illiterate countryside, it quickly became difficult to furnish them with qualified staff. Countless reports claimed that local Red Teahouse directors did not even know how to read. In 1933, for example, *Yosh Leninchi* (*Young Leninist*) reported that 35% of G'ijduvon Raion's Red Teahouses were staffed by illiterate people, and even more Red Teahouse directors were only semi-literate.[107] In Yangi Yo'l raion, the regional director for the Commissariat of Enlightenment was accused of lying, saying he had trained twelve Red Teahouse directors, when in fact no training had happened at all.[108]

Whether qualified or not, some Red Teahouse staff seemed to consider the job a sinecure. Newspaper correspondents observed that teahouse directors, often barely supervised, could get away with drawing a salary while doing little agitprop or cultural work.[109] In addition to having easy access to teahouse revenues, some collective farm teahouse directors benefited from a day off from work in the fields in order to "tend to the teahouse."[110] For example, one agrotechnician employed by a Red Teahouse spent all his days drinking tea, but according to a frustrated correspondent, had never actually conducted agronomy consultations.[111] The cadres who ran these failed teahouses seem to have understood their role to be much more similar to that of "black" teahouse-keepers. They were providers of hot water and rudimentary furnishings, not the curator-cum-reference librarian-cum-programming directors that Red Teahouse managers, in theory, were supposed to be.

Correspondents complained that even Komsomol and Party activists did not always engage in Red Teahouse work with enthusiasm, suggesting that sabotage lurked even within Party ranks. When a *Young Leninist* teahouse inspection drive began in 1933, the editorial board reported that only eight raion Komsomol cells took up the charge immediately, while no one in the Ferghana Valley had paid the drive any attention at all.[112] Other Komsomol members, such as those at Stalin raion's redundantly named Stalin Collective Farm, spent hours lazily drinking tea at the Red Teahouse.[113] At a 1932 conference for Central Asia's "agitational and mass workers," a certain Comrade Israilov complained that the Communist Party and Komsomol had failed appropriately to apportion their cadres. Too often, he argued, the best Party and Komsomol members were assigned to teahouse duty, when they should really have prioritized production. Despite his activist pedigree, Israilov lacked a vision for teahouse work, preferring to send the most highly qualified individuals to the fields. "Any collective farmer can handle teahouse work," continued Israilov, "even a woman."[114] His statement reflected both his assumption that women were less competent than men, and that teahouse work was unimportant.

Red Teahouse Media Publics

Red and "black" teahouses differed in large part because the former stocked periodical publications, especially newspapers. In practice, however, teahouse correspondents and Party activists denounced bureaucrats across the administrative hierarchy for inhibiting public access to the mass circulation press. Their complaints began at the source: according to a Central Asian Bureau commission on the press, publishers consistently failed to publish newspapers and journals on schedule. Once they made it off the presses at the few towns that had printing presses, newspapers had to be sent to their destinations by rail, at least in part. However, railway administrators were not always cooperative. Newspaper editorial boards lacked qualified staff to manage distribution and subscription.[115] Even the most dedicated agitprop staff, such as a certain Comrade Kamalov of Namangan, might pay for and subscribe to a publication, only for it never to arrive.[116] It was almost a cliché for correspondents to excoriate a teahouse for stocking only out-of-date books and periodicals; in 1934, one teahouse was accused of stocking books from 1924 at the most recent.[117] From teahouse managers to newspaper editors and typographers, incompetent men (or were they wreckers?) inhibited the access of the masses to the mass press, and hence, to belonging in the Soviet public.

Even when the correct newspapers arrived at Red Teahouses in a timely manner, they frequently just lay around gathering dust. Reports bemoaned the fact that books and newspapers were used for all kinds of things other than reading, including wrapping meat and rolling cigarettes.[118] Another teahouse headline stated gaspingly, "newspapers are being burned instead of wood!"[119] Similar complaints applied to other media as well. The magazine *Madaniy Inqilob* (Uzb. *Cultural Revolution*) reported that, at many teahouses, radio receivers and film projectors cluttered the space, neglected and in a state of disrepair.[120] In Urgut, no fewer than 100 radio receivers lay about unused.[121] Circles for political reading, theater, music, etc., all too often fizzled out for lack of enthusiasm or dedicated leadership. Readers were too exhausted after a day of work.[122] In a context when many visitors felt that the mere presence of Soviet media was sufficient to make a teahouse red, Soviet activists were hard-pressed to show that it was imperative also to *participate* in those media. *Mushtum* (*The Fist*), the Uzbek satirical journal, addressed the problem of media indifference in 1933, with a cartoon showing a Red Corner at a so-called Red Teahouse, fenced off and locked (Plate 3). In the caption, when a collective farmer challenges the teahouse manager about this state of affairs, the manager retorts, "Our raion cultural base (Rus./ Uzb. *kul'tbaza*) instructed us to make the teahouse's Red Corner just like a club!" In other words: clubs were unpopular, and teahouses were popular—not *because* they provided access to the media, but *despite* that fact.

In other contexts, newspaper readers could take out individual subscriptions, but in Soviet Central Asia very few readers encountered the newspaper at home. In 1933, an activist from Patta-Gisar Raion (Termez region) indicated that only 10–15% of local Party members and candidates subscribed to national newspapers.[123] Other regional activists corroborated the concern that Party members rarely subscribed to newspapers; some even indicated that nonparty individuals were more likely to take out subscriptions than Party members.[124] Instead, institutional subscriptions were the norm: an Uzbekistani reader was more likely to encounter a Soviet newspaper at a library, a school, or a worker's club than in a private home. Institutions like the Red Teahouse were thus crucial venues for Central Asians to encounter the media. When a teahouse patron did not engage the periodical press or did not engage it properly, then, he undermined the teahouse's function as a venue for building a Soviet public. Hence Shcherbakov's panic about the newspapers hanging from the ceiling of a Red Teahouse. Instead of building a state public that stretched beyond the face-to-face, the Red Teahouse had become a space for purely local sociability.

Consumption at Red Teahouses

Teahouse correspondents worried that rather than promoting a sense of mass publicity through the periodical press, some Red Teahouses instead facilitated the reverse: a drug-addled sense of the suspension of time. Teahouses were often accused of being opium dens (*ko'knorixona*)[125] or cannabis houses (*nashaxona*).[126] Tobacco was also widely used at teahouses.[127] Smoking was so closely associated with teahouse life that the 1927 Red Teahouse handbook argued that if it was banned altogether, patrons would simply take their business to a "black" teahouse.[128] Instead of a blanket ban, then, the brochure proposed a harm-reduction policy. Provide a "Red Pipe" (*qizil chilim*), the brochure said, making sure to sanitize the mouthpiece between users.[129] This would keep customers coming, while also inculcating them with modern practices of everyday life. Although such a level of tolerance for drug use did not continue into the 1930s, the approach shows just how difficult it was for Red Teahouse activists to eradicate established social practices around teahouses. The brochure's section heading says it all: "It is terrifying to eradicate the *chilim* from teahouses."[130] Somewhat less traditional, but no less widespread, was the consumption of alcohol at Red Teahouses.[131] Correspondents claimed that many teahouse directors spent the day drinking.[132] In a countryside Red Teahouse in Tashkent raion, the director, one Akbarov, spent his time drinking and playing a game called "pasha-pasha."[133] Another alcoholic teahouse worker, whose establishment was located near a train station, reportedly drank daily and harassed the women who got off the train there.[134] In

Khorezm, one Red Teahouse had no newspapers; instead, most patrons spent their time playing cards and drinking vodka.[135]

Soviet policy strongly discouraged the use of narcotics. But most teahouse visitors just wanted to drink tea and talk—and in the new context of socialist time-discipline, those behaviors obstructed socialist construction. At the Red Teahouse, not just *what* patrons did, but *when* they did it was of pivotal importance. Behaviors that Red Teahouses permitted, even encouraged after work hours, became intolerable when they conflicted with the prescribed regimented schedule for socialist labor and cultural enlightenment. From the activist perspective, the culture of tea-drinking became particularly problematic during the Islamic fasting season of Ramadan.[136] Because they could not eat or drink during the day, Central Asian Muslims were accustomed to resting for much of the day and socializing at teahouses by night. In order to combat this when Ramadan fell during important seasons for cotton production, the Party called upon Red Teahouses to close promptly in the evening and to hold anti-religious lectures when they were open.[137] But even during the rest of the year, teahouses kept people from their work. Propagandists put down their propaganda; cotton pickers abandoned their fields.[138] It was only in the context of the battle for cotton autarky that mere tea-drinking and chitchat could become the most egregious form of civic neglect. In Soviet Uzbekistan of the 1930s, after all, the best expression of civic engagement was not to vote, but to work the cotton fields.

Gender and the Red Teahouse Public

In the above, I have used the masculine pronoun advisedly. Uzbek pronouns do not identify gender, but in reports where the gender of a teahouse offender can be identified, he is invariably a man. Indeed, after reviewing over a hundred teahouse reports in multiple Central Asian newspapers, I have not identified a single complaint about a woman teahouse patron or teahouse organizer. To the contrary: women and girls appear in teahouse reports exclusively as the victims of incontinent men: drinkers, smokers, harassers, layabouts. Despite the official rhetoric about women's emancipation, and despite the print by Mal't discussed at the beginning of this chapter, the emphasis on women as victims reified their position under the protection of the state and its representatives.[139] In the Soviet context, despite the state's official ambition to eliminate the private sphere, in practice even women who entered the state public sphere were represented as less public than men, and therefore, more in need of protection from "enlightened" activist men and, more broadly, from the patriarchal state.[140]

The Red Teahouse amplified this dynamic. Teahouses were, and long had been, spaces exclusively for men. Red Teahouses, in contrast, were expected to welcome women, but in practice they rarely did so. The gendering of the Red Teahouse is best exemplified in an episode Fannina Halle, a German traveler, recorded during her journey through Central Asia in the 1930s. On a village market day in winter, Halle claims she encountered a group of women vendors who had given up on selling their wares in the midst of a hard freeze. Business was bad because of the weather, and many men had gathered to stay warm inside a Red Teahouse near the market. According to Halle, the women gazed through the window of the warm teahouse in envy as the men enjoyed tea and conversation: women were not welcome there. Gathering behind a woman, Mastura, who had just been elected village elder (*oqsoqol*), the women vendors decided as a group to go into the teahouse to warm themselves. But when they stepped onto the threshold and announced their intention to enter, the men inside responded with laughter and mockery. Even the young Party secretary responded to Mastura, "Have you ever known women sitting in a *chaikhana*, that is meant for men?" Unperturbed, Mastura responded, "This is a new *ksyl* [sic] *chaikhana*, a Red *Chaikhana*, and nobody has said that it is only for men..." Halle reports that the men were sufficiently cowed by this confrontation that they abandoned the teahouse en masse, leaving it for the women. She concludes the story with a promise from Mastura: "By the next bazaar we will have our own *chaikhana*."[141]

The dialogue Halle reports is likely semi-fictionalized, but it exemplifies a common dynamic in Red Teahouses. To be sure, some particularly active Red Teahouses hosted events that included women; but most frequently, women attended single-sex events, while the default, "co-ed" programming attracted mostly men.[142] Men and women simply were not accustomed to socializing in mixed company, and it was a massive overreach to assume that dubbing a teahouse "red" would automatically facilitate women's inclusion on an everyday level. Furthermore, while women's clubs were widely visible in cities and in the press, their number totaled less than one percent of the number of Red Teahouses. Despite persistent rhetoric about emancipating women, outreach to women remained a lower priority for administrators in Central Asia than that addressed to farmer men; or, at best, the administrators who spearheaded the growth of Red Teahouses made a grave miscalculation in assuming that calling a teahouse "Red" would immediately overturn centuries of gendered norms around teahouse sociability.

Conclusion

The worker correspondents' reports I have discussed show that, for every exemplary teahouse, there were many other Red Teahouses where older norms of teahouse sociability prevailed. At these teahouses, men who cared little about the latest issue of *Qizil O'zbekiston* (*Red Uzbekistan*) shirked their civic duty—cotton production—in favor of whiling away the afternoon at the teahouse, chatting, smoking and drinking tea. Red Teahouses, as a result, had quite the opposite of the desired effect in many cases. According to frustrated administrators, teahouses lured men away from socialist construction, leaving women to work the fields, care for the children, and run the collective farm. Some even rejected modern furniture, such as tables and chairs. One observer complained that a certain teahouse lacked enough chairs for people to sit down and read—but what did that matter if everyone was sitting on the floor anyway?[143] Published at the peak of the cotton-picking season, a 1931 cartoon from Uzbek-language newspaper *Kolxoz Yo'li* (*Collective Farm Way*) exemplifies the anxiety around delinquent teahouse men. In the image, a group of women hunch over at work in a cotton field, while in the foreground, three men relax on a teahouse rug, smoking a hookah, drinking tea, and enjoying *dutar* music (Figure 1.2). The caption drives the point home: "At the Ferghana region's Stalin Collective Farm, women work while the men never leave the teahouse."

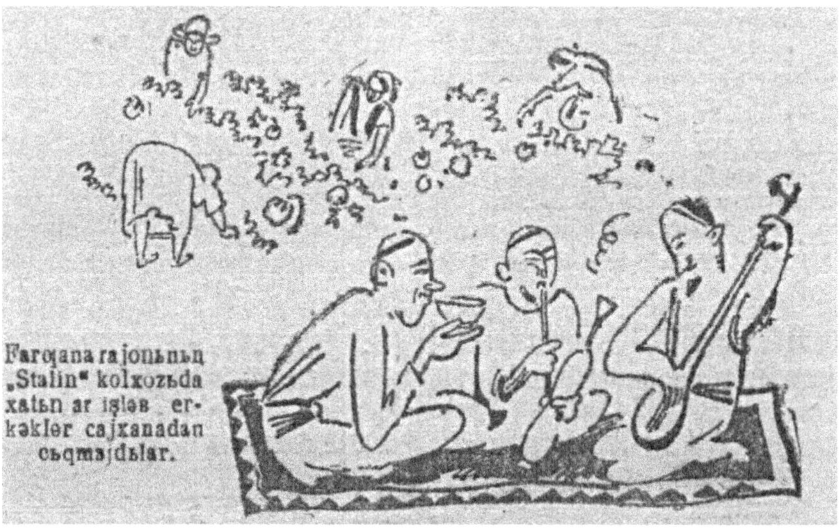
Farƣana rajonьnьꞑ
„Stalin" kolxozьda
xatьn ar işləʙ er-
kəklər cajxanadan
cьqmajdьlar.

Figure 1.2 Editorial cartoon, "The Men Don't Leave the Teahouse," uncredited, *Kolxoz Yo'li,* Oct. 13, 1931, 1.

Red Teahouses were essential institutions for building a Soviet public in Central Asia. At exemplary Red Teahouses, women learned to read, collective farmers brushed up on agronomy, and young people acquired the habits of Soviet modernity—reading the newspaper, playing billiards. Quite often, however, Red Teahouses functioned much as teahouses had before the revolution—they were a space for men to gather and converse, to beat the heat during the summer midday, to listen to music—but these habits were not consistently compatible with Bolshevik publicity. Correspondents' reports pathologized normal teahouse behavior, offering it up as evidence of incompetence, incontinence, or, worse, insubordination. Importantly, while some "black" teahouse behaviors such as harassing women and smoking were intolerable prima facie, others—resting, chatting, listening to music—were not inherently incompatible with socialist modernity. Their main crime was a failure to accord with European norms of time-discipline and the practices of Soviet everyday life.

This chapter has examined the Red Teahouse as a state-run institution of mass publicity. Unlike other Eurasian states, which ignored or suppressed the teahouse, the Soviet state public in Central Asia co-opted the teahouse as its premiere institution. In so doing, Soviet activists tapped into longstanding cultural and social norms that both boosted the Red Teahouse's popularity and undermined its goals for mass mobilization, modernization, and "culturedness." The Red Teahouse legitimized the Soviet project as national, gender-integrated, and proletarian—as a project rooted in a self-organized public sphere rather than a top-down hierarchy. At the same time, the discourse around the Red Teahouse reinforced new social hierarchies between cultural mediators and the non-compliant men who used the teahouse in un-Soviet ways. At the Red Teahouse, "culturedness" became Central Asians' ticket to participating in the state public, while mediators like workers' correspondents policed its boundaries, relegating the "uncultured" beyond the pale.

Socialism Mediated: The Making of Soviet Culture in Central Asia. Claire Roosien, Oxford University Press.
 DOI: 10.1093/9780198971153.003.0003

2
Pens

Introduction

When Husayn Shams was fired, he did not learn about it as one might expect, from a stern typewritten letter or in a face-to-face meeting. No: when the Writers' Union that had employed him for the better part of a decade voted summarily to expel him, Husayn Shams learned of it from the newspaper. Like the names of many of his co-workers, friends, and drinking buddies in the dark fall and winter of 1937, Shams's name appeared in *Qizil O'zbekiston* (*Red Uzbekistan*) in a clipped summary of the most recent meeting of the Writers' Union.[1] Much of the report was mundane: the Union was working on translating a Central Asian epic poem into Russian and writing a screenplay for a film about cotton autarky. It was gathering historical materials about the Revolution and admitting new members. Shams's name appeared almost as an afterthought: at the end of the meeting, the committee responsible for purging the Writers' Union ranks had finally confirmed its resolution to expel him. Within weeks, Shams lost access to all the privileges that accrued to him as a Responsible Secretary of the Writers' Union—the company car, the well-appointed dacha, the subsidized housing, the publication support. In a five-page letter he wrote in Uzbek to appeal the decision, Shams entreated that he had risen from his working-class origins, only to be plunged again into destitution: along with his four children, he was reduced to peddling at the bazaar.[2] Shams's career and his reputation never recovered, and he died under unknown circumstances in 1942. Still, he was one of the lucky ones: he escaped the summary executions and long imprisonments that befell many of his colleagues.

Shams's experience, however particular to him, reflects core paradoxes in the Party-state's project to build a Soviet public that would organize, address, and mobilize Central Asia's masses. Not least among these is the unhappy fact that the Soviet newspaper, the very medium that made his career, turned out to augur his demise. Equally ironic is the way that Shams's humble origins both facilitated his ascendance and hurried his fall. Shams's career rose astronomically: he began his upward path in a workers' literary circle in the provincial Ferghana Valley city of Kokand and soon reached the halls of power in Tashkent and even Moscow. His star fell just as precipitously when, during the Terror, his own former colleagues accused him of ensconcing himself an elite, hard-partying clique and neglecting to support writers from among the masses.

This chapter examines the Writers' Union of Uzbekistan as the leading institution for making mediators in Uzbekistan and for imagining them as representatives of a broader public. Mediators could be found in many institutions. But in Soviet culture, literature held pride of place. Writers consequently took on an outsize role in shaping the effort to integrate the masses, in all their complicated diversity and potential incompatibility, into a universal public. At the same time, I show, their effort to cultivate a universal public also actually created or reinforced social hierarchy. The material conditions of Soviet cultural production, namely, that the Party-state financed writers as highly qualified specialists, inducted Writers' Union members into an emerging specialist elite. I focus on four leading members of the Writers' Union in Uzbekistan. These individuals were leading figures in Uzbekistani literature at the time, but they also exemplify broader trends. Sadriddin Ayni became the face of Tajik, and indeed, of Central Asian literature at the Moscow Congress of the Writers' Union. As a denizen of the multilingual Persianate cultural sphere of the newly "Uzbek" cities Samarkand and Bukhara, Ayni's biography shows how Central Asian culture shifted from a polycentric Persianate milieu to a centralized national public with a newfound separate discipline of "literature" (*adabiyot*). Abdulla Qahhor and Husayn Shams exemplify the turn to "proletarian" cultural production in the late 1920s. They crafted narratives about themselves as worker-writers, but their status as Tashkent-based literary professionals both facilitated their status as mediators and distanced them from the "working masses." Finally, during the 1930s Oydin Sobirova became the most prominent woman in the Uzbekistan Writers' Union in her role as Responsible Secretary. Oydin's position as a token woman in a male-dominated institution ultimately shored up accusations that she was a traitor to her sex rather than its vanguard.[3]

Union writers like these four addressed the "masses" they claimed to represent: editing journals, publishing adult primers, directing circles for aspiring young writers, and leading brigades to visit collective farms. At the same time, I show, the Writers' Union paradoxically yielded a new professional elite, organized around a Tashkent-based inner circle of official writers with immense cultural capital and material privilege, answering, in turn, to Moscow. This inner circle constituted a "shadow public sphere," possible only because of the patronage of the state but operating in ways it could not predict or control.[4]

The Writers' Union plucked representatives (or claimed to pluck them) from among the "working masses"; but those representatives came to enjoy the uncommon cultural capital and material advantages that official propaganda claimed now accrued to *all* Uzbekistan's workers. Soon, however, they were punished for not being sufficiently representative of the masses they claimed to represent. To tell this story, I examine the Terror in the micro-context of the Soviet Writers' Union of Uzbekistan. Terror, I argue, functioned as the apotheosis of the system of Soviet publicity that created a new cohort of mediators from among the masses and then, subsequently, punished them for that selfsame status as mediators.

The Writers' Union of Uzbekistan took shape in a moment when writers and other cultural producers were attaching themselves to newly formed bureaucratic institutions, both in the Soviet Union and beyond. The institutionalization of national writers at the turn of the century had long roots in romantic nationalism, which had begun creating national mythologies around the "people's" poets: Pushkin for Russians; Goethe for Germans. By the mid-nineteenth century, it became natural for Europe's writers to think of themselves in national terms, and they began advocating for professional societies to defend their own interests already in the mid-nineteenth century.[5] In the early twentieth century, professional organizations began to emerge for American writers, Czech writers, Bulgarian writers, and so forth. These institutions self-consciously created a myth of the writer as national hero, both calling into being a nascent national public and setting writers up as special mediators between the untutored, indifferent "masses" and the nation they learned to represent.[6] National literatures could teach the "people" to behave as properly national subjects.

In organizing a dedicated institution for national writers, the Soviet Union was thus following a well-established precedent, but this time under the direct tutelage of the state. In 1932, a resolution of the Politburo formed the Writers' Union that became the umbrella organization for a cascade of national chapters. The Politburo claimed that far from forcing conformity, the Union would facilitate a diversity of viewpoints by uniting all writers under a "big tent," including both Party and nonparty members.[7] According to the Politburo decree, independently organized groups such as the Association for Proletarian Writers had produced a chilling effect in the arts by insisting on a narrow and exclusionary definition of "proletarian" culture. In its rhetoric, if not in practice, the Writers Union was supposed to loosen the grip of narrow ideological strictures, not to tighten them. Ultimately, the "cliquish insularism" of APP would give way to a universal publicity, organizing and addressing "new writers and artists...from industrial plants, factories, and collective farms."[8] To their role representing the toiling masses, writers in the national chapters of the Writers' Union added the burden of national representation. Although the Uzbekistan Writers' Union comprised a maximum of only about fifty members in the 1930s, membership in the Writers' Union entailed an unprecedented burden of universal representation and mass address.[9]

The basic contours of Uzbek literary politics in the 1920s and 1930s are known in broad strokes.[10] In the years immediately following the Bolshevik revolution, the Soviets struggled to obtain a solid foothold in Central Asia. In order to build their local base of support and to legitimize themselves as an authentically anti-colonial government, the Soviet Party-state made allies among a range of local elites and intelligentsia. Given the absence of Party cadres who spoke Muslim languages well enough to censor works in those languages, the early-mid 1920s marked a moment of relative polyphony in Soviet Central Asian culture. This discursive heterogeneity mirrored a relatively decentralized institutional culture. Jadids ran discussion groups in their homes, Muslim clerics spoke out on behalf of women's "emancipation," and ephemeral publications proliferated.[11] Projects exploring the deep history of Uzbek and Turkic cultural identity in Central Asia were particularly prominent; the "Chaghatay Conversation," a literary circle devoted to recovering a distinct Turkic literary language for Central Asia and building connections throughout the Turkic world, exerted significant influence even after it was disbanded in 1922. State violence was targeted primarily against those who explicitly opposed Soviet rule, not against the ideologically diverse range of cultural producers who made common cause with the Bolsheviks.

After the 1927 Hujum and the launch of the Five-Year Plan in 1928, this dynamic began to change. Youthful "proletarian" critics viciously attacked the ex-Jadids and their associations as expressions of "bourgeois nationalism," and for the first time, they created a state-backed literary organization, the Red Pens (*Qizil Qalam*). Also in the mid-1920s, an Association of Proletarian Writers emerged in Tashkent under the auspices of the all-Soviet organization devoted to advancing an authentically "proletarian" culture. In 1929, as part of an all-Soviet campaign against "bourgeois nationalists" in every republic, both the Red Pens and the Jadids were roundly denounced as anti-Soviet conspiracies, and many of their members were shot or imprisoned or, at best, retreated from public life in ignominy. Like all its counterparts Union-wide, the Association of Proletarian Writers (APP) was also shut down as an expression of "left deviationism." In 1932, all independent literary organizations officially closed when the Writers' Union was promulgated as *the* institution for literary activity in the Soviet Union. To become a writer (or a scholar, folklorist, musician, poet, or editor), one had to join the Writers' Union.

Particularly in the west, scholars of Central Asian cultural politics have stressed the Writers' Union's role in asserting Moscow control over the region's culture. Edward Allworth, the founding father of scholarship on Uzbek literary politics, described the Writers' Union as a "bureaucratic device for controlling Uzbek and other Soviet writers." As evidence for this characterization, he adduces the literary brigade that came from Moscow in 1934 to inspect the work of the Writers' Union and the ideological control it embodied.[12] The Writers' Union made it much easier to surveil the activities of local cultural producers and subjected it, in particular, to unprecedented oversight of European cultural arbiters. Ingeborg Baldauf claims that in the 1930s, "literary life was turned into an allegedly inclusive, yet in fact monopolistic, state-controlled, centralised and Sovietized social phenomenon."[13] Likewise, Adeeb Khalid describes the Writers' Union as an engine of "steadfast party control."[14] Yet particularly in the early years, the Writers' Union was not a faceless institution, but a group of embodied individuals whose position as mediators put them in a position of both uncommon privilege and extraordinary risk. This chapter reconsiders prior studies of Soviet Central Asian culture in the 1930s by demonstrating that the Writers' Union created new hierarchies *within* Central Asia and *among* Central Asians as well as *between* Uzbekistan and the Soviet metropole. In so doing, it raises questions about the broader effects of state patronage among national and regional publics.

The Writers' Preschool

When the Party called the Writers Union into being in 1932, Central Asia's literary leaders were, by and large, extremely young. Teenage radicals experimented with futurism; schoolgirls published poems in top Soviet journals. So youthful were the writers of Uzbekistan's Writers Union that a 1933 editorial cartoon represented them as the charges of what it mockingly captioned a "Writers' Preschool named after the Uzbekistan Soviet Writers' Union" (Plate 4). In the cartoon, Ayni and Oydin appear as buxom middle-aged nannies, nurturingly patting the heads of leading writers. The bespectacled G'ofur G'ulom, who today is remembered among the most venerable of Uzbek litterateurs, wears short pants and plays with a toy tractor—a miniature emblem of socialist construction. More writers play nearby, using, respectively, a train, a miniature cotton plant, and a set of blocks with Latin-script letters. A large red banner above their heads reads, "Children! Instead of memorizing words like *samo* and *ufq*, play with these [toys] and do not break them. When you reach maturity you will not regret it." The cartoon implies a stark break with the cultural traditions that had come before. If Central Asia's elders practiced Sufi meditation (Uzb./Arabic *samo*) and fixed their minds on things above (Uzb./Arabic *ufq*, the firmament), the youthful members of the Writers' Union would turn their attention to the temporal world, the tractors, cotton plants, and radio broadcasts of socialist modernity. If the oppressive religious traditions of the past trafficked in Arabic scrawlings, the new writers would operate exclusively in Latin script. There is much to say about this cartoon, but I will begin by pointing out one most obvious point: the cartoon makes Ayni the only adult man in the room. This representation was rooted in the stark fact that at fifty-five, Ayni was positively geriatric when compared to the other leading members.

Historically, in Central Asian cultures, age was a badge of honor: old men, in particular, earned pride of place at community events. Seated at the head of the table, elders offered, and today still offer, the blessing before and after meals. No major decision could be taken without the permission of family and community elders. Indeed, the term for local community leaders—what became an official bureaucratic position in tsarist Turkestan—was *oqsoqol*, literally "white-beard."[15] In Soviet Central Asian literature, Ayni had special credibility because of the combination of his venerable age and his background as an old-guard revolutionary. Born in a village outside Bukhara, Ayni was orphaned at a young age, but managed to put himself through a *madrasa* education in Bukhara. Ayni became involved in Jadid reform movements well before the Russian revolution. In February 1917, he joined a coalition of reformers in an abortive attempt to overthrow the Bukharan Emir with support from a Russian Red Army commander. When the Emir prevailed, Ayni and many of his collaborators were imprisoned and severely beaten in the Emir's palace.[16] The photograph of his bare, scarred back appeared frequently in publications about Ayni from this time onward. Nevermind that the Ayni of 1917 was fighting on behalf of a Muslim reform project: his scars proved his devotion to revolution, and he successfully parlayed his backstory into proof of his credibility as a revolutionary. After his elder brother was killed by the Emir's men in 1920, Ayni officially allied himself with the Communist Party, and it would seem he never looked back.[17] Over the course of the 1920s, he developed a robust bilingual body of literary work in both Uzbek and Tajik, establishing himself as the father of the Soviet

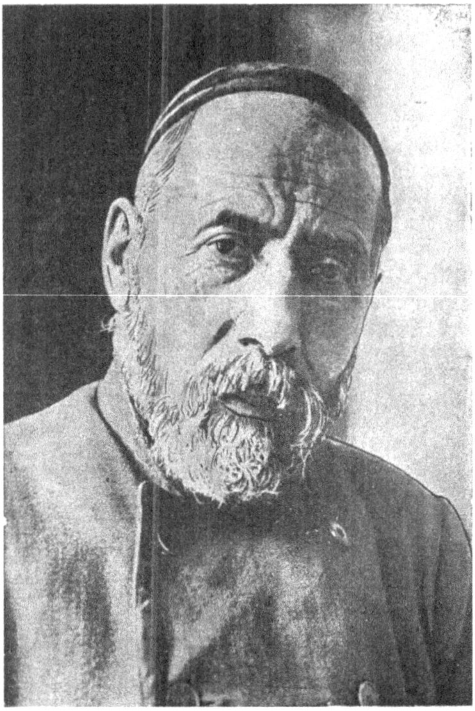

Figure 2.1 Sadriddin Ayni, frontispiece of *Qullar* (Tashkent: O'zdavnashr, 1935).

Tajik literary language despite remaining in Samarkand almost until the end of his life.[18]

By 1933, then, Ayni should have been coming into his own as the grandfather of Central Asian literature and politics (Figure 2.1). Ayni did indeed play a major role in cultivating generations of writers in both Tajikistan and Uzbekistan, and for decades afterward, many would refer to Ayni as a formative mentor. For the cartoonist and the captioner, however, Ayni's age was less an honor than an embarrassment. The European cartoonist, Mikhail Reikh, assigns Ayni a low-status position as a childcare worker, and to amplify the insult, feminizes his figure.[19] The captioner, likely of Central Asian heritage due to his intimate familiarity with Central Asian literary and religious tradition, makes Ayni not a venerable sage, but a glorified nanny.

Age was a liability in the early Soviet Union. By the 1930s, Soviet educational institutions had managed to turn out their first cohorts of educated "proletarian" specialists—engineers, technicians, artists, and writers. Those who had risen in the ranks through "bourgeois" institutions were automatically suspicious. Often emerging from non-proletarian class backgrounds, older generations had to work doubly hard to "re-educate" themselves along Bolshevik lines.[20] The gray beard and decades of experience that would once have earned Ayni honor now became smudges on his reputation.

Ayni leaned into this tension in the speech he delivered at the Writers' Union Congress of 1934, as the representative of Tajik national literature. His Russian translator renders the beginning of his speech thus:

> Comrades! A sincere, fiery greeting to the Congress of Soviet Writers from an old man now become young. Yes, comrades; I am an old man, who in our days has become a young man. I have worked in literature for over 40 years. I was an eyewitness of the feudal period in Bukhara and the epoch of Jadidism, and I personally participated in the literature of that time. But in that time I was unable to produce a work of even the slightest significance. Everything in my oeuvre that deserves attention, I wrote after October. That's why I say that from an old man I have become a young man. The dictatorship of the proletariat returned my youth to me.[21]

Ayni's speech taps into the Soviet cult of youth, minimizing his prerevolutionary experience in order to stress his legitimacy as a Soviet writer, rather than a bourgeois nationalist holdover. In so doing, he implicitly situates himself in a lower-status category when compared to his fellow writers from Moscow, St. Petersburg, Odesa. Ayni may be advanced in age, but in terms of the historical dialectic, he suggests, he is little more than an adolescent. According to the Leninist-Stalinist line on nationality, the more "backward" nations of Siberia, Central Asia, and the Caucasus needed support from the more "advanced" European or historically Christian nations to progress beyond both feudalism and bourgeois nationalism. In this narrative, then, the "dictatorship of the proletariat" encodes the leadership of the European working class, bringing new life to the decrepit societies of Soviet Central Asia. The chronotope of Soviet modernity maps literary progress onto the imperial metropole, where Ayni delivered his address; and backwardness onto the periphery from which Ayni came. In this respect, Ayni's speech can be placed in a long, trans-imperial tradition: the colonized subject thanking his colonizer for the "gift" of civilization.[22]

But if Ayni's introduction lent itself to a Eurocentric narrative of linear progress, the remainder of the address implied a more disjointed chronotope. "Tajik poetry has a rich history. Persian poetry, which disappeared in connection with the conquest of Persia by the Arabs, was reborn after 250–300 years during the age of the Sasanians [sic] in Bukhara."[23] Despite Ayni's avowed commitment to a Soviet modernity emanating from Moscow, he also appealed to another, *indigenous* literary mastery emanating not from Moscow, but from Bukhara, and before that, from Persia. In attributing the perceived "decline" in Persian culture to Arab hegemony, Ayni tapped into revisionist narratives then taking root in a nationalizing Iran, thereby implicitly linking Tajikistan to a broader cosmopolitan Persianate sphere that spanned well beyond Soviet borders.[24] He insisted that Tajikistan's young poets needed to learn this illustrious tradition of poetic mastery from their more skilled elders. Despite the way that Ayni's speech lent itself to a narrative of linear progress when it came to *socialist content*, then, it also offered a narrative of temporal rupture with respect to *national form*—one that transcended Soviet nations insofar as it was a Tajik-language tradition rooted in the now Uzbekistani city of Bukhara and emanating from outside the borders of the Soviet Union.[25] The speech thus walks a precarious line: it proposes Soviet modernity as the ultimate goal, while also legitimizing Ayni's project for Tajik literature through appeal to the distant past. To be legitimately Soviet, the Central Asian public had to "catch up" to the dictatorship of the proletariat; to be legitimately Central Asian, for Ayni, it had to be rooted in the historic legacy of Persianate culture.

Why, if Ayni traced his career to the historic city of Bukhara—now in Uzbekistan—did he speak as representative of the Tajik tradition? Why, as a self-identified Tajik writer, did the cartoonist represent him as a leading mentor for the *Uzbekistan* Writers' Union? Ayni's unique status *across* Soviet national literatures, and his career through a range of institutional and aesthetic forms, tells a much bigger story of a long process of disciplinization and nationalization. Born in 1878, Ayni represented the oldest generation active in Soviet culture, and he brought his lifelong experience to bear as a leading member of the Writers' Union chapters of both Tajikistan and Uzbekistan. In particular, Ayni became the national writer par excellence, representing Tajik literature at the highest levels. Ayni's story thus reflects the consolidation of an idea of literature as answerable to a *national* public, and of himself as a cultural intermediary on behalf of the Tajik nation. At the same time, his position as a *Bukharan* intellectual, one that he maintained to the very end of his life, undermined this strictly national understanding. Ayni's persona embodied a cosmopolitan understanding of the literary public that drew in equal parts on the Persianate cultural sphere in which he was raised and on an emergent Soviet conception of internationalism.[26] His position as a Tajik writer in Uzbekistan, and as a representative of a Persianate cosmopolis, came into tension with the Writers' Union as a national institution centered in a single national capital.[27] Ayni's affiliation with the Writers' Union both lent itself to the centralization of Soviet cultural production and complicated its straightforwardly national organization.

When Ayni began his education in Bukhara, he entered the most prestigious system of education then available to a boy in Transoxania, and indeed, throughout much of the Muslim world. Bukhara was a prominent hub in a network of centers for Islamic learning and Persianate culture across Eurasia. James Pickett describes this "Persianate cosmopolis" as an *oikoumene* that transcended political boundaries, tapping into a long history of cultural production in multiple languages, and spanning a vast geographical and temporal scope. In Central Asia, Bukhara was the most prominent cosmopolitan center; scholars traveled to Bukhara from towns and cities throughout Transoxania, the Ferghana Valley, East Turkestan, and northern Afghanistan. Bukhara competed with other regional centers—in Iranian and South Asian cities like "Qom, Basra, Lahore, and Delhi,"—but when it came to prestige, "Bukhara the Noble" held pride of place.[28] It was in such institutions that students like Ayni would have learned spiritual-philosophical vocabulary like the terms the cartoon mocked. Bukhara was just one node in a polycentric cultural sphere, with scholars traversing centers of learning in cities across Eurasia. When Ayni joined the *madrasa*, he was inducted into this rich network of cultural ties and textual legacies.

By the time Ayni attended the Writers' Congress, in contrast, his conception of literature had shifted dramatically. Around the same time as the capital of Uzbekistan shifted from Samarkand to Tashkent, the market town of Dushanbe was renamed Stalinobod and designated the first capital city of Tajikistan. At the time, Stalinobod was far from a city, but the state administration plunged furiously into construction, from building electrified European-style houses to modern administrative buildings. As a corollary to Stalinobod's designation as capital, the Tajikistani leadership made strenuous efforts to woo leading Persephone intellectuals from the territory of what was now known as Uzbekistan. Writers, scholars, and other intellectuals were promised housing, jobs, and other benefits as an incentive to relocate to what initially seemed like a country backwater.[29] Despite Dushanbe's less-than-illustrious reputation, Stalinobod must have seemed promising as the site of a socialist modernity-under-construction in Central Asia. The early 1930s thus saw a significant "brain drain" from the historic hubs of Central Asian culture—Bukharan, Samarkandi, and Ferghana Valley intellectuals who now identified as "Uzbeks" relocated to Tashkent, while those who subscribed to the Tajik national project turned to Stalinobod. Only a few lingering holdouts, Ayni among them, remained in the old cosmopolitan centers.[30] This put

Ayni in the unique position of reporting to and working for the Writers' Union representing Uzbekistan, while also embodying allegiance to a pre-Soviet Persianate literary lineage.

Tashkent-Bound

In recentering Uzbekistan's cultural capital in Tashkent and demarcating Stalinobod as the center of a nascent "Tajik" literature, the Writers' Union displaced the Persianate cosmopolis that had shaped cultural hierarchies among sedentary Central Asians for centuries. Ayni's continued appeal to that legacy thus represented something of a departure from the emerging Soviet national narratives. Indeed, when the capital moved to Tashkent, Ayni remained in Samarkand, where he lived almost until his death.[31] His residence in Samarkand held together a vanishing vision of a Persianate cosmopolis, which persisted in literary culture well into the late Soviet period, even as its institutions were rejected.[32] The cartoon's representation of Ayni as a nanny, and his speech in which he demotes himself to a "youth," can thus be read as a cipher for the way that Soviet literary institutions both absorbed the Persianate cosmopolis and rendered it impotent; likewise, they both destroyed the Jadid public sphere and appropriated its legacies.

This story holds up from a material as well as a representational perspective. The Writers' Union marginalized literary life outside the capital city. The Persianate *imaginary* may have persisted under the auspices of official internationalism, but the institutional structure of literary patronage undermined it. Literary production in 1920s Uzbekistan had been multicentric and multilingual, with major cultural centers in Samarkand, Bukhara, Tashkent, and the Ferghana Valley. In 1930, however, the republican administration abruptly moved the capital from Samarkand to Tashkent, citing Tashkent's industrial significance and proximity to the cotton-producing Ferghana Valley region as justification.[33] In the context of the first Five-Year Plan, industrial production clearly mattered, but the capital transfer also resulted from Moscow's intervention in the competing national projects of Tajikistan, Uzbekistan, and Kazakhstan's elites. Tashkent and its environs were the subject of intense conflicts between the leaders of the Kazakhstan ASSR and the Uzbekistan SSR, and allocated by Moscow to Uzbekistan at the Thirteenth Party Congress in 1924.[34] Thanks to Moscow's mediation, and the Uzbek nationalists' successful manipulation of it, the republic of Uzbekistan thus emerged victorious in multiple struggles over major Transoxanian cities.[35]

By 1930, the republic of Uzbekistan could assert Tashkent as its capital—maintaining regional control over the populous and productive Ferghana Valley and the culturally prestigious cities of Bukhara and Samarkand alike, and submitting the republic to the Moscow-facing institutions that were well established in Tashkent.

The Writers' Union followed the same process of regional hierarchicalization. By the mid-1930s, the Writers' Union met exclusively in Tashkent. Most of Uzbekistan's officially recognized writers relocated to Tashkent with the capital, leaving the other regions to languish and creating a "brain drain" to the capitals—Tajiks to Stalinobod, Uzbeks to Tashkent.[36] According to a 1933 article, of the eighty-four administrative regions (*raion*) in Uzbekistan, only twelve had a chapter of the Writers' Union.[37] On paper, the Writers' Union at least maintained chapters in major cities, but the central administration generally ignored requests for financial and administrative support from regional chapters.[38] Over the course of 1934, for example, the chapter of the Writers' Union in the far southern city of Termez registered multiple complaints to Tashkent about Tashkent's lack of support for its work—Tashkent offered little publication support, and issued so little funding that the chapter's head secretary went without pay for nearly a year.[39] In response, the central Writers' Union responded with mockery: in 1934, a *Red Uzbekistan* cartoon represented the Termez chapter of the Writers' Union as a supplicant in a suit, his hands folded in entreaty, his head replaced by an open coin purse (Figure 2.2). The cartoon was accompanied by an article claiming that the Writers' Union chapter in Termez was a pathetic burden on the Tashkent-based Union.[40] And Termez was far from the only regional center to be marginalized. In 1937, one Writers' Union member was even accused of gathering up all publication submissions from the border region of Xorezm and stuffing them in a file, dignifying them with neither response nor publication.[41]

One could perhaps claim that, if any Writers' Union chapters were to be neglected, the distant Afghan border city of Termez and culturally distinct Xorezm would be first. But complaints abounded even from the historic hubs of Transoxanian culture. Reports from the Ferghana Valley abounded during the 1930s, often complaining about the meager resources given to cities like Namangan and Andijan when compared to Tashkent. In a four-part 1933 article series on Writers' Union youth outreach, one writer complained of "the Uzbekistan Soviet Writers Union Organizing Bureau's lack of lively support for other cities and regions (*raions*)."[42] One author reported that it was possible to get his work published by the Uzbekistan State Publishing House (O'znashr) only if he visited Tashkent and pulled strings with his friends

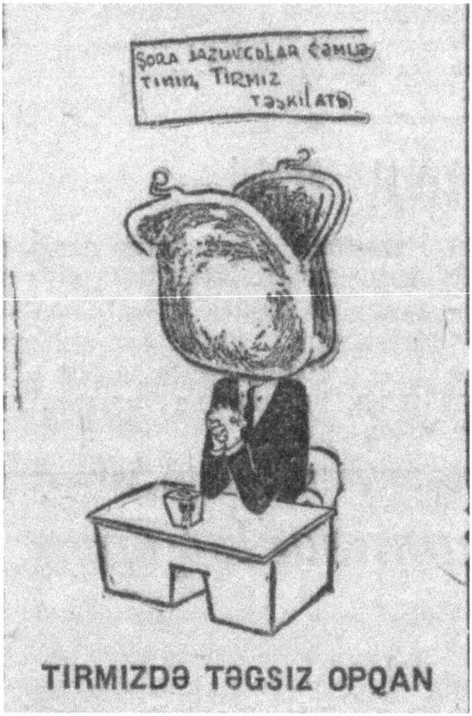

Figure 2.2 Editorial cartoon, "An organization in disarray," *Qizil O'zbekiston*, March 4, 1934, 3.

there.[43] In 1934, the Andijon Cultural Propaganda division wrote to the Writers' Union, claiming that the Andijon chapter existed "in name only."[44] The chapter had no desk, let alone an office, so the chapter's supplies were kept at its secretaries' homes.[45]

Despite Ayni's presence there, the historic cosmopolitan hub of Samarkand fared little better. In an article in 1934 *Qizil O'zbekiston* (*Red Uzbekistan*), one Ismoil Akram proposed making Samarkand's Soviet literature like the literature of "Uzbekistan's Leningrad."[46] The implication that Samarkand *could potentially become* Uzbekistan's second city after Tashkent if it only worked hard enough was myopic to the extreme. Never mind: Samarkand was now a "regional" city, a distant second to Tashkent. In April 1936, Ayni petitioned the Uzbekistan Writers' Union on behalf of Samarkand, pointing out that his chapter had received no money from the central Union during that year.[47] Apparently he received no response, because in March 1937 he telegrammed Tashkent in an even more exasperated tone: "Either close the Samarkand chapter or support it financially...Local organizations are not financing us. Respond by telegram."[48] The Writers' Union in Tashkent produced and distributed content to the regions; but it offered little financial support for cultural activity elsewhere than Tashkent, and it did not, generally, promote the work of regional authors on a republican level. To succeed as a writer on the republican level, one had to move to Tashkent. Ayni was the exception who proved the rule.

But this is not just a story of failure or of marginalization. Ayni's presence in Samarkand, like the in-name-only presence of Writers' Union chapters in many Uzbek cities, served to produce an *imaginary* of public participation distributed evenly across the republic of Uzbekistan—even when it did not exist in practice. Ayni's petitions reflect a new understanding of Uzbek literature as a coherent, unified discipline, organized through an official institution, and centered in a capital city. If cultural capital in pre-Soviet Central Asia could be represented by a "heat map," showing interdependent but ultimately autonomous cultural hubs, the new literary order took on a hub-and-spoke form. The capital city, Tashkent, was now expected to underwrite cultural production in the regions, and the regions situated themselves as dependents of the central national authority. In petitions and newspaper articles, Ayni and the other regional Writers' Union officials position themselves as mediators between the central Writers' Union, based in Tashkent; and their local chapters in Samarkand, Bukhara, the Ferghana Valley, or other cities. The newfound hierarchical organization of Central Asian letters—subordinating Samarkand to Tashkent, and Tashkent to Moscow—also cast some writers in the role of intercessors on behalf of their regional or minoritized national communities, such as Uyghurs or Tajiks.

Ayni's biography thus represents a pivot point among three modes of imagining the Central Asian literary sphere—between the Persianate cosmopolis, centered around the historic cities of Samarkand and Bukhara; the Jadid public sphere, rooted in a local national project; and the Soviet state public, which, in literature and culture, answered to the Writers' Union headquarters in Tashkent (for Uzbekistan) and Stalinobod (for Tajikistan), and above that, in Moscow.

Going Pro

Ayni's biography makes it clear that literacy was a rarefied pursuit in pre-Soviet Central Asia. Those who attended Bukhara's madrasas were the *crème de la crème*—all men, all with access to a limited number of hand-copied manuscripts and face-to-face mentoring relationships with their teachers. While some men of lower status made their way to madrasas, they were a minority among the students. Women learned to read and write largely in domestic spaces; while early modern Central Asia produced its share of women poets, the ones whose names have survived emerged largely from courtly circles.[49]

As they became leading members of the Writers' Union, writers crafted their personas as representatives of Central Asia's public: spokespeople for the oppressed nations of Central Asia; the downtrodden workers of Uzbekistan's factories and fields; the oppressed Muslim women of Turkestan. These lives convey the tensions inherent in Soviet publicity. On the one hand, Uzbekistan's writers represented their public; they spoke for the "millions" who had never had a voice before. On the other hand, in setting themselves up as representatives, they also became members of a new elite, a rarefied circle of professional writers, with unique access to state resources and official publication. Writers' Union members enjoyed a level of privilege far greater than any teahouse manager or local agitprop worker.

These hierarchies had material origins. Eight months after the Writers' Union was formed, in December of 1932, the Uzbekistan Soviet of People's Commissars made a resolution to offer a select list of thirty writers and visual artists the same privileges enjoyed by other professional specialists, such as medical and sanitary personnel, engineers, and technicians.[50] These benefits included access to high-quality housing and food, as well as higher salaries.[51] In 1936, the Writers' Union received approval to move its offices to a new space while retaining their old building as apartments for the leading writers, and the Soviet of People's Commissars allocated 61,500 rubles toward remodeling the building.[52] As a shorthand, I call the writers who earned the specialists' stipend members of the "inner circle" of Uzbekistan's writers. It is difficult to document by precisely what process the recipients of special benefits were selected (Figure 2.3). Possibly, the principle of selection had something to do with the personal relationships of Fayzulla Xo'jayev, Chair of the Soviet of People's Commissars of Uzbekistan.[53] According to the resolution, the measure was intended to improve the everyday life (*byt*) of Uzbek writers, thereby, theoretically, improving their ability to carry out outreach to the masses. In reality, it had precisely the effect on Uzbekistan's writers that the Writers' Union had in Moscow: it created an elite group of Uzbek writers who enjoyed visibly higher living standards than most other people in the republic, including the collective farmers, students, and factory workers they were called upon to write for and about. In the Soviet Union, including in Uzbekistan, literature became a salaried, full-time job at precisely the moment it was supposed to be closest to the working masses.[54]

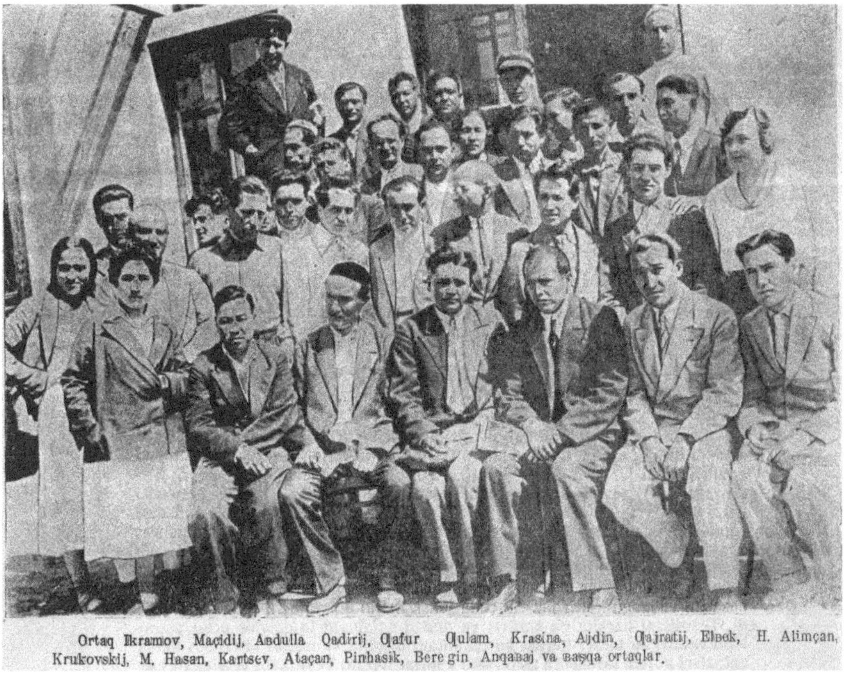

Figure 2.3 Writers' Union members with Uzbekistan First Party Secretary Akmal Ikromov: Majidiy, Abdulla Qodiriy, G'ofur G'ulom, Krasina, Oydin, G'ayratiy, Elbek, Hamid Olimjon, Krukovskii, M. Hasan, Kartavev, Otajon, Pinkhasik, Beregin, Anqaboy, and others, *Guliston* (no. 5), 1935, 2.

In reality, of course, the Writers' Union made Uzbekistan's writers into a new elite, but also placed them in a highly precarious position. Rather than controlling the distribution of resources, the writers now merely enjoyed resources that the upper-level Party administration directed their way. Uzbekistan's leading writers consequently worked under a double burden—that they represent and address the toiling masses at the same time as they work as privileged professional "engineers of human souls."[55] As a result, they relied heavily on narratives about their formation as writers that emphasized their representativeness: their working-class origins.

Abdulla Qahhor and the Jadid Public Sphere

Born in 1907, one such writer, Abdulla Qahhor, crafted an autobiographical narrative of belonging to a liminal generation of Soviet writers: old enough to remember a time before the Revolution, but young enough to grow up Soviet

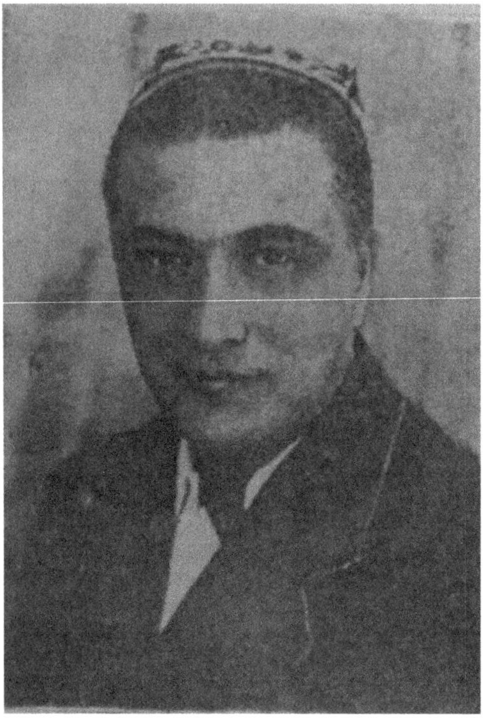

Figure 2.4 Abdulla Qahhor, *Sovet Adabiyoti*, no. 10 (1935), 70.

(Figure 2.4). Indeed, later in life Qahhor described the Bolshevik ascendancy as a coming-of-age story. In his 1960s memoir, as the Bolsheviks fight for ascendancy in his native Kokand region, Qahhor experiences the new regime as an educator. He sings songs of revolution, studies Russian, and eventually joins the Komsomol.[56] His Russian translator, Konstantin Simonov, amplifies Qahhor's representation of the revolution as a coming of age, ending the text with a physical marker of his maturing: "It seemed that week that my voice was beginning to crack. I was beside myself with joy."[57] Simonov was notorious for his free approach to translation, and the Russian text implies a finality that is not present in the original. Regardless of the translation, Qahhor's memoir echoes Ayni's metaphor about his "second youth": for both authors, Soviet rule inaugurates a (second) adolescence, placing them in the position of a student and situating them as the vanguard of a new culture, rather than the backward legatees of the past.

Qahhor was the sole surviving son of a blacksmith's family in the Ferghana Valley. The biography he fastidiously crafted over his long career functioned as confirmation of many Soviet narratives. Eight of his siblings died in infancy, and his parents' desperation in the absence of "modern" medicine served to prop up Soviet biomedicine. Qahhor learned to read at an early age from his father, and like Ayni, he attended lessons at the home of an *otin*.[58] After 1917, Qahhor entered a Jadid school in the town of Oqqo'rg'on taught by a Qur'an reciter named Muhammadjon Qori.[59] Among the first texts he read were works of classical Turkic and Persian poetry, and the first contemporary works he read in school were the poetry of Jadids Abdulla Avloniy and Tavallo. When his father moved to Kokand and enlisted in the Red Army, Qahhor entered the Soviet school there. At the House of Knowledge (*Bilim Yurti*) in Kokand, the institute of higher education where he matriculated in approximately 1923, he frequently associated with the Jadid luminati Cho'lpon and Rafiq Mumin. He met Hamza Hakimzoda, a prominent Jadid-affiliated playwright and activist whose zeal would soon make him a martyr for the cause of reform.[60] It was only as an older teenager that Qahhor began to learn Russian, and even later that he gained any extensive familiarity with the works of Chekhov, Gogol, and Gorky that he would hold up as models for his own later works.

Qahhor represented a transitional generation of Uzbek intellectuals. Early in his career, he did not belong to the old *madrasa* elites from which Ayni emerged, but solidly to the Jadid milieu. Even though he disavowed the Jadids later in life, he brought some of their sensibilities with him throughout his career. From the Jadid institutions where he got his earliest education, the young Abdulla moved smoothly on to Komsomol activism and Bolshevik institutions, where he made his first forays into literary work with feuilletons and satirical verse on superstition and everyday backwardness. Qahhor's publications in the Uzbek satirical journal *Mushtum*, as well as short works in women's journal *Yangi Yo'l*, distinguished him enough to earn him an invited position with *Red Uzbekistan* in Tashkent, beginning in 1925. While in Tashkent, Qahhor earned a degree from the Eastern Faculty of the Central Asian Communist University. Then, in fall 1929, he transferred to a position as managing secretary and editor of the satirical column, "Chig'iriq" ("Cotton Gin"), at *Yangi Farg'ona* (*New Ferghana*) newspaper in his home region, the Ferghana Valley.[61]

1929 was a tense moment in the Ferghana Valley. The Bolsheviks fought long and brutally there for control during the early years after 1917, and local resentments were stoked again by the increasingly interventionist Soviet policies of the mid-late 1920s—the launch of land reform in 1925, the Hujum unveiling campaign in 1927, and the inauguration of Stalin's First Five-Year Plan in 1928.[62] In August 1928, an active correspondent for *Yangi Farg'ona* (*New Ferghana*) was killed along with his wife by opponents of the Bolsheviks.[63] Another Communist activist, G'ani, was murdered in December of the same year, and in March 1929, Qahhor's old mentor Hamza was stoned to death.[64] In this tendentious time, Qahhor's work as a newspaperman solidly positioned him as a representative of Soviet power.

At the same time, however, he continued to associate with the earlier generation of pro-Soviet Jadids. Like Ayni, Qahhor began his career in the institutions of the Jadid public sphere, joining a *gap* affiliated with former Jadids soon after his return to Kokand. *Gap* denotes a social gathering for men, usually held in an individual's home, and often dedicated to the discussion of an agreed-upon topic. *Gap* literally means "talk," and *gaps* typically involved men in the same trade or from the same neighborhood. For Jadids, the *gap* became a type of *salon*, in which members debated cultural and political issues they read of in the periodical press. These "modern" gaps, as Khalid calls them, became hubs for a shared Jadid discourse; before the Revolution, Qahhor's teacher, Munavvar Qori, led a large and influential *gap* in Tashkent.[65] The *gap* destabilized the institutions of the Persianate cosmopolis, shifting the center for public discourse from the *madrasa* to the home of the Islamic modernist.[66] While *gaps* were not inherently oppositional, nor were they ideologically marked as exclusively Jadid, they demarcated a kind of public sphere independent of the state, and therefore became a liability as the state public gained ground.

The demise of the Kokand *gap*, then, marked the demise of the Jadid public sphere. In January 1930, Qahhor was arrested along with the other members of his *gap*, ostensibly for conspiring against Soviet power. The secret police claimed the *gap* had a name—the "Brave Debaters" (*Botir Gapchilar*)—and an agenda to overthrow what they called Soviet "colonial" hegemony and establish an independent state based in the Ferghana valley.[67] The denunciations claimed that the Kokand branch of Red Pen was linked to a "conspiracy" at *Yangi Farg'ona* (*New Ferghana*) newspaper.[68] The OGPU's accusations of conspiracy, like most such accusations of the time, should not be taken seriously. There is no indication the so-called "Brave Debaters" actually had any intention to carry out an uprising, that they had the organizational capacity to do so, or that they were anything other than a group of friends that occasionally complained about politics.[69] Still, the OGPU's description of the "seditious" speech taking place in the group likely contains some grain of truth. The secret police report indicates that the group's primary orientation was not ethno-nationalist, but rather, in some sense, anti-colonial. Participants spoke in terms of "Europeans" or "Russians," who were variously opposed to the interests of "Uzbekistan," as well as those of "Uzbeks" and "Turks." According to the report, *gap* participants even used some class language derived from the Soviet playbook, arguing that Soviet agendas were destructive to the "broad peasant masses."[70] The *gap* was ultimately denounced as a "bourgeois nationalist" conspiracy, but if the denunciations were at all valid, it merely continued the pro-Bolshevik, class-based but also anti-colonial rhetoric that had been tolerated in post-revolutionary Turkestan less than ten years before.[71] Qahhor's denunciation as a member of the "Brave Debaters" marked a transition in his career between the Jadid public sphere and the Soviet state public.

Husayn Shams and the Imagined Proletariat

The *Yangi Farg'ona* purge was just part of a major operation to "unmask" supposed anti-Soviet conspiracies throughout Uzbekistan, particularly in courts and educational institutions.[72] Many former Jadids were taken into custody, and almost all were roundly denounced in the press. The majority of those arrested in the purge did not live out the year—many were shot after being transferred to Moscow—but Qahhor was released under mysterious circumstances, and permitted to return to his journalistic work under the auspices of a reorganized literary establishment. By the mid-1930s, Qahhor would wind up back in Tashkent. Qahhor's formative experience in the *gap* around *Yangi Farg'ona* and his narrow escape in the purge that followed would comprise the kernel of his first novel, *The Mirage*, which I discuss in the next chapter.

Qahhor's early career represented a temporary truce between the Jadid reformist program and the Bolshevik revolutionary one. By the late 1920s, a new cohort of cultural producers emerged, claiming, for the first time in Central Asia's history, the class identity of "workers." If the "dictatorship of the proletariat" was to have any legitimacy under the Soviet nationalizing regime, then, "proletarians" of Central Asian descent were of particular importance for culture and propaganda work. One such young national proletarian, Husayn Shams (1903–43), emerged from the minuscule non-European working class in Kokand (Figure 2.5). Very little is known about his early life, but we do know that he began work as a typesetter at the Kokand publishing house at age eleven, and spent the 1920s climbing the ranks of typography and printmaking.[73] Shams apparently began writing in his hometown of Kokand as early as 1922. In 1924, he was invited to Tashkent to work at the First Exemplary Typography, and in 1927 transferred to the Uzbek State Publishing House in Samarkand and then Tashkent. Probably because of his pedigree as a trade unionist, at the First Congress of Soviet Writers in 1934

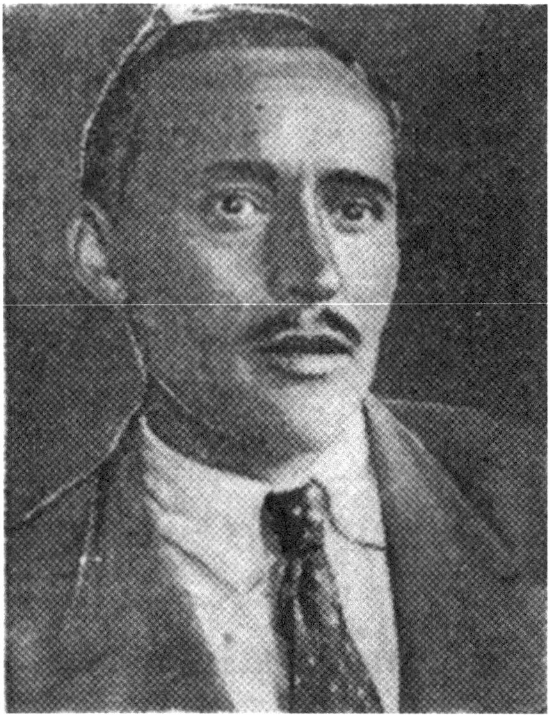

Figure 2.5 Husayn Shams, *Sovet Adabiyoti*, no. 10 (1935), 71.

Shams was one of only three Uzbek delegates who claimed the class identity of a "worker" (Rus. *rabochii*).[74]

Shams was perhaps the single most prolific author in 1930s Uzbekistan. His first volume of poetry, *The Bell* (Uzb. *Gudok*), appeared in 1930. Between the publication of that collection and his temporary repression in 1937, Shams published at least thirty volumes, including multiple novels, pamphlet editions of his short stories, poetry anthologies, "Workers' Library" abridgments of his longer works, plays, and children's literature.[75] He also published frequently in official periodicals. Critics commented on the naïveté and flatness of his work, but praised him all the same for his willingness to take on the most challenging "proletarian" subject matter. Immediately after discussing Qahhor in his overview of Uzbek literature, for example, leading writer Hamid Olimjon also mentioned Shams as a major prose writer who had "bravely" taken on the topic of collectivization in a "voluminous" work that was ultimately "successful."[76] By comparison to Olimjon's rhapsodies about Qahhor as a virtuosic prose stylist, this amounted to a damnation by faint praise. Yet no one else had dared to attempt an entire novel about Uzbek factory workers, as Shams did in 1933. Shams was a bona fide worker-writer, likely the only industrial worker in the inner circle of the Writers' Union, and it could not afford to lose him. At the First All-Union Congress of Soviet Writers, Majidiy specifically mentioned Shams as evidence of the Writers' Union's success at bringing young workers into literature.[77]

Husayn Shams was an early participant in a push for a "proletarian" literature among non-European Central Asians.[78] This trend paralleled patterns elsewhere in the Soviet Union: in 1923 a cohort of radical writers established the Tashkent Association of Proletarian Writers' (TAPP) in imitation of the Moscow-based Russian Association of Proletarian Writers (RAPP), but the Uzbek-language section of TAPP, directed by a teenaged Sotti Husayn, remained largely inactive.[79] For the remainder of the decade, TAPP was overwhelmingly dominated by Russian-speakers.[80] Instead, Central Asia's radical writers followed a precedent set in Baku, where a literary organization, Red Pen, was founded in 1925 at the instigation of the Council for Propaganda established at the Congress for the Peoples of the East. In 1926 in Samarkand, then the capital of Uzbekistan, a group of Young Communists announced the creation of their new literary society, Red Pen (*Qizil Qalam*), under the leadership of Shokir Sulaymon. Sister chapters soon opened in Ferghana and Namangan.[81]

Because Red Pen was so short-lived and so aggressively denounced, very few of its publications remain accessible today. Much of what we know about their work comes from criticisms against them. For example, one 1929 review of a Red Pen literary anthology welcomed Red Pen's turn away from the "hopelessness and pessimism" of previous literature. Although it did not mention them by name, the critique of "pessimism" was a clear reference to the Jadids.[82] It welcomed the publication's newfound emphasis on the short story (Uzb. *hikoya*). At the same time, the critic argued that the group's young writers could have benefited from better mentorship from their elders, and called for it to establish separate sections for experienced and young writers, in order to facilitate mentorship.[83] The writers published in the compendium clearly belonged to a younger generation: post-Jadid writers Hamid Olimjon, Uyg'un (Rahmatilla Otaqo'ziyev), Oybek (Musa Toshmuhammedov), Botir (Nosir G'ulomov), Davron (Vohid Ibrohimov), Mirtemir (Mirtemir Tursunov), and Oydin (Manzura Sobirova), among others, all contributed to the issue.

Although Red Pen consolidated Uzbek literature in a new way, the institutional base of literary production remained diffuse. Membership in Red Pen did not foreclose membership in other literary or intellectual organizations. Parallel to Red Pen, several Uzbek cities also hosted prominent literary circles, often organized around institutions of higher education or regional publications. Most notable among these were the literary circles formed around *New Ferghana (Yangi Farg'ona)* newspaper, the regional newspaper for the Ferghana valley, and based in Kokand; and the literary circle formed around *Young Leninist (Yosh Leninchi)*, initially in Samarkand.[84] Unlike elsewhere in the Soviet Union, then, the Moscow-centric Association of Proletarian Writers (APP) played a very small role in the development of Uzbekistan's non-European literary scene.

By the late 1920s, the alliance between Jadids and proletarian writers became untenable. In 1928, the twenty-four-year-old poet Botu, an active member of the Red Pens, expressed the mood of disequilibrium in an article for *The Flame (Alanga)*, the official magazine for propagating the new Latin script and a major literary outlet. Full of contradictions, Botu's article claimed that the Jadids were a mouthpiece for the wealthy (Uzb. *boi*) class and relics of "feudalism." At the same time, Botu argued that some Jadids, such as the Chaghatay Group of which he had once been a member, had spurned the most regressive wing of the Jadids and fostered a promising "proletarian" agenda. To many young writers of Red Pen, desperately in search of guidance, the Jadids were both feudal relics and proletarian vanguard, literary mentors and false guides.[85] By spring 1929, these concerns spurred an investigation from the Division for Agitprop and the Press (APPO).[86] In the fall, the first rumblings of lasting reorganization began—the director, Shokir Sulaymon, was ousted, and a new organizational bureau was appointed for Red Pen, incorporating primarily Young Communists.[87] In 1930, a collections of articles in radical cultural journal *Alanga* viciously denounced both the New Ferghana "conspiracy" and the Red Pens.[88] The accusations tapped into a repertoire of ideological errors that corresponded to the changing political winds spanning the entire Soviet Union. At the forefront of the accusations against the Jadids was "bourgeois nationalism"; the other stock accusations—"left opportunism," "right opportunism," denoted cultural producers who respectively veered too radical or too conservative for the Party line. To give one example of the granular critiques that upheld the accusations: writers who had recommended creating an "Uzbek Revolutionary Writers' Union" were condemned for attempting to clothe a nationalist wolf in proletarian clothing—by naming their organization after the nationality (Uzbek) rather than the republic (Uzbekistan).[89] At the end of their denunciation, the former members of Red Pen formally disbanded their organization and proclaimed that they were reconstituting it as the "Uzbekistan Association for Proletarian Writers."

The triumph of the proletarian vision in literature inaugurated a new era in literary publicity in Central Asia. Just as Ayni's petitions had reified a hub-and-spoke model for Central Asian literary hierarchy, the rise of "proletarian" culture created new expectations that literature was to be reoriented as of and for the *masses*—for agricultural workers as much as for Islamic scholars, for women as well as men, for factory boys as much as merchant elites. As Soviet Uzbek culture consolidated around the "proletarian," Husayn Shams's career began to take off. Shams became a member of the Uzbekistan Association of Proletarian Writers in 1930.[90] UzAPP may have been the first formal literary institution to which Shams belonged. He later claimed, in fact, that when he began writing in the early 1920s, there were "no literary organizations in Uzbekistan."[91] This was, of course, patently false. But it reflected a narrative that surfaced first with the denunciations of 1929–30 and quickly became commonplace: before Soviet institutions invited them in, so-called "workers" and peasants were excluded from literature altogether. As Rahmat Majidiy put it in his speech at the First Congress of the Writers' Union in Moscow, before 1932, literary organizations existed only in "Tashkent, Samarkand, and Kokand." Majidiy's speech had the calculated effect of writing pre-Soviet letters out of the story of Central Asian literature.

Ayni, Qahhor, and Shams's masculinity suffused their personas as national-proletarian writers. Ayni's autobiography stresses not only the "backwardness" of traditional *maktab* education, but also the way it feminizes him: the only way he can get a decent education before the revolution is to join a group of girls. Qahhor's adolescent voice, cracking as the Revolution enters his city, serves as proof not only of his *maturation* with the revolution, but also of his *masculinization* through Revolution. Still, by and large the masculinity of these writers goes without comment. Their masculinity, like the Russianness of the Party's leading members, is the default, unmarked category. Indeed, the joke in the "Writers' Preschool" cartoon hinges on femininity as a marked category, as a divergence from the masculine norm.

Oydin and the Women's Public

This brings us to Oydin, the other caretaker in the "Writers' Preschool" and one of Uzbekistan's leading writers throughout the 1930s (Figure 2.6).[92] While a small number of other women were active in publishing, Oydin was the only one to make it onto the specialists' stipend list. Over the course of the late 1920s and 1930s, she developed her persona as a woman-writer and leading

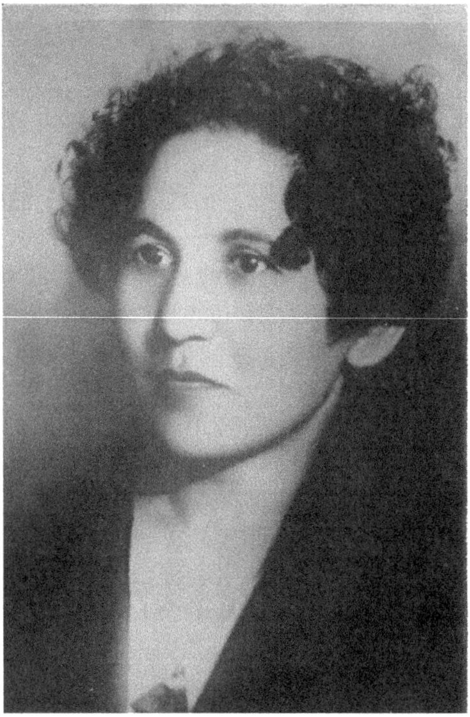

Figure 2.6 Oydin Sobirova in the 1930s, courtesy of Alisher Navoiy State Literature Museum Archive, Tashkent, Uzbekistan.

representative for a broader public of Uzbek women. Unlike Qahhor, Shams, and Ayni, Oydin (Manzura Sobirova) came from an intelligentsia (*ziyoli*) background.[93]Although she had participated in Red Pen, she escaped denunciation and transitioned smoothly to the Writers' Union, where she served from 1932 to 1937 as Responsible Secretary.[94] During the 1930s, Oydin participated on the editorial boards of most journals that published literature, including *Mosholo/Guliston* and the women's journal *Bright Life* (*Yorqin Turmush/ Yorqin Hayot*). She attended the first meeting of the Writers' Union's Organizational Committee, held in 1932 in Moscow, as well as the 1934 Congress of Soviet Writers and almost every other major Moscow literary event to which Uzbekistan sent a delegation. At the 1934 Congress, Oydin was one of only two women attending on behalf of Uzbekistan, alongside her longtime collaborator Sobira Xoldarova. Oydin was used to being the only woman in the room. According to the meeting protocols of the Uzbek Writers' Union during the 1930s, she was the only woman participating in the leading Presidium of Uzbekistan's Writers' Union until at least the end of the Great Terror.[95]

As an accomplished poet, prose writer, and organizer, Oydin certainly deserved this recognition; but given the importance of Muslim women's "emancipation" as a propaganda narrative in the Soviet center, her visibility in Moscow may also be ascribed, at least in part, to tokenism. In reality, participation in public literary life was punishingly difficult for women. According to a biography by Oydin's protege, the woman poet Zulfiya, Oydin had unveiled in the late 1920s at a Moscow conference and then, fearing the social repercussions of appearing in public unveiled, re-veiled on the train back to Tashkent. When she published an early literary piece as a young woman, her father was so upset to see her name and portrait in print that she stopped publishing under her given name and patronymic, Manzura Sobir qizi, and took on the pen name Oydin. She failed, however, to follow her father and uncle's instruction to stop publishing altogether.[96] It is unclear whether Oydin ever fully reconciled with her male relatives. Possibly, Oydin was able to participate so widely in Writers' Union events because she was "free" from the tutelage of her male relatives. This combination of factors, especially the rejection by her family, could explain why Oydin seems never to have married. Regardless of the real outcome of Oydin's break with her father or her presumed marital status, we know for sure that ultimately she unveiled permanently. By the 1930s, not just her (pen) name, but also her photographic portrait appeared regularly in the mass press. Although she was highly unusual for an Uzbek woman of the time—attending nighttime events alone, rejecting the protection of her male relatives—Oydin owned her position as a spokesperson for all Central Asia's women.[97] Indeed, in her work from the 1930s, she frequently ventriloquized a cast of everywomen, speaking on behalf of, say, a collective farm mother of six, a working girl at a factory, or a young student.[98] As one award citation said of her, "Oydin Sobirova's biography is the biography of all Uzbek women and girls."[99]

Reaching the Masses

As they made increasingly ambitious claims to represent the "wide working masses," Soviet institutions poured resources into inducing those masses to participate in Soviet culture. Beginning in the late 1920s, many institutions began sponsoring literary circles under Party patronage: schools or newspapers facilitated groups of young writers under the mentorship of more senior ones; factories and collective farms sponsored circles for young workers to learn to read and write literature.[100] Circles grew vastly in number as Red

Teahouses began to mushroom after 1929, especially after the Association for Proletarian Writers initiated a concerted effort to organize them. And once APP was disbanded, the Writers' Union took over: the 1934 charter for the Writers' Union specifically mentioned "circles" as a core component of their work among workers, collective farmers, and Red Army soldiers.[101] In a 1931 speech, young writer Anqaboy claimed that writers were just beginning to emerge directly from among the "proletarians," and mentioned Husayn Shams by name as an example. By the time the Writers' Union was formed in 1932, it was taken for granted that any legitimate literary institution would conduct outreach to the "masses."

Literary circles had two main functions: to train young writers in the practical skills they needed, and to cultivate their sense of belonging to an imagined Soviet public.[102] The curricula focused on writing Central Asia into a shared literary history, situating it in a historical progression from bourgeois to socialist literature, modeled on a simplified interpretation of the Marxist-Leninist narrative about the cultural history of western Europe. European culture was assumed to have transitioned from "feudalism" to "capitalism" and thence to socialism. As ill-suited as that story may have been to a Central Asian setting, the curriculum applied it nevertheless. In 1935, the first detailed curriculum for literary circles appeared in *Soviet Literature of Uzbekistan* journal, the official organ of the Uzbekistan Writers' Union.[103] Geographically, the curriculum progressed from Moscow to Tashkent. The initial session of the curriculum was dedicated to unpacking Gorky's speech at the 1934 First Congress of the All-Soviet Writers' Union. The curriculum was laden with borrowed words, entirely new to the Uzbek language: "burzhuaziya" (bourgeoisie); "folklor," "meshchanlik" (petit bourgeois); "kapitalizm." As if to acknowledge how distant Gorky's language was from the lived experiences of Central Asia's collective farmers, the writers of the curriculum conceded that it would likely be overwhelming for literary circles to examine Gorky's speech in detail; instead, circle facilitators were instructed to describe a few brief examples of "bourgeois" literature and move on. The curriculum's second installment followed the outline of the Writers' Congress speech by the chair of the Writers' Union of Uzbekistan, Rahmat Majidiy.[104] Whereas Gorky's narrative focused entirely on nineteenth-century Europe and Russia, Majidiy's speech mapped those categories onto the social setting of Central Asia, adding a critique of "bourgeois nationalism": the so-called "Jadids" were the ideological servants of the "national bourgeoisie." In Majidiy's account, the Red Pens and APP had failed to fulfill their popular mandate, and the Writers' Union opened the way for true Party leadership. Still, in this case as well as in others, the instructions assumed few groups would make it through the curriculum. In fact, the curriculum offered a vastly abridged summary of Majidiy's text, specifying that circle directors would do best to read the original speech, but again acknowledging that participants in many circles would likely find it too difficult.

The contrast between Majidiy and Ayni's speeches at the Congress is particularly instructive. If Ayni stressed the novelty of Soviet cultural construction—his newfound "youth"—he also emphasized his rootedness in the centuries-old literary tradition in which he received his earliest training. In practice, in Uzbekistan no such "grandfathering in" occurred on a broad scale. Majidiy did not acknowledge any prerevolutionary works from Central Asia as elements of a canon worthy of redemption in the Soviet period. The ensuing installments of the Writers' Union curriculum, both published in 1936, bear out this blinkered view of the literary past. Two installments of the curriculum appeared in 1936; both were designed to support a year's worth of literary circle programming. While the first targeted less educated and less literate groups, the second was designated for "upper-level" literary circles at higher education institutions and workplaces with educated staff. Both curricula shared introductory material: a unit on "the importance of literature" and another on "folklore and its significance." After the two opening units, the curricula completely diverged. The "lower-level" curriculum focused entirely on short works—short stories, poems, and novellas (*povest*).[105] After units dedicated to short works by Maksim Gorky, Dem'ian Bednyi, and Vladimir Mayakovsky, the curriculum turned entirely to Uzbek writers: Qahhor, Oydin, Shams, Qodiriy, among others. Proportionally, the amount of Soviet Uzbek literature in the "lower-level" curriculum was nearly triple the amount of Russian literature. The "upper-level" curriculum reversed this proportion by significantly dilating its treatment of Russian literature.[106] It began with a long, albeit spotty journey through nineteenth-century Russian literature: Pushkin's *Captain's Daughter*, Tolstoy's *Hadji Murat*; short works by Gogol and Nekrasov, and Gorky's *Mother*, presented in full. All told, Russian literature comprised about 60% of the instructional hours in the "upper-level" curriculum.

In both cases, the effect was to write Soviet Uzbek literature into a longer Russian tradition, whether that began from the revolutionaries of the early twentieth century or from nineteenth-century "critical realism." The curriculum framed that tradition not in national terms, of course, but in universal ones: as an expression of transhistorical linguistic virtuosity (Pushkin) or revolutionary verve (Gorky). All Central Asian literary production from before the 1930s was surgically excised from the narrative. Ayni may have successfully written *Persophone* literature into a Tajik canon and into a Persianate international, but in early Soviet Uzbekistan, particularly in the aftermath of the purges of the late 1920s, the safer bet was to deny the existence of any preexisting Turkic literary history. Pushkin, Tolstoy, and Gorky made the cut, but not nineteenth-century poets Muqimiy or Nodira or Jadids like Fitrat and Munavvar Qori, let alone the classical Persian-language poet Rudaki, whom Ayni was now appropriating for the history of Tajik literature and a broader Persianate "international."[107] While the curriculum excised both the Persianate and Turkic heritage of Central Asian literature from the canon, it also began the process of building a new canon of modern Uzbek literature. Most of the works included in the curriculum and some of the authors—Oydin, Shams—have been forgotten by the Uzbek establishment. Still, a high proportion of the authors, if not their works, have become canonical—Oybek, G'ofur G'ulom, Abdulla Qahhor—and continue to be widely anthologized in post-Soviet Uzbekistan today.

More than the canonical works themselves, then, the curriculum cultivated in aspiring writers a new hierarchy of genres. Genre had been a focal point for literary reform since well before the Revolution, as the Jadids pioneered new prose and dramaturgical forms. By the mid-1920s, genre categories became a major preoccupation in mass education initiatives. In 1927, for example, Red Pen member Anqaboy's *How to Write News, Articles, Poems, and Stories*, offered basic, practical instructions on how to write in unfamiliar genres: a futurist poem, a feuilleton, a newspaper article.[108] The curricula of the mid-1930s amplified the preoccupation with genre. The 1936 curriculum began with a discussion of "genre markers," and as the year proceeded, students systematically worked through a range of new literary genres. Pushkin's *Captain's Daughter* and Qahhor's "The Village Has Awoken" exemplified the novella (*povest'*) form; Yashin's *Honor and Love* represented plays; G'ofur G'ulom provided models of short stories, sketches, and feuilletons. The Russian literary tradition modeled prose forms; in poetry, in contrast, the curriculum offered a brief nod to Central Asian literary history by presenting a distinction between Persianate prosody (*aruz*) and Turkic folk meter (*barmoq*). Facilitators were to ask participants to identify the features of each genre and to attempt to reproduce them and then to workshop those efforts. The circles thus trained participants both to recognize and reproduce emerging genre categories.

The aims of these curricula were ambitious, but in fact, it is quite difficult to determine what effect any of these initiatives had in Uzbekistan during the 1930s. Based on the limited statistics available, music, choral, and basic literacy circles far outnumbered literary circles in Uzbekistan's clubs and Red Teahouses. One set of statistics from 1936 indicates that at Red Teahouses, basic literacy and music circles exceeded the number of literary circles *tenfold*.[109] By the mid-1930s, the number of active worker-participants in official literary circles may have numbered in the low hundreds. Still, the mass circulation press generated great fanfare about the few circles that did function. In May 1934, *Komsomol of the East* reported eleven functioning literary circles in Tashkent, although it also complained that some of them were under poor direction.[110] Earlier in the same year, a forty-three-year-old factory worker was one of three circle participants who spoke to *Literature of Central Asia* about it: he was a "highly qualified carpenter," but with support from his local literary circle, he said he hoped also to become a "master of words." He mentioned meeting Abdulla Qahhor, who had visited his construction site to start a literary circle there.[111] A select number of literary circles exerted an outsize influence on the ensuing development of Uzbek literature. The young woman poet Zulfiya, who would become a major cultural ambassador to the Third World later in life, started her career at a literary circle at her school in Tashkent under the tutelage of Hamid Olimjon, who would later become her husband and the leader of the Writers' Union. It is no coincidence, of course, that the most influential literary circles were organized in Tashkent.

A report from early 1935 enumerated all the efforts the Uzbekistan Writers' Union had made to attract the masses since its creation in spring of 1932.[112] As a report to the center, it probably exaggerates the amount of "mass work" the Writers' Union had conducted, but nevertheless provides a rough description of its activities. The Union reported it had hosted literary evenings on the work of seventeen writers, including beneficiaries of the specialists' stipend, but including also some from among non-titular minorities and four "young" writers. It claimed to have hosted a series of seminars, at which beginning writers could familiarize themselves with the materials produced at the All-Union Congress of Soviet Writers and learn from the experiences of more senior writers. Twenty-six young writers had attended a three-month-long course that the Writers' Union sponsored, where they were taught "literary theory, Soviet literature, the history of the underground revolutionary movement in Central Asia, Marxism, Leninism, language, etc." The report acknowledged that an "office for worker-writers" (*kabinet rabochego avtora*) had been opened only recently, but it had already managed to assist forty writers from a variety of national backgrounds in person. The official Consultation Bureau of the Writers' Union had corresponded with 286 beginning writers about 494 works, 222 of which were in Uzbek.[113] Fifty-five youth writers had also received oral consultations.

The report acknowledged that much remained to be done, pointing out in particular that the active members of the Writers' Union were extremely overburdened with outreach work. Nevertheless, the report attached a plan for the second half of 1935 that promised to increase outreach to the masses.[114] For example, two writers were delegated to organize "exemplary libraries" at Chirchiq, a river near Tashkent where a major project to construct a hydroelectric station had just begun; and at several clubs and factories in Tashkent. Regional chapters of the Writers' Union were also asked to do the same for collective and state farms. Consultations, seminars, literary evenings, conferences, and literary circles were also all on the agenda for 1935. For example, the report called for a discussion of "one of the most relevant works of Soviet writers," the precise work to be discussed as yet undetermined, at two Tashkent factories and a collective farm, also as yet undetermined. "Writers' corners" were to be opened at a variety of locations around Tashkent, as well as the state libraries in Andijon, Samarkand, Bukhara, Kokand, and Ferghana.

In Uzbekistan, workers and beginning writers had never participated in official culture so systematically, and this early organizational work represented a sizable investment in mass work across the republic. Still, the vast majority of Writers' Union-sponsored events and organizations were based in Tashkent. The exemplary works mentioned in the Plan were written by members of the inner circle, and many of the literary evenings were focused on their works. The primary effect of all this organizational frenzy, then, was not to create a functional network of mass-level literary institutions throughout the entire republic. Instead, it created an imagined *norm* for a broadly distributed network of participants even in the absence of a broadly functioning literary sphere. The literary circle, the mass circulation newspaper, the literary journal—all these technologies functioned to create an *imaginary* of mass participation even in its absence, and to produce a small but significant cohort of worker-, woman-, or national representatives who would demonstrate the triumph of the Soviet order.

Purges and the Pedagogies of Publicity

During the early years of the Writers' Union, Ayni, Shams, Oydin, Qahhor, and the rest of the Writers' Union inner circle walked a fine line between their status as representatives and their material position as members of a new elite.

When the Great Terror swept through Central Asia in 1937–38, however, these contradictions came surging to the fore.[115] In this section, I argue that Terror denunciations, while often demonstrably false or unverifiable, apotheosized the universalizing agenda of mass publicity in Uzbekistan. The Terror relied on participation in the institutions and media of the state public: the Writers' Union and its circles and congresses, newspapers and journals. It operated through the literary circles and institutional networks that had been established in the years leading up to the Terror. As Wendy Goldman has convincingly argued with reference to factories in Russia, the Terror was a highly participatory mass movement, taking place as a result of campaigns from the top down but quickly spiraling out of control on the ground level.[116] The Terror in this micro-case cannot, therefore, be reduced to Moscow control, but can only be understood as the outcome of participation from writers on the ground. It follows then that the Terror was a manifestation, not a violation, of state publicity. Writers who had been celebrated and even financially rewarded for their role in establishing a new literary culture, were now suspect for benefitting from the Party-state support that made their work possible. While intervention from the center could be decisive, serving as angel of death, it also, at times, arrived as *deus ex machina* overturning the inexorable weight of mass denunciations.

In its rhetoric, the Terror also articulated the norms of state publicity in an unprecedented way. Terror denunciations served as a pedagogical technology, articulating and reinforcing the norms of participation in the state public, which was at once highly participatory and deeply constrained by the state's monopoly on violence. In this respect, my analysis of the Terror in the Uzbek Writers' Union draws on Gail Kligman and Katherine Verdery's characterization of Terror denunciations as a pedagogical tool. Producing, presenting, and observing political denunciations were powerful methods for inculcating political norms in a largely untutored and often unsupportive population.[117]

While it is difficult to parse Terror denunciations for social-historical information, they are useful documents of the cultural narratives that had triumphed by the end of the 1930s in Central Asia. My goal here is not to tell a complete history of the Terror, then, nor to enumerate the many accusations that were leveled against Uzbekistan's intelligentsia or the subterranean and often undocumented dynamics of patronage and punishment that determined who lived and who died. Instead, I expose the narratives of publicity and its violations that undergirded the discourse of state violence. I argue that the discourse of universal publicity paradoxically served to justify the most brutal state repression. In each case I examine, Uzbekistan's writers were (ostensibly) punished and punished others for their supposed offenses against the universal public: for elevating the specific over the universal, for pandering to an elite while excluding the masses. The Terror thus laid bare the paradox at the heart of Soviet publicity: that it created a national elite that in turn was supposed to pretend it was not, in fact, an elite, but merely the vanguard of an ostensibly mass movement.

In the Writers' Union, Terror accelerated in the spring of 1937, beginning with attacks on the former Jadids. On April 5, the Writers' Union held a meeting at which many members of the inner circle came under attack, along with many ex-Jadids who had been begrudgingly tolerated during the 1930s.[118] Cho'lpon and Qodiriy, both notable ex-Jadids, were excoriated in the press for holding themselves aloof from the public (*jamoatchilik*), sequestering themselves in secretive, inbred circles of "bourgeois nationalist" enemies of the people.[119] At one point, Cho'lpon found himself in the preposterous position of defending himself for accepting a gift of mulberries from a "class enemy" while relaxing at his *dacha*. He needed the mulberries to treat his diabetes, he explained. He argued that it was difficult to reinvent oneself, and that he needed more time and more help to become truly Soviet.[120] After ongoing interrogations and press denunciations, deliberations on many members of the Writers' Union's inner circle continued at another long meeting in August.[121] Cho'lpon was arrested on July 13, Fitrat on the 23rd, and Qodiriy at the end of the year. By the end of 1938, they would all be dead.[122]

The crimes that ex-Jadids were accused of were just the earliest example of the violations of Soviet publicity that came to the fore in the Terror denunciations, the targets of which rapidly expanded beyond the Jadids to the members of the Writers' Union inner circle. One denunciation against Oydin, for example, claimed that she actively turned younger women away from literature. "Once Oydin dies," her (male) accuser represented a number of supposedly disgruntled women writers as having said, "We will come to the Writers' Union to visit her," implying that one day, they hoped the hierarchies would reverse and that Oydin would become supplicant to *them*.[123] Oydin repudiated these claims almost flippantly, pointing out that she had spent years working to support young women, and claiming she had never actively discouraged anyone.[124] Essentially, Oydin's offense was to have set herself up as a token woman, a placeholder for the women of the universal Soviet public, rather than as their representative and champion. It is impossible to verify the claim that Oydin actively discouraged other women; certainly, her literary and especially her editorial work from the mid-late 1930s would indicate the reverse. Nevertheless, Oydin suffered the consequences, albeit much milder ones than the Jadids: the accusations about women joined others about her connections to "nationalists" such as Elbek, and the Writers' Union temporarily expelled her from its rolls.[125] Her career never again reached the heights it had attained in the mid-1930s.

In July 1937, the Union held a special committee meeting focused on investigating another member of the inner circle, the young writer Elbek. If the accusations against Oydin revolved around gender, Elbek's focused on nationality. Of the eight writers listed as present at the meeting on Elbek, Abdulla Qahhor gave the most extensive testimony about conversations he had had with Elbek, another member of the inner circle.[126] Elbek's supposed violations were, similarly, betrayals of the universal public. If Oydin had ostensibly to promote women, Elbek was accused, like many other Uzbek intellectuals, of bias against Tatars, some of whom had historically served as colonial intermediaries before the revolution. In the stenographic report of his conversation, Qahhor mentions some anti-Tatar comments he claimed to have heard Elbek making. In response, Qahhor's interrogator, writer and playwright Komil Yashin, put words in Qahhor's mouth: "So you say there is an anti-Tatar group (*guruh*)?" Later at the meeting, Qahhor participated in interrogating Elbek. Elbek acknowledged that he had studied with Jadid Munavvar Qori as a youth, and admitted that, while socializing with "bourgeois nationalists" like Qodiriy, he had sometimes said things that might be construed as nationalist. He denied condemning Tatars. Elbek was imprisoned and died in a prison camp in February 1939.

The denunciations against Oydin, Elbek, and Shams represent a broader set of assumptions that lay at the heart of the Terror. The writers' (purported) crimes against the people were really, more specifically, crimes against the public. Ostensibly, mediators excluded the masses from Soviet publicity, while in turn appropriating state resources for their private pleasures. Indeed, the accusations against Oydin were just one example among a broader set of denunciations that painted the inner circle of the Writers' Union as violators of Soviet publicity. The accusations along these lines, mostly from fall 1937, followed scripts about cliquishness (*semeistvennost'*) and conspiracy that must be read against the grain, although they do appear to contain some kernels of fact. For example, beginning in July 1937 many members of the inner circle were accused of holding frequent gatherings in the Union-sponsored writers' vacation lodge (*dom otdykha*) or in private residences, such as the home of Elbek.[127] They supposedly made pilaf and served astonishing amounts of wine on the Union's dime, or, when the bureaucracy could not be prevailed upon to pay for the alcohol, through individual contributions.

Oydin and her co-secretary, Shams, used the Writers' Union's official car and driver for transportation to and from such events, as well as for carting around their own relatives.[128] Purportedly, they rarely showed up for work before midday, but on weekends and holidays they worked the Writers' Union driver "mercilessly."[129] Once, G'ofur G'ulom supposedly appeared drunk at the Writers' Union office on a work day and began swearing at Oydin, for which he received no consequences.[130] At least some of these denunciations contained a grain of truth: the culture of excessive drinking in Tashkent publishing circles has also been corroborated by Party activist Saodat Shamsieva, who ultimately separated from her husband, Husayn Shams's brother Zokirjon, due to his heavy drinking.[131] Later, these accusations were parlayed into spurious evidence of a nationalist, Fascist, or Trotskyite conspiracy, which all the defendants strenuously denied.[132] But they did "confess" to socializing primarily with a core group of Union members, albeit a group they claimed was neither exclusive nor conspiratorial.[133] If they spent time partying with one another using official resources, the inner circle was also accused of shunning public events. At the Writers' Union Plenum in early August 1937, speakers attacked several of the Union's leading members of the inner circle—Olimjon, Fathullin, Shams, and Yashin—for skipping artistic meetings, and therefore depriving young writers of important ideological guidance.

It is demonstrable that literary success on a republican level coincided, generally, with participation in the Tashkent inner circle. Those who appeared in the attendance lists from Tashkent Writers' Union meeting protocols during the mid-1930s overlapped with the purportedly hard-partying purge-era "conspirators," as well as the most frequently published names in Union publications. From the perspective of many writers outside the inner circle, centering the inner circle marginalized everyone else. In his testimony in October 1937, for example, the poet Davron described what he perceived as the Writers' Union's neglect of aspiring writers. He began by describing the process by which a journal's editorial staff were supposed to cultivate young writers. "Writers gather around journals, write letters to them, and mature through those journals. We know from the past that all writers come of age by gathering around journals."[134] Davron went on to argue that the editors of the illustrated cultural-literary *Guliston*, including inner circle members Rahmat Majidiy, Anqaboy, A'zam Ayyub, and Oydin, had failed to encourage young writers in this way. Instead, he pointed out, accurately, that month after month they had almost exclusively published works from established Writers' Union members. Davron also attacked them for publishing works from long-discredited Jadids, including Cho'lpon, whose works were appearing in

Guliston as late as 1935, and whose novel *Night and Day* (*Kecha va Kunduz*) was published in 1936.[135] The poet Davron also claimed that as editor of *Yosh Leninchi* newspaper, Anqaboy had created such an unsupportive environment that Davron almost left.[136] Davron argued that these facts evidenced a widespread bourgeois nationalist conspiracy ultimately reaching all the way up to the discredited First Secretary of Uzbekistan's Communist Party, Akmal Ikromov.

As a non-beneficiary of the specialist's stipend who nevertheless circulated among members of the inner circle, Davron may have felt personally excluded and therefore more willing than most to offer damning denunciations. But his claim that republican-level literary publications did not prioritize young writers as much as they could have, despite Party injunctions to do so, is certainly grounded in fact.[137] Until the Great Terror, which eliminated most of the older generations, young writers rarely appeared in the national press. There is no evidence that the neglect of aspiring writers outside Tashkent was part of some concerted conspiracy. Rather, it seems to have resulted from a combination of limited funding and a Writers' Union culture that revolved around face-to-face networks among the members of the inner circle.

In the absence of evidence for organized conspiracy, the more likely explanation for these accusations is structural to the discourse of mass publicity. By positioning writers as cultural intermediaries whose primary responsibility was to the masses, it placed those writers in a fundamentally unstable position, in which they were called upon to represent the mass public even as they comprised a privileged new elite. The *imaginaries* of mass publicity these writers produced rendered them vulnerable to exposure for their fundamentally un-public behaviors. While they succeeded in constructing that imagined public with their carefully narrated biographies and their fictional writings, that imaginary proved more enduring than many of the writers themselves. The writers were key mediators of the imaginary public, but the professionalization of those writers became a marker of their betrayal. During the years of the Terror, this delicate balance became the open justification for expelling a large portion of the members of Writers' Union. Many, particularly those with connections to the Jadids during the 1920s, were imprisoned or killed. When an investigatory brigade led by Aziz Niallo came to Tashkent, it held Shams, Oydin, and Hamid Olimjon up to intense scrutiny for their associations with "enemies of the people" like Young Communists Anqaboy and Botu, as well as the ex-Jadids.[138] Oydin, Shams, and Hamid Olimjon were all expelled from the Writers' Union in the fall of 1937.[139]

Ayni's fate uniquely dramatizes the paradoxes of state publicity during the Terror. For much of 1937, Ayni was away from Central Asia, in Moscow and on an extended sabbatical in Sochi. Upon returning to Samarkand, he learned that he was being attacked as an "enemy of the people" in Samarkand newspaper *Lenin Yo'li* (*Lenin's Way*).[140] His ties to a brother-in-law who had been exiled to Siberia on grounds of conspiracy were particularly damning, and Ayni began to realize how serious things were when rumors began to circulate that he had been arrested. Ayni appealed for mercy by reminding the authorities of his sacrifices for the revolution: the death of two of his brothers, one at the hand of the Emir, the other at the hand of *basmachi* fighters.[141] The bodily infirmity that made his name as a Soviet writer also helped to save his skin: Ayni reminded his readers of the seventy-five lashes that still scarred his back and of his old age, the mark of long years in service of the cause. Like Pavel Korchagin from the Socialist Realist novel *How the Steel Was Tempered*, Sadriddin Ayni bore in his mutilated body the proof of his boundless devotion to the revolutionary cause.[142] It was in his bodily weakness, not the "restored youth" he had once proclaimed at the Writers' Congress, that Ayni sought salvation.

Ultimately, according to Tajikistani scholar Abdulnabi Sattorzoda, Ayni escaped imprisonment and death only by appeal to the very top: he wrote to his friend and patron, Iranian Soviet writer Abu'l Qasem Lahuti, who called for the intercession of Orientalists Igor Diakonov and Evgenii Bertels, who in turn gained the ear of leading Russian writer Alexander Fadeev, who called on Viacheslav Molotov, who won the support of Stalin himself. By early 1938, the First Secretary of the Writers Union of the Soviet Union traveled to Tashkent, where he interceded personally on Ayni's behalf. Ayni, unlike so many of his comrades, had survived the Terror.

Conclusion

In the wake of the fall of 1937, the Writers' Union was almost completely depopulated. In early spring 1938, a trickle of reinstatements began. Ayni had never been excluded from Writers' Union membership, but he was formally cleared of the accusations only in February, after he had acknowledged the "mistakes" of his Jadid youth.[143] Oydin, Shams, and Olimjon were all reinstated to the Writers' Union in March 1938, while Qahhor, after participating in some denunciations but largely lying low during the Terror, never experienced any censure.[144] The old-guard Jadids were completely gone. Only Ayni and

Qahhor regained their previous stature; both authors are now recognized as "national" authors even in post-Soviet Central Asia. Although Oydin and Shams survived the Terror, their legacies were permanently tarnished. While all four were equally prominent in the 1930s, today reams of monographs cover the life and works of Ayni and Qahhor, while Oydin and Shams appear mostly in brief tangential references and scattered dusty archives. Through the pedagogies of publicity, including their apotheosis in Terror, Central Asia's writers were now thoroughly inducted into a Soviet state public—one that reified its own "massness" while at the same time creating new, unspoken hierarchies of its own.

In many ways, the Terror marked the end of an era. The ex-Jadids who lingered in the wings through the 1930s were effectively eliminated, and the "class of 38" that emerged after the Terror would dominate cultural life through much of the Soviet Century.[145] From this perspective, the 1920s and 1930s appear an ephemeral moment in Soviet cultural life in Uzbekistan. But the dynamics of representation and publicity that the Writers' Union forged in the 1930s cast a long shadow over cultural life thenceforth. It was in the early 1930s and through the first cohorts of the Writers' Union that cultural life shifted from the old geographical centers to the Tashkent center. The Writers' Union created a new cohort of writers who claimed gendered, class-based, and national legitimacy as representatives. Those writers carefully crafted narratives about themselves that made them spokespeople for entire categories of massness, and they worked to build organizations that, at least in theory, would make Soviet culture the provenance of the "working masses," from cotton farms to silk factories. At the same time as the masses came under the purview of mass publicity in a new way, the Writers' Union made writers into a professional class and literature into a specialized discipline. Among themselves, the few dozen members of the Writers' Union participation cannot be reduced entirely to those in "support" of or "resistance" to these new regimes of social life. Instead, they made use of state resources to facilitate a kind of "shadow public sphere" that operated with state patronage, but with a tenuous relationship to state control.

Socialism Mediated: The Making of Soviet Culture in Central Asia. Claire Roosien, Oxford University Press.
 DOI: 10.1093/9780198971153.003.0004

3
Novels

Introduction

On March 27, 1933, the Uzbek People's Commissariat of Enlightenment (Narkompros) announced the fledgling Union's first major programmatic undertaking, a competition for literary works to be administrated by the Uzbek Soviet Writers Union. Fayzulla Xo'jayev, the Narkompros Chairman who made the announcement, claimed that Uzbek literature had failed so far to illuminate "Uzbekistan's heroic workers' struggle for proletarian dictatorship and socialist construction," and the fight against Central Asia's anti-Soviet *basmachi* fighters.[1] Xo'jayev continued that the Party needed such works to help "educate the masses in the spirit of socialism." In Uzbek literature, Xo'jayev specified, prose lagged behind poetry and drama." Poetry, not prose, had historically been the prestigious literary mode in the region, but Russocentric Soviet genre hierarchies reversed that order. Now, long prose works—novels—would receive special consideration for the prizes: large sums of cash—10000, 7000, and 5000 rubles for first, second and third prizes respectively; but also highly coveted all-expenses-paid professional development trips (*komandirovki*) to the central cities of the USSR, ranging in length from two to six months.

A cartoon published on the back cover of *Mushtum* in August 1933 vividly represented the stakes of the novel competition (Plate 5). In the cartoon, by an unknown European cartoonist named Bondarevich, the competition becomes a steeplechase race, and writers become runners, using their pens as pole vaults to surmount the hurdles on the racetrack. The caption reads, "The one who walks will fall behind, the one who runs will reach the end, and the one who jumps in time and keeps the tempo will be first!" The cartoon leaves the race in a state of indeterminacy, with the crowd eagerly waiting to recognize the winner. The crowd looks on as the racers struggle comically. A man on a donkey, an animal then associated with rural Central Asian "backwardness," lags pitifully behind the pack of runners; his mode of transportation is clearly not up to the task at hand. Even the best runners struggle to traverse the course of obstacles: one competitor struggles so much to surmount a hurdle that he accepts an undignified boost from a female assistant. The runners in the cartoon, like the writers in the competition, were all men, but they all reckoned with the reality that women were visible in their world in a new way. All these embarrassing contortions happen in front of a huge, cheering crowd, comprising Russians and Uzbeks, men and women, and workers of all stripes. In the *Mushtum* cartoon, the viewer takes the vantage point of the crowd, looking down on the race as if from the highest row of bleachers.

The cartoon represents the competition as a spectacle for the masses. At the same time, Xo'jayev's prompt made it clear that the crowds in the stands were more than mere fans. They represented the novel's proposed public in two senses. First, they comprised the aspirational readership for the novels the competition would produce: it was these "masses" that the novels would "educate" for the future. Second, they were the novels' proposed object of representation. The sought-after novels would portray the proletarians' "heroic struggle," producing a historical novel about the recent past that would lend itself to a clean narrative arc for its collective hero, the proletarians of Uzbekistan: from feudal backwardness and capitalist oppression to socialist emancipation. The novels were to represent the public in the Andersonian sense, according to which the novel is an "imaginative" technology—in his case, for the modern nation; in ours, for the national public and the multinational, gender-integrated global proletariat.

This chapter examines the novel competition of 1933–34 as a study of the construction of the Socialist Realist novel in Central Asia, and more broadly, as a key moment of imaginative public-formation in Uzbekistan. Some scholars have represented the making of national literatures as a process of consolidating central control over the Soviet periphery.[2] In many ways, the novel competition of 1933–34 would seem to confirm that representation. Socialist Realism in Uzbekistan adapted the "master plot" from Russian socialist literature, and particularly, from the works of its paragon and demiurge, Maksim Gorky.[3] Each of the three novels under consideration, in fact, can be read as adaptations of major Gorky novels.[4] The three novels—which became the first Socialist Realist novels in Uzbek—were published "to order" in response to a directive handed down from the state. Aside from one or two Jadid works, they were the first novels to be published in a newly consolidated literary Uzbek and as representations of an Uzbekistani national republic, replacing the multilingual, supranational literary field that had previously reigned in Central Asia. The novels imposed ideological conformity and repressed the cultural ferment that had flourished in the region just a few years before—or so it would seem.

When the aspiring winners got down to writing, however, nothing turned out to be quite so simple. Xo'jayev's prompt assumed a great deal. It presumed an already-existing proletariat in Central Asia—the "heroic workers"—and a shared understanding of the nature of their historic "struggle" for socialism. In fact, both these premises were far from given in Central Asia: who could these "heroic" Central Asian workers struggling in behalf of socialism actually be, given that most of the earliest Bolsheviks in the region had been European? What did that struggle look like, when in fact a large proportion of the Central Asians who had fought alongside the Bolsheviks had now been condemned as Jadid class enemies and "bourgeois nationalists"? Things became still more complicated when considering the audience. If Uzbekistan's *writers* resisted long prose forms, its *readers* struggled with them even more. Xo'jayev spoke as if the masses were ready and waiting for novels; in fact, the vast majority of Uzbekistan's readers were newly literate, perhaps able to parse a newspaper article or a poem, but hardly prepared to tackle Gorky's *Mother* or anything like it, no matter what language it was published in. Even the most well-educated Central Asians tended to prefer poetry over prose. One Uzbek author had even complained in 1930 that Uzbekistan's writers were beset with "poetry sickness," at once denigrating poetry from an official perspective and acknowledging its undimmed popularity among Uzbekistan's literati.[5]

The prompt may have sounded straightforward, then, but in fact the task it assigned was enormously difficult. In the end, the selection committee, helmed by Oydin, decided that *none* of the novels deserved top honors. The two novels the jury deemed best—Sadriddin Ayni's *Slaves* and Abdulla Qahhor's *Mirage*—shared the second prize, while the third novel—Husayn Shams's *The Law*—earned third place. (To be fair, we might attribute this snub to less lofty causes: the Soviet of People's Commissars delayed disbursement of prize funds, and without that allocation the sizable grand prize may have been beyond the means of the cash-strapped Writers' Union of Uzbekistan.)

The competition illuminates the history of the Soviet novel in Central Asia. I argue that we might read these early Socialist Realist novels as documents of a fraught process of public-formation, much as Jochen Hellbeck and others have argued that we might read ego-documents as artifacts of the building of a Soviet subjectivity.[6] In writing these novels, Qahhor, Shams, and Ayni attempted to imagine Central Asians as a public participating eagerly in socialist construction, rather than as a hodgepodge of passive imperial subjects. As they did so, however, they also articulated contradictions at the heart of the project for Soviet public-formation.

Even though Qahhor's *Mirage* purported to satirize those who held on to the relics of the past, the affective tone of the novel undermined that ostensible satire, registering a profound ambivalence about a project of Soviet publicity at the expense of everything that had come before. Ayni's *Slaves* situated agricultural collectivization within a sweeping family history going back more than a hundred years. In doing so, it indigenized the socialist revolution, in the process decentering both the nascent nation and the emergent narrative of European leadership. Finally, while Husayn Shams set out to imagine an internationalizing Central Asian proletariat, the emotional fulcrum of his novel pivoted not around class warfare but gendered "respectability." I begin with a discussion of the theory of the novel as it took shape in the Soviet 1930s, demonstrating how for Soviet theorists, novels presented a tension between a totalizing vision of revolutionary development and the dialectical contradictions inherent to socialist construction. Through analyzing each of the competition novels, I then show how the three central categories of difference—gender, nation, and class—produced tensions that none of the writers ever managed to fully resolve. In my reading, the first Socialist Realist novels in Uzbekistan thus present an archive of the unresolved tensions of Soviet public-formation.

Socialist Realism and the Soviet Novel in Uzbekistan

Why was the novel so important to Xo'jayev? By the late 1920s, the novel had become the preeminent Soviet literary form.[7] This was far from a foregone conclusion: the novel form was associated with bourgeois culture, and for Soviet theorists, it reflected the contradictions inherent to capitalist society. Early Soviet literary theorist Mikhail Bakhtin developed a robust theory of the epic with relation to the novel form. For Bakhtin, epic posited an "absolute past," characterized by unalterable completeness and linguistic homogeneity.[8] The novel, in contrast, undermined the absolute and totalizing vision of the world presented by the epic. Instead of homogeneity, heterogeneity; instead of monologism, Bakhtin argued, the novel put forward polyphony; instead of absolute truth, the novel offered parody. Georg Lukács, who would become the leading Soviet literary theorist in the 1930s, put it succinctly in his earliest attempt to theorize the genre: "The novel is the epic of a world that has been abandoned by God."[9] The novel, for young Lukács, was an expression of the loss of totality under the conditions of modernity. Epic, in turn, was the artifact of a world in which a unifying macro-narrative made sense. In 1936–37,

Lukács would update that theory in socialist terms, arguing that novels—and historical novels of the eighteenth and nineteenth century in particular—expressed the social tensions between "feudal survivals" and the emerging bourgeoisie. The drama of the historical novel emerged from the contradictions between the survivals of the past and the emergent social order.[10] The historical novel was an artifact of the social conflicts inherent to capitalism.

Lukács and Bakhtin both focused most of their analyses on the novel as it took shape under capitalist modernity. Despite the novel's associations with bourgeois culture and its contradictions, however, Soviet theorists argued that under the conditions of socialist construction, the novel would take on new social significance as it gradually converged, again, with epic. Although Lukács was instrumental in debates about Socialist Realism, in *The Historical Novel*, Lukács explicitly left Socialist Realism outside the scope of his study. In the final pages of the text, however, Lukács gestured toward how the historical novel would be transformed in what he called the "popular and democratic spirit of our time."[11] If the very best bourgeois historical novels articulated the inner contradictions of capitalist society, Lukács suggested, the novel form would transform as socialism came into its own. The contradictions of capitalist society would vanish, and likewise, the "antagonism of contradictions" would cease to animate the novel. This, in turn, would lead to a "tendency towards epic" in the novel form.[12] After separating from epic totality with the rise of capitalism, the novel would again converge with the epic as the contradictions of capitalism were overcome.

Lukács's theory of the historical novel coincided with the formulation of Socialist Realism as the preeminent mode of Soviet cultural production. Socialist Realism emerged as the culmination of both political process and aesthetic debates. In the late 1920s, as purges rocked the national republics for their patronage of "bourgeois nationalists" like the Jadids, a parallel set of denunciations, spanning from the centers to the peripheries of the USSR, attacked "left deviationists" and "formalists" because their artistic visions purportedly lacked the requisite mass appeal for true Soviet culture. Vicious polemics emerged about the future mode of socialist art: would it take the shape of "revolutionary romanticism," which would inspire workers with dreams of a bright future; or of a "proletarian realism," which would galvanize them through representations of the world as it was, with all its imperfections?[13] These debates culminated in the emergence of the aesthetic program of Socialist Realism, which was supposed to bring together the future-oriented revolutionary zeal of revolutionary romanticism with legible representations of reality. To quote Andrei Zhdanov's famous speech from the

First Congress of the Writers' Union, socialist realism was to "represent reality in its revolutionary development" (*izobrazhat' deistvitel'nost' v ee revoliutsionnom razvitii*).[14] Scholars usually identify tendentiousness (*ideinost'*), class-mindedness (*klassovost'*), and Party-mindedness (*partiinost'*) as "ideological postulates" of Socialist Realism, although other formulations were common, and accessibility to the "people" (*narodnost'*) became particularly important in the context of what David Brandenberger has termed National Bolshevism in the mid-1930s.[15] Of course, all these slogans were notoriously vague, and writers struggled to put them into practice in specific works. In practice, they often turned to imitating a body of canonical texts, many of which predated the official promulgation of Socialist Realism.

Consequently, as Uzbek national writers forged their national "forms" during the early 1930s, Soviet writers were in the process of consolidating a theory of Socialist Realism, which would ultimately become, at the First Congress of the Soviet Writers' Union in 1934, "the basic mode of literature and literary criticism." In Uzbekistan, writers were discussing Socialist Realism well before the Congress: in spring 1933, for example, poet Hamid Olimjon led a public meeting on Socialist Realism for all of Tashkent's writers and poets.[16] Even without referencing Socialist Realism by name, we might refer to a nascent aesthetic of Socialist Realism already by 1930. Jadids and their interlocutors tended to write in a critical mode, using satire as the dominant mode to lampoon irrationality, superstition, and backwardness. While Uzbekistan's prose writers in the 1920s articulated great enthusiasm for a revolutionary project, they often prioritized the critical process of sweeping away the vestiges of the past, rather than imagining a positive future or developing a program for its implementation.[17] After the Writers' Congress concluded in 1934, *Soviet Literature of Uzbekistan* published several of the gathering's documents in Uzbek translation: a *Pravda* article emphasized the Zhdanov quote about "reality in its revolutionary development," while also stressing Socialist Realism's imperative to critically appropriate the literary heritage (*meros*) of the past. While the article was translated from Russian, in the context of 1934 Uzbekistan, it clearly implied that Uzbekistan's writers' main task was to respond to and remake recent literary norms (the Jadids) as well as the longue-durée literary history of the region. In practice, however, Socialist Realism was a nebulous aesthetic project, lacking clear specifications and offering a relatively wide latitude for cultural experimentation—at least until the works that passed for a time as "Socialist Realist" were condemned as counterrevolutionary ex post facto, as happened to much of the literary production of the mid-1930s. Ultimately, Socialist Realism became not a set of prescriptive norms but a discursive and institutional field, rooted in an accepted canon of works that predated its promulgation (Gorky, Gladkov, Fadeev, and so forth).[18]

It is highly unlikely that the writers in the Uzbekistan novel competition read or substantively engaged with the theories of Lukács and Bakhtin, some of which were not fully articulated until the competition had ended and none of which, to my knowledge, were translated into Central Asian languages at the time. But Bakhtin and Lukács articulate some of the unresolved problems with the novel form in the context of Uzbekistan's effort to promote Socialist Realist novels. To what extent could novels reflect social contradiction, and to what degree, in the context of socialist construction, should they instead express a "tendency towards epic"? Certainly, literary works that emphasized the unresolved tensions in Soviet society over its "victories" were frequently criticized as counterrevolutionary, and the competition novels were no exception. The Narkompros prompt for Uzbekistan's novelists clearly tended toward the epic: rather than works that accommodated and reflected social contradictions, the prompt implied that the winning works would offer a heroic sense of the past, an absolute metric of right and wrong, and a clear division between heroes and antiheroes. The judges, likewise, seem to have expected a totalizing vision—one that, if achieved, would have differed significantly from many of the most familiar bourgeois novels. In many ways, Stalin-era literature embodied the tendency toward epic totality; Katerina Clark argues that in many novels of the time, "there is no collision in the novel between 'is' (or 'present') and 'ought to be' (or 'epic past'—or future)."[19] For Clark, the Soviet novel embodied a synthesis between the novel form and the epic's transcendent totality. In fact, however, the competition novels did not achieve the epic mode that Lukács posited would soon emerge in socialist literature or that Clark describes for Soviet novels in other parts of the Soviet Union. The novels strive to represent a unified Soviet public, subsuming proletarian men and women, Muslims and European workers, but instead they archive the tensions produced by the project of Soviet public-formation.

The contradictions that Qahhor, Ayni, and Shams articulate fall along the three key axes of difference with which this book began: nation, gender, and class. More precisely, the competition prompt framed the desired novel in class terms—as the story of "Uzbekistan's heroic workers"—and the three novelists endeavored to represent the proletariat as a unified historic subject. But in every case, the expression of that collective agency runs up against resistance emerging from the ongoing realities of empire and patriarchy.

The dynamic reflected in these novels might effectively be compared to what Fredric Jameson describes in his much-critiqued article, "Third-World Literature in the Era of Multinational Capitalism." Writing at the sunset of the Cold War, Jameson claimed that Third-World novels must, almost without exception, be read as "social allegory." Jameson's argument has rightly been criticized as Orientalist and reductive, but as Rossen Djagalov argues, it is possible to partially appropriate it not as a blanket statement about all non-western writing, but as pertaining to literature that emerged from the Third World as a *project* of the Cold War rather than an essentializing category.[20] For the texts Djagalov examines, national allegory is not an unconscious effusion but a self-conscious political agenda.

A similar argument can be made with respect to Uzbekistan's competition novels. The presence of a national novel, like the presence of a national opera, functioned as a litmus test for the success of the Soviet project in a national republic. The prompt explicitly called for novels about the "heroic workers of Uzbekistan," or in Jamesonian terms, for plots that functioned as both national and class allegories. With respect to the Uzbekistani competition novels, if not with respect to all "Third-world texts," we might thus concur with Jameson that "even those which are seemingly private and invested with a properly libidinal dynamic—necessarily project a political dimension in the form of national allegory: *the story of the private individual destiny is always an allegory of the embattled situation of the public third-world culture and society*."[21] The fact that each novel gravitates toward interrupted love plots thus not only reflects the challenges of forging Soviet masculinity and femininity, but also encodes the broader conflicts inherent in making Central Asia Soviet.

My reading of the Socialist Realist novel in Uzbekistan also draws on a broader scholarship on the novel in Turkey and other post- and anti-colonial contexts. Nergis Ertürk reads modern Turkish literature as an archive of the "violent effects" of phonocentrism, or "the programmatic privileging of spoken language over its written forms."[22] Phonocentrism posited a one-to-one correspondence between objective reality and its mediation in written language, which was ideologically identified with the spoken word, however different written and spoken language might actually be. The phonocentric worldview depended on a rational conception of modernity and presumed national community to be natural and self-evident.

Such was the ideological program of phonocentrism, but in practice the novel troubled these simple myths of modernity. The rise of Turkish phonocentrism produced a novelistic discourse that *both* articulated essentialist national identity politics *and* was haunted by the nation's uncanny others.[23] The colonial, postcolonial, and anti-colonial novel thus became a site of contestation and contradiction: for Lukács, on class grounds; for Ertürk, as for Jameson, on the grounds of the nation and its uncanny others. My reading, in turn, argues that the earliest Socialist Realist novels both articulated ideology from the center and exposed its unexpected inner tensions.

Qahhor's *Mirage*: The Phantom Public

Abdulla Qahhor's *The Mirage* opens in the busy lobby of the main building of Central Asia State University.[24] The novel's protagonist, a student and aspiring writer named Rahimjon Saidiy, encounters an attractive young woman named Munisxon. I quote the passage at length, because it is one of the novel's few scenes set entirely in a Soviet public space:

> From the first floor lobby came the smell of a train station: crowding, heat, dust. Sweaty people flowed toward the outside—not to the fresh air, but to the front of the lobby, toward the announcement boards. Even when bread was handed out for free in the famine year, things hadn't been like this.
>
> Here were the girls; here were the young women, blooming like flowers, as if in the presence of a favored bridegroom. Too bad for their dresses made from silk and marquisette—they stuck tightly to the girls' sweaty bodies. Hair that had been brushed smooth and laboriously, attentively braided was now untidy and disheveled. Perfume, sprayed excessively in honor of the occasion, now melded with the smell of sweat, producing a scent that was neither repulsive nor pleasant to the nostrils. The young dandies—who had carefully buttoned their vests and shirts, anticipating being in the presence of girls—now sported crooked ties and hairstyles that resembled crabgrass stuck to a shoe. Their frequently worn, carefully cared-for shirts were as wrinkled as dishrags and disgusting as bath towels.
>
> The lobby really was just like a train station. There were all kinds of people there: Tajiks from Hisor, Ko'lob, Badakhshan and the environs; youths from villages and nomadic settlements; workers and all kinds of other people.
>
> Looking briefly into the lobby, the girl [Munisxon] laughed: "The university really is a joke these days..."
>
> Saidi politely joined in on her laughter, and then commented, "There's the Workers' Faculty (*rabfak*) too. These people belong at the Workers' Faculty.

> There are twenty-nine different nations enrolled at the Workers' Faculty these days. I saw the chart yesterday.[25]

In official terms, the passage about the university gets a lot of things right. It shows students from all around the young Soviet Socialist Republic of Uzbekistan gathering in their new shared capital. Those students include both men and women, thanks to new Soviet policies on coeducation and unveiling. The students belong to the nations-in-construction that populated Uzbekistan—not just Uzbeks and Russians, but Tajiks too, along with the unnamed other twenty-six non-titular nations. They came from cities, villages, and the countryside—even from nomadic settlements.

And yet, the passage does not celebrate the moment unequivocally. A certain disdain is expressed throughout the passage, in Munisxon and Saidiy's mockery of the riffraff assembling at the university: readers are meant to identify both Saidiy and Munisxon immediately as class enemies. But a more sympathetic sense of ambivalence seeps through already in the opening sentence. The "train station," that emblem of Soviet modernity, here appears as an unfavorable comparison, conveying the crowding and chaos in the university lobby. The simile about bread in a famine year conveys real desperation, and the aspiring co-eds and their classmates are both charming and pathetic, with their perfume and their neckties. The text does not imply open *opposition* to the project of Soviet modernity, but a sentiment rooted in literary realism: that life is complicated and, sometimes, uncomfortable.

Abdulla Qahhor was commended in his lifetime as a fine prose stylist, and the passage exemplifies his attention to sensory detail and the material world.[26] In his autobiographical writings, Qahhor attributed his stylistic approach to his engagement with the Russian realist classics, and Anton Chekhov in particular. In large part, Qahhor's vocal protestations of indebtedness to Chekhov functioned as insurance against accusations about other types of influence—namely, the Jadid satirical tradition, his debt to which Qahhor publicly disavowed.[27] Praising Chekhov gave Qahhor cover for his often critical (as opposed to positive) tone, and lent itself to incipient cultural hierarchies that prioritized Russian culture above all others.

Still, Qahhor's citation of Chekhov is not mere propagandistic window-dressing; it reflects a substantive engagement with the realist prose tradition. In this respect, his attention to detail—and specifically, his judicious mobilization of concrete material objects—recalls Lukács's famous distinction between narration and description.[28] For Lukács, realism, as opposed to naturalism, represented material objects not just out of a desire for flat verisimilitude, but because when properly mobilized, objects have the power to articulate social relations in concentrated form. Realism, for Lukács, is about selecting the "poetically significant" object as a tool for narration—he cites Daniel Defoe and Leo Tolstoy—rather than bombarding the reader with undifferentiated description like Emile Zola.[29] "Anything which plays a meaningful role in the activity of a man about whom we are concerned becomes poetically significant," Lukács argues in favor of narration as opposed to description, "precisely because of its relationship to the character's activity." In Qahhor's novel, the young men's crooked ties and unkempt hairstyles do more than just paint an accurate picture of everyday life in 1930s Uzbekistan; they articulate something more significant about the social world that Saidiy and Munisxon inhabit. Realism is a double-edged sword: it accords with the calls for "realism" emanating from the Writers' Union, but in its evocative reflection of a broader social order, it also complicates the rosy picture of socialism ascendant.

Certainly, that is how Qahhor's readers interpreted his attentive eye for detail. In 1939, over five years after the passage was first published in serial form in the journal *Uzbek Soviet Literature*, and two years after it appeared in book form, it became the topic of an intense debate at a meeting of the Uzbekistan Writers' Union dedicated entirely to *The Mirage*.[30] Qahhor's harshest critic, Habib Musaev, complained, "Qahhor compared a university lobby to a stinky train station." In response, Qahhor feebly retorted, "Where do you see the word 'stinky'?"[31] Musaev's critique may seem petty, and Qahhor's response pedantic. But their conflict touches on a much larger problem than how precisely the Tashkent university smelled on admissions day: the problem of how to render a socialist public attractive.

Like the passage about the university, *The Mirage* as a whole ostensibly defended the Soviet project of public-making. It portrays a young Uzbek student and aspiring writer, Rahimjon Saidiy, attempting to make his way in the world of Soviet journalism. He visits a Red Teahouse, participates in Party meetings, tries to get published in the official newspaper. But rather than integrating himself in the Soviet public, Saidiy instead becomes ensnared in a counterpublic: a bourgeois nationalist conspiracy that has infiltrated the world of Soviet letters, aspiring eventually to overthrow Soviet power, create an Islamic state, and sell off Central Asia's natural resources to the British.[32] In the novel's melodramatic denouement, Saidiy dies when he ventures blindly into a snowstorm after realizing that the entire conspiracy was nothing but a "mirage." The novel's bare-bones plot—its *siuzhet*—lends itself to a straightforward reading of Saidiy's life as a moralistic fable, warning readers of the dangers of fraternizing with class enemies.

For some of Qahhor's readers, though, the novel had quite the opposite effect. Shortly before the meeting where he denounced Qahhor, critic Habib Musaev penned a harsh review criticizing *The Mirage* because, he argued, it engendered sympathy for counter-revolutionaries and disdain for Soviet workers.[33] According to Musaev, the malodorous lobby was just one symptom of Qahhor's failure to render Uzbekistan's proletarian community attractive. Musaev was not the only critic to react this way. In November 1937, another critic, Yusuf Sultonov, concluded an otherwise positive-seeming review of the book's first edition with fighting words, concluding that *The Mirage* was an "enemy work" (*yot asar*) because it caused the reader to sympathize (*achinish*) with bourgeois nationalists.[34] And yet, in the opening scene of *The Mirage*, Qahhor merely articulated what many eager young students must have experienced: that Soviet New Men, too, had body odor; that mass education in Central Asia, especially in its early, formative years, was often loud, crowded, and disorganized.

In large part, Qahhor's critics in the late 1930s were simply responding to the changing times. In 1934, *The Mirage* won the novel prize. At the time, the judges were already demanding that Qahhor revise it, even as they agreed that it was among the best novels ever written in Uzbek. By 1937, at the nadir of the Terror, what the judges had once dismissed as minor imperfections became evidence of precisely the type of conspiracy that the novel purported to expose and condemn. Even though Qahhor made significant revisions to the novel before it appeared in book form in 1937, critics of the Terror era deemed even the updated version of the novel intolerably sympathetic to the "enemy."

To the extent that they pointed up the novel's fundamental polyphonicity, the critics of Qahhor's novel were not entirely wrong. The novel comprised more than the heroic narratives it was supposed to put forward: it stressed the *difficulty* of Soviet public-making much more than it celebrated the triumph of that project. In *Mirage*, two types of (counter)public do battle for Saidiy's loyalty: the Soviet state public and the Jadid counterpublic. Qahhor's novel traffics in propaganda tropes about lascivious NEPmen and traitorous internal enemies, transnational Islamic conspiracies and bourgeois Jadid merchants. But that propaganda narrative rests lightly on the surface of the *siuzhet*. In its *fabula*, the novel introduces a degree of instability that, while hardly constituting the degree of insubordination his critics assigned, indicates a deep tension in the project of Soviet publicity: in *The Mirage*, the "bourgeois" counterpublic is far more affectively compelling than its "proletarian" counterpart.

For most of *The Mirage*, Saidiy straddles the divide between bourgeois and proletarian, much as Qahhor himself had in his early life. Saidiy comes from a "bourgeois" family—his father was a merchant who died by suicide after the 1917 revolution—and was educated at a Jadid school. Invited by the brother of his love interest Munisxon, Saidiy begins participating in anti-Soviet *gaps* (the similarity to Qahhor's own biography is unmistakable) and becomes slowly enmeshed in a bourgeois nationalist conspiracy. At the same time, Saidiy is not a lost cause from the start. He is, after all, fatherless, and therefore distinctly amenable to reeducation in a Soviet vein. His closest friend, Ehson, comes from a proletarian background, and encourages Saidiy's early efforts to produce poetry for the local literary journal. When the novel begins, Saidiy is a Komsomol member, and visits a village on assignment to assist in the collectivization process. He participates in the debates put on by local literary organizations—debates about, for example, how best to portray land reform in literature. Throughout the novel, Saidiy builds his career in the world of Soviet journalism, holding editorial positions in local and national newspapers, much like those Qahhor himself had held. As Saidiy's allegiances shift from the Soviet to the counter-revolutionary, however, he retreats into a conspiratorial dreamworld, an imaginary republic with a green Islamic flag, based in the fertile Ferghana Valley and governed from an Ark, or Central Asian fortress. It is this seductive "mirage" that dances before Saidiy's eyes in the tragic conclusion of the novel, when a blizzard buries Saidiy alive as the Red Army takes his co-conspirators into custody.[35]

Clearly, the novel was meant to indict the ephemerality of bourgeois aspirations. But the novel's sensuous portrayals of bourgeois public spaces belie this interpretation. Early in the novel, for example, Saidiy has a relationship-defining conversation with Munisxon in a workers' park where the two have come to study. Readers learn that the Soviet public park has taken the place of a prominent pilgrimage site. Munisxon disdained the university as a "mockery" in the stinky lobby scene, but as Munisxon and Saidiy discuss their relationship, she uncharacteristically praises the Komsomol for condoning public relationships between unmarried men and women, like hers with Saidiy. And yet, despite the benefits of the Soviet order for her personal life, Munisxon pines for her pre-Soviet childhood. "We are children of the old way of life [*turmush*]," agrees Saidiy, triggering Munisxon to a reverie about outings with her late father:

> Munisxon knew the place where she was sitting from those [childhood] days. In those days, this place was a site of pilgrimage. The roots that twisted and

> criss-crossed as they emerged from the ground; the crooked doors that shone in the rain that washed them; the wagon beds that lay helter-skelter, forming a stairway to the pavilion; the wheel hubs; the many-colored broken clay pots; the rusty bits of iron; the old mulberry tree with flags tied to its branches; the sycamores, and the withered grave markers beneath them; the bushes that grew like no other—there had been a unique pleasure [*gasht*] for people here, specific only to this place. There was no pleasure in today's standard buildings, built as if according to a plumbline; no pleasure in the young city, young garden, young air, young trees and flowers. For Munisxon, a single broken clay pot, a single withered grave marker from that old pilgrimage site was greater, more beautiful than all those things—the symbol of a sweet way of life. Tears came to her eyes again, but this time she quickly blinked, swallowed her tears, and involuntarily, quietly sighed.[36]

Munisxon's reverie assembles a multitude of objects: not as a museum of description, but in Lukács's terms, as a shrine of narration. More powerfully than any expository dialogue, the objects Qahhor assembles here evoke the melancholy of a way of life suppressed. In place of "superstition"—venerating saints, tying prayer rags to twisted trees—Soviet power brings modern medicine and technology. Instead of rust and rot, Soviet power offers steel and concrete. Instead of everything crooked, narrow, and decrepit, Soviet power builds right angles and spacious boulevards. But in this moment of free indirect discourse from Munisxon's perspective, Qahhor again permits a moment of polyphonicity: a moment of mourning for all the "pleasures" lost to the project of Soviet modernity. It does not make rational sense, in the world of *The Mirage*, for anyone to reject the promises held out by the Soviet project—let alone Munisxon, who is able to study with Saidiy only because the Soviet educational system has made it possible. But when the alternative is a smelly, crowded "train station," the old world may not be sensible, but it is sensual.

Munisxon and Saidiy's encounter at the garden/pilgrimage site is sensual in more ways than one. By this time, Munisxon and Saidiy have been "studying" together daily, although Saidiy is far too preoccupied with flirting with Munisxon to tutor her on Marx and Darwin.[37] Flouting social censure, they have even begun holding hands, and Saidiy is thinking of marrying her. Spring foliage adorns the garden, and a brilliant blue sky looks down from above. Saidiy and Munisxon banter flirtatiously. In a richly Freudian exchange, Munisxon gives Saidiy a red flowerbud in exchange for a snack of green apricots.[38]

The conversation quickly turns serious, however, when Munisxon announces that, if she were given the garden, with all its "standard buildings," she would begin by surrounding it with a clay wall and installing a pavilion in the middle. In describing a garden with a pavilion at its center, Munisxon evokes an image with historic roots in Central Asian political culture. Beginning with the Timurids—a sedentary dynasty with historic nomadic roots—it had been customary for Transoxanian royalty to hold court in covered garden-pavilions, a way of bringing non-urban nature into an urban or suburban environment. Garden pavilion scenes became a common trope in miniatures from the region, an icon of princely grandeur.[39] From the official perspective, then, Munisxon's garden pavilion fantasy thus identifies her as an atavistic political reactionary while again presenting an attractive alternative to the rectilinear Soviet park.

This political vision carries with it a gender hierarchy, but also paradoxically for Saidiy, a threat of castration. Saidiy responds to Munisxon's fantasy by reminding her that hers is a fantasy of masculine domination. "No matter how regal the pavilion you build, you would still end up sitting at the threshold, pouring tea for your prince (*amir*) seated in the place of honor." Munisxon responds by doubling down on her fantasy: "If he were worthy, I wouldn't mind." Saidiy, in turn, asks Munisxon if she would ever take the place of honor herself. "There'd be no pleasure in it," she says, and follows up, "Would you put me in that place of honor?" For Saidiy, even though "his entire body said yes," he is unable to reply. Munisxon shouts in response: "I would not marry you anyway!"

This scene is ambiguous. Later in the novel, Munisxon admits her attraction to Saidiy: her apparent rejection does not express her true feelings. Perhaps Munisxon rejects Saidiy because, as a woman beholden to the wishes of her male relatives, she is ashamed to openly communicate her desire and accept his proposition. Conversely, perhaps Munisxon is so committed to her atavistic vision of the garden pavilion that she refuses to tolerate anyone who would question the gender hierarchies it entails, no matter how harmful those hierarchies may be for her. Some readers have suggested that Munisxon rejects Saidiy because, as the privileged daughter of a wealthy merchant, she sees him as too poor for her.[40] One might even read the exchange between Munisxon and Saidiy as a kind of kink. Regardless of the reason for Munisxon's outburst, however, Saidiy experiences it as an emasculation. The seditious fantasy for which he is willing to relinquish his privilege appears to be one of male domination and feminine abjection, but the exchange places

Saidiy in the position of a supplicant, willing to subordinate himself before Munisxon by granting her the place of honor.

Saidiy's sedition is both a capitulation to his treacherous sex drive and a symbolic castration. This plays out dramatically in the remainder of the novel. After Munisxon's rejection, Saidiy eventually marries Soraxon, the cruel, childish, and sickly daughter of his anti-Bolshevik mentor. Munisxon marries a much older wealthy counterrevolutionary, and ends up profoundly disappointed with her lot. When a dejected Munisxon tries to orchestrate a tryst with Saidiy after their marriages to others, Saidiy proves impotent—even though he admits that he can only think of Munisxon every time he embraces his wife. Munisxon and Saidiy never see each other again: Munisxon shoots herself in her husband's cellar. Deeply depressed after his failed tryst, Saidiy stops visiting Soviet public spaces and retreats into his home, becoming, in Qahhor's words, a "house girl" (*uy qizi*).[41]

Eric Naiman has identified anxieties about the enervating force of bourgeois sexuality for the Soviet proletariat as a hallmark of NEP-era culture.[42] For the Russian texts Naiman analyzes, making the Soviet man is a process of sublimating disordered bourgeois hypersexuality, marshaling it instead toward socialist construction. The *siuzhet* of Saidiy's story indicates something else: the narrative arc of *The Mirage* suggests that bourgeois sexuality is all smoke and mirrors, and that the counterrevolutionaries' much-vaunted masculine dominance is nothing but empty show. And yet, the garden scene with Munisxon is so suffused with sexual energy that it resists such a flattening. In moments of crisis, Saidiy returns to his conversation with Munisxon as a symbol of what could have been. The scene cannot be reduced to a comfortable story about a counterrevolutionary temptress, because Munisxon's appeal, like the appeal of the world she represents, is sensual in a way that far exceeds the Soviet public.

The rectilinear park or the crooked pilgrimage site: Munisxon and Saidiy's momentous encounter articulates a profound "affect gap" between the state public and the counterpublic. Another such counterpublic space is the school Saidiy attended in the early Soviet years, which the novel indicates is one of the many schools founded by former Ottoman prisoners of war in the aftermath of WWI.[43] In a chapter-long flashback to Saidiy's youth, Saidiy recalls his time there in the present tense, and with sensory detail—including the clanging of the bell used to wake students during Ramadan, the splashes of water used to wake the students who oversleep, and the darkness of a teacher's room where students once gathered around a table for the purpose of divination. Over a decade later, Saidiy's ears still "hear" the wistful songs he and his classmates sang at school, accompanied by a grand piano: "The stars on the sky's face / Shine down on this world of vanity..."[44] Clearly, these and other details indicate, the school is linked to a transnational community of Turkist intellectuals, committed both to Islam (the Ramadan ablutions) and to European modernity (the piano).

For readers, Qahhor makes it clear that the school is a place of injustice. The most wealthy—those with merchant fathers, connections to the Ottoman glitterati, and the resources to study abroad—enjoy special treatment from their instructors, while many of Saidiy's worker classmates are expelled for insubordination. But despite the obvious injustice of the school order, Saidiy remembers the place with intense feeling. Indeed, Saidiy's recollection of his school days is spurred by another set of evocative objects—a collection of photographic portraits, belonging to Munisxon's conspiratorial brother, that he finds at her house. When Munisxon shows him several of the images—of a Turkish officer (*zabit*) Saidiy recognizes, of intellectuals who used to visit his school—the photographs attract him irresistibly. Apparently concerned about betraying the conspiracy, Munisxon attempts to hide the photographs by covering them with a newspaper. But during a moment when Munisxon is distracted, Saidiy snatches several and takes them home.[45] It is these photographs—wormholes to the seductive past—that spur Saidiy's fit of nostalgia for his childhood school. His encounter with the portraits is his first step into the world of bourgeois nationalist conspiracy.

Munisxon's attempt to hide the counter-revolutionary portraits with a newspaper underscores in two significant objects the primary conflict in *The Mirage:* between the bourgeois nationalist counterpublic and the proletarian public, between transnational Turkist discourse and the Soviet media. But the two do not meet on equal terms: the nationalist counterpublic functions underground, while the Soviet public operates openly with the patronage of the state. According to official state policy, "old" gathering spaces such as pilgrimage sites, mosques, and religious schools were supposed to be replaced entirely by Soviet institutions. In the long run, in fact, the Soviet public was to subsume even the private sphere, forcing everything outside its purview into the underground.

Despite that clear ideological imperative, for Qahhor, the underground spaces are suffused with sensuality and saturated with music, textures, scents, and tastes. The guest room of Abbosxon, Saidiy's conspiratorial mentor, exemplifies such an underground space. The walls of the room are adorned with portraits of writers in lushly decorated gilded frames, and mesmerizing landscapes with sunsets and rising moons. The soft couch is upholstered with black velvet, while the bed frame, adorned with a silk comforter and a feather pillow, is coated with shiny nickel. A seductive statue of a nude woman "calls" Saidiy to work at the finely decorated desk, while a thick rug muffles his footsteps.[46] Munisxon's brother, Salimxon, holds weekly meetings in his warm, hospitable guest room, where alcohol flows freely and the walls are so thick that the "Komsomol cell cannot reach in."[47] On the piano that furnishes this room, Saidiy again hears the music he first heard as a child in the Jadid school: militant Arabic marches (*mashq*) and lilting Turkish songs.[48] Such bourgeois luxury forms the backdrop to the conspiratorial meetings Saidiy begins attending.

For Saidiy, then, the seduction of sedition has little to do with rational argument. Instead, it emerges from the embodied, interpersonal experience of counter-revolution: face-to-face encounter, first with photographs, and then with the people they represent in richly sensuous spaces. The sexual subplot with Munisxon only amplifies this dynamic. Compared to the sensuous spaces Saidiy inhabits with the bourgeois nationalists, the "proletarian" public sphere is bland at best. In fact, the university lobby is perhaps the most tactile of all Soviet spaces Saidiy enters. The level of detail Qahhor offers in the lobby scene compares only to the description of a village Red Teahouse where Saidiy is sent to help enact land reform. Although less overtly unpleasant than the university lobby, the Red Teahouse is crowded with villagers, noisy, and furnished only with a coarsely hewn wooden table. Otherwise, Qahhor offers few descriptions of the university's lecture halls, the newspaper's editorial office, the Komsomol meeting room, the university library, or other ostensibly proletarian public spaces Saidiy frequents.

In part, we learn so little about Soviet public spaces because Saidiy quickly begins avoiding them. Every time he enters the Workers' Faculty (*rabfak*) hall, for example, he feels as if the room echoes with the voices of his fellow Komsomol members, chastising him for his failure to attend meetings and his negligence as a Komsomol activist.[49] Eventually Saidiy's feeling of inadequacy becomes so intense that he prefers to remain in the "warm embrace" of his father-in-law's courtyard, rather than going out in public.[50] By the end of the novel, the meetings of the nationalist cell cease under pressure from the government, effectively shutting down the counterpublic sphere that once seduced Saidiy. But Saidiy still prefers his exclusive dreams of bourgeois life—idyllic gardens, publication in Hearst journals, a retreat to nature "like Thoreau"—to the harsh realities of Soviet public life.[51]

Soviet public spaces repulse Saidiy, and in *The Mirage*, the denizens of the Soviet public are little more appealing than the spaces they inhabit. Qahhor rarely offers physical descriptions of Soviet men, including Barat and Kenja, eager Komsomol poets, and Saidiy's newspaper colleagues, Tesha, a miner and Saidiy's Komsomol mentee; or Ehson, Saidiy's childhood friend and a Moscow-trained doctor. These men appear far less frequently in the plot than the bourgeois conspirators. In fact, Ehson, the most well-rounded of all the "positive" characters, is away for his studies in Moscow for the vast majority of the novel; readers get to know him primarily in absentia, through the letters he writes Saidiy. In the 1939 debate about *Mirage*, an otherwise sympathetic critic addressed this issue: "Why did the positive types, like Ehson, Barat, and Tesha, turn out as dry and soulless (*jonsiz*) as mannequins?...The reader has a right to demand that [Qahhor] give blood and a living (*jonli*, lit, 'ensouled') organism to the novel's skeletons dressed in positive costumes."[52] The absence of any pro-Soviet female character is equally glaring.

This was not the first time Qahhor had been criticized for his failure to portray positive heroes, despite his vividly drawn antiheroes. In 1935, soon after Qahhor won the novel competition, critic Saidg'ani Valiev argued that Qahhor's short stories had exhibited "mastery" in their representation of "negative types," but showed positive characters in a "one-sided" manner.[53] The Writers' Union's official assessment of *Mirage*, which supported its second-place victory in the novel competition, acknowledged Qahhor's mastery of prose style but chastised him for his failure to represent a "positive hero."[54] But if Saidiy was an antihero, it was only because of his incapacity to integrate himself into a Soviet public: he represented less an anti-Soviet *subjectivity*, than a counter-Soviet *publicity*.

Qahhor began responding to such criticisms almost immediately after the novel was published. Between the original version, published in serialized form between 1934 and 1936, and the first book edition, from 1937, Qahhor made significant changes to help correct the imbalance between the unappealing proletarian public and seductive bourgeois nationalist counterpublic. Early in the 1937 edition, for example, a still-uncorrupted Saidiy visits a literary journal's office, where the editor Kenja offers kindly advice ("Write a short story about land reform") and helps Saidiy investigate why his earlier submissions were rejected with no comment (a conspiracy member-cum-journal editor blocked their publication).[55] This chapter did not appear in the earlier journal run.[56]

Still, although the proletarian public is a key theme in the novel, readers encounter it more through its absence than its presence. In the second half of *Mirage*, Saidiy no longer attends Komsomol meetings, proletarian literary discussions or university lectures. He stops working as a newspaper editor and avoids his worker friends. And yet, the proletarian public continues to crop up. Unaware of Saidiy's betrayal, Ehson tracks him down when he returns from Moscow, inviting him to the new opera house—the last proletarian public space the reader sees. Afterward, Ehson regales Saidiy with accounts of the site of Uzbekistan's new hydroelectric power plant, where Ehson has been invited to assist with public health initiatives. Ehson is full of enthusiasm about the power plant's new "workers' city," but as readers, we never encounter it. For the future, Ehson imagines a sterile scene: "peaceful buildings and laboratories, silent as the grave; countless glistening instruments; rabbits and dogs lying on top of experiment tables." But even Ehson describes the site as, for the moment, nothing but a dusty, smoky construction site, crowded with people and full of noisy machines.[57] Saidiy finds himself at an impasse: he is caught between a conspiratorial dreamworld that is highly seductive and intensely tactile, but lacking in real substance; and a rectilinear Soviet dreamworld that repulses him both aesthetically and sexually. In *The Mirage*, the bourgeois public pulses with life, while the proletarian public sphere is as ephemeral as a phantom. The anti-Soviet activists may be a dying breed, but they bleed red, while proletarian men are skeletons with no flesh. Bourgeois public spaces bring warmth, music, texture, while the proletarian public languishes under construction, destined anyway only for sterility and right angles.

Responding in 1938 to the barrage of criticism he had begun to receive, Qahhor wrote a letter in his own defense, addressing it to the editors of *Pravda* and the USSR Writers' Union. He admitted that, from the very beginning, he had known the topic of bourgeois nationalism to be "slippery and very dangerous." Still, he defended his decision to focus on counterrevolutionaries rather than "positive heroes":

> I considered thus: bourgeois nationalists are the enemies of the Uzbek people—that much is true. If that is the case, then why should I not tell people what I know? If a pig stands before me grunting, why can't I call him a pig?...One of Chekhov's characters says, "Look the devil straight in the eyes, and if he is the devil, then say so."[58]

In his self-defense, Qahhor leans into realism as a defense for his intensely sensuous representation of bourgeois nationalists. But Qahhor's defense flattens the novel's deeply ambivalent representation both of the proletarian public and the bourgeois counterpublic. The conspiracy, for Qahhor, was both beautiful and terrible; the Soviet public, equitable and desirable as it may be, is a pale shadow of the bourgeois counterpublic in all its sensuality.

When he republished the novel—in 1957, as the second volume in his *Collected Works*, and again in 1967, as part of another *Collected Works*, Qahhor significantly revised it.[59] In 1957, the chapter about the Jadid school, the paragraph about the pilgrimage site, and many of the most detailed descriptions of the conspirators and their agenda disappeared. In comparison to the original 1937 publication, the new edition lacked a full five chapters, most of which had added depth to Qahhor's representation of the anti-Soviet conspiracy.[60] Some of the redactions can be explained as an effort to tighten up the sometimes meandering narrative arc, but most of them clearly hark back to the complaints of the late 1930s: that Saidiy, despite being an anti-hero, elicits too much sympathy from readers, and that Soviet spaces and characters come off as anemic when compared to the full-blooded anti-Soviet spaces. When it became possible to talk about the redactions in detail, during perestroika, critics argued that the more artistically meritorious edition was, in fact, the 1937 version.[61] "Sympathy" for the counterpublic, it seems, is precisely what made the novel so effective.

Ayni's *Slaves*

If the readers of Uzbekistan's competition novels were expecting the winning works to cover the nation-state of Uzbekistan, Ayni's novel would have disappointed them. Readers first encounter the protagonists of *Slaves* not in Tashkent or Kokand or even Dushanbe, but in nineteenth-century Herat, in modern-day Afghanistan. The protagonists are fruit farmers, growing melons, grapes, and most importantly, apricots. It is fall, and Hasan's large extended family, men and women alike, are busy harvesting the fruit and laying it out to dry in the sunshine. Their numbers have diminished since a Turkmen slave raid the previous year, but there are still enough hands to do all the work, if they are sufficiently industrious. That work brings them renown far beyond Herat. According to a brief narrative digression, these dried apricots are famous in distant lands: Iranians call them "Bukharan apricots"; while in Bukhara, Samarkand, Ferghana, and Tashkent they are called "Herat apricots." From his opening pages, then, Ayni situates the historic cities of Uzbekistan not with reference to the Soviet Socialist Republic to which they now belong, but in a network of the historic hubs of the Persianate cosmopolis, including both cities within Soviet Uzbekistan and cities far beyond its borders.[62]

But these heroes appear only in Chapter 2—and Chapter 2 is not the first time we hear of Herat. Chapter 1 of *Slaves* begins by introducing readers to the enemy. Somewhere in the desert, surrounded by sand dunes, in a Turkmen settlement shielded from the evil eye by the skulls of camels, goats, and sheep, an old man named Qilich Khalifa concludes his prayers and turns to his guest: a trader named Abdurahmon. Between pots of tea and opium pipes served by silent women, Abdurahmon states his business. Trade is bad these days, Abdurahmon says; he is not making much money off the rugs and blankets his slaves and wives weave, and wool is hard to come by in these parts. Can Qilich Khalifa offer any advice? The old man responds that he can. The wars in Afghanistan have made its borders porous, and Herat might be a good place for Abdurahmon to try his fortune with a raid. The agrarian idyll and the desert haunt; the industrious family and the grizzled patriarch; the sedentary workers and the rootless nomadic parasites: these are the binaries that structure the opening chapters of *Slaves*. The two worlds collide when Abdurahmon's horsemen descend on Hasan's fruit farm, capturing his entire family and carrying them away as slaves for sale in the renowned market at the Ark of Bukhara.

The rest of *Slaves* is a historical epic in five parts, tracing this family, other slaves, and their descendants through a series of episodes that span generations. Many aspects of the workers' lifestyle change across the novel's long chronological scope. There are, however, a few constants. Whether they grow fruit, grain, or cotton, they are always farmers. When they do raise livestock, such as sheep, the text notes that they supplement herding with grain cultivation. In contrast, the class enemies are "parasites," nomadic herders who survive by exploiting the agricultural labor of the working class. Over the course of five books, the Herati fruit farmers become Manghit Bukharan slaves, Turkestani sharecroppers, Red Army soldiers, and, finally, farmers on a collective cotton farm as the vanguard of Central Asia's working class.[63] Likewise, the Turkmen raiders of Book I are progenitors for the antiheroes of the later books—the Bukharan Emir, the greedy landowners and tax collectors, the clergy and the Tatar capitalists, the *bosmachi* rebels, and the wealthy peasants who attempt to bring down the collective farm.[64]

Agriculture is not the only thing that defines Ayni's workers. When Ayni imagined the Central Asian "proletariat," he characterized it not just in terms of an agrarian community, but also with reference to a shared Persianate cultural sphere, spanning Soviet nations and extending beyond the borders of the Soviet Union.[65] In contrast, the "class enemies" are not just opponents of proletarian agriculture, they are violators of proletarian (Persianate) culture. Ayni links agriculture to the learned literary culture of the great cities of Bukhara, Samarkand, and Herat that frame the novel. The novel is studded with shorter forms produced by the worker: stories, fables, aphorisms, jokes, and, most of all, lyric verse. For Ayni, verse—memorable and accessible, even for the illiterate masses—was the most proletarian of forms. As Samuel Hodgkin has observed, Ayni inaugurated an era in which the image of "the good, politically-conscious Tajik citizen...was an instinctive singer of ghazals, [or lyric poems], which spontaneously poured out at moments of high emotion."[66] Accordingly, in moments of great pain and great desire, in situations of combat and romance, Ayni's working-class heroes break out in poetry and song. Working the fields for a cruel master, they trade verses; in breaks from work on the collective farm, they hold an extemporaneous poetry contest (*askiya*), a kind of Central Asian rap battle. Early in the novel, verse functions most often as a form of protest. For example, when the master of an older slave concubine named Qolmoq supplants her with a younger slave wife, she effortlessly composes a quatrain while tending the kitchen fire:

> Thistles are good for the fire
> Qolmoq is good for a wife
> What an unmanly (*nomard*) thing
> To take a new lover alongside another."[67]

Later, when the same master instructs his foreman to arrange liaisons among childless female slaves and healthy male slaves, Qolmoq responds by changing the final line of the song:

> Thistles are good for the fire
> Qolmoq is good for a wife
> What an unmanly thing
> To force your own lover to marry.[68]

For Qolmoq, a powerless enslaved woman whose days are spent in drudgery and nights in sexual slavery, composing verses is the only way to register her protest. By repeating the word "unmanly," Qolmoq shows class enmity to be more than just a breach of economic justice; it is a pathology of masculinity as well.

But poetry is not just a tool of protest for Ayni. It reveals the slaves' humanity even in the face of their subservience. In the context of their forced "breeding," for example, a slave woman named Gulsum avers that women are not just for men's pleasure and childbearing; she dreams of building a companionate home with her lover, Neqadam. Stealing away in the night, they take turns composing quatrains. Gulsum begins, telling Neqadam she composed her verse while sitting along a dried-up irrigation canal:

> As water does not flow through the Suvoqar [canal],[69]
> So dry words do not quench the soul.
> I have a rose, all wilted;
> My nightingale does not even look at it.

The verse is no naive ditty: although composed using a *barmoq* meter, in using the motif of the nightingale and its beloved rose, the verse taps into a long lineage of Persian love poetry. Traditionally in Persian lyric, the love-struck nightingale sings of unrequited love for the cruel and inconstant beloved rose, whose thorns pierce the nightingale and cause it anguish. Here, Gulsum inverts the motif, turning the rose into the lover, left to wilt away, and the nightingale into the inattentive beloved. By changing the motif, Gulsum converts a lyrical mode that had almost always presumed a male speaker into one that can accommodate a feminine voice.[70]

Through its use of long-established verse forms and imagery, the poem places Gulsum in a broader Persianate tradition. This pattern continues throughout the book, with workers making references to the Iranian calendar, Central Asian history, Islamic cosmology, and Persian literary tradition. Drawing on his extensive research in Bukharan archives and classical texts, Ayni arrays the text with footnotes explaining everything from Manghit dynastic history, to local topography and meteorology, to pre-Soviet bureaucracy. Ayni's decades of scholarship and erudition do not go to waste, at least in the novel's Uzbek and Tajik versions. These references are so culturally specific that they proved very difficult to translate, and the 1977 Russian translation of *Slaves* omits many of these annotations.[71]

In *Slaves* to a much greater degree than in his early works, Ayni makes a serious effort to conjure a Central Asian "proletariat" over and against a parallel construction of an "elite." Gulsum's vocabulary is simple although sophisticated, and Ayni's working farmers, although illiterate, show familiarity with the movements of the stars, the basics of Islamic cosmology, and the types of windstorms that might affect their crops. Nowhere is this effort to construct a working-class Persianate culture more evident than in Ayni's representation of the Jadids to whom he once belonged. In Part III of the novel, which covers the period from 1917 to 1920, Ayni introduces a Jadid character, Shokir, who encounters a group of farmers while traveling in disguise in 1917 on a secret mission, working in opposition to the Bukharan Emir. In the course of their conversation, it becomes clear that Shokir is completely ignorant about the real plight of the "working class." He waxes eloquent about the value of universal education for raising the welfare of the nation, and, referring to the recent reforms undertaken in Iran and the Ottoman Empire, he excoriates the Bukharan Emir for his crimes against freedom (*hurriyat*). Shokir's speech reads like a caricature of Jadid catchphrases.

The shepherds humor Shokir by listening to him, and even agree that it is wrong to attack the Jadids as infidels. Nonetheless, they reject his transnational Islamic modernist program, replacing it, instead, with a new kind of internationalism. Drawing on their boundless reserves of folk literature, the shepherds tell parables articulating their suspicion that Shokir is not really interested in workers' advancement at all. Just as a foolish farmer might cut off his bull's head to prevent damage to its horns, they say, so Shokir is willing to sacrifice the workers for the sake of his misguided ideas about education and freedom (*hurriyat*). As one former slave, Qulmurod, argues in response to Shokir's claim that education will solve all his problems, "So you'll make everyone a mullah, but isn't it the mullahs that are driving us crazy already?"[72] As for "freedom," Qulmurod says, "Go ahead and rejoice from afar about your Turkey and Iran that have turned into paradise, but don't hope to see them in reality—you'll be disappointed." "All I know is what I've seen," continues Qulmorod, "and if Iran has become free and turned into a paradise, and if every citizen (*fuqaro*) can enter that paradise, then why are so many city-dwellers (*hamshahri*) coming here from there, seeking bread?"[73] Effectively, then, Qulmurod replaces Shokir's elite, Jadid cosmopolitanism with another type of cross-border connection: international worker solidarity.

But this is no stereotypical Soviet internationalism, linking the oppressed urban workers of, say, Moscow, Berlin, and New York. Ayni integrates Qulmurod not into a European proletariat, but into a Persianate one, embracing the migrant workers, sedentary pastoralists, and peasants of Turkestan, Iran, and the Ottoman Empire. Ayni's proletariat is international not only in the spatial sense that it crosses Soviet borders into Iran, but also in the sense that it incorporates Turkic and Persian speakers, Tajiks and Uzbeks. Although Ayni devoted considerable effort into constructing a Tajik national culture, in *Slaves* it is often unclear whether even the Soviet-era characters should be considered Tajiks or Uzbeks, especially in light of the fact that Ayni published his own Tajik translation just one year after the Uzbek version. Furthermore, although Ayni was surely aware that the abolition of the slave trade had been a key (false) justification for the Russian conquest of Central Asia, for Ayni, Russian "emancipators" are entirely absent. Indeed, Ayni passes over the entire Russian imperial conquest without comment, as it falls between the temporal scope of the novel's Books 1 and 2.

Ayni's decision to write Russians out of the novel can be read in two ways. First, it might be seen as his effort to indigenize the revolution, aligning it with his experience as a reform-minded intellectual who saw the Soviet project as the best way to enact his and his local comrades' vision of reform. Alternatively, Ayni's choice might be read more cynically, as part of an effort—whether forced or voluntary—to erase the histories of colonial violence in Central Asia. Indeed, it is well established that by the mid-1930s the histories of colonial empire in the Russian nineteenth century were being elided in official Soviet historiography, instead being replaced by a narrative that the Russian conquest had been a "progressive" historical force for the "backward" peoples of Central Asia. Arguably, the two narratives were both at play—Ayni was at pains to emphasize his own personal agency and that of his community, while those who had the power to publish or disappear his novel had made it clear that certain aspects of Russian imperial history were now unspeakable.

In the context of a Stalinist nationality policy for which language was key for the definition of nation, the language of the novel also serves to drive home the Tajik–Uzbek linkage. When Ayni's workers compose poetry and tell stories, their vocabulary is the shared idiom of Persianate culture, regardless of the language. In the slave woman's verse about the nightingale and the rose, for example, the words "nightingale" (*bulbul*) and "rose" (*gul*) are cognates in Uzbek and Tajik, as is the word "soul" (*jon*). We should not be surprised by a high proportion of cognates in verse forms that developed in a Persian-dominated context. But even in normal dialogue, as well as in the narration of the novel, the language is Persian-inflected. Analyzing *Slaves* in Ayni's Uzbek original and Tajik translation, linguist H. Tursunova has identified 705 "parallel" phrases in *Slaves,* in addition to the wide variety of cognate Tajik-Uzbek vocabulary. According to her analysis, about two-thirds of these phrases are direct cognates; the other third consists of a combination of calques and near-equivalents.[74] The novel blurs the distinction between Uzbek and Tajik as much as possible.[75]

But Ayni's choice to elevate the international Persianate community does not efface all national boundaries; it merely shifts them. By maximizing the Persian vocabulary in the Uzbek version of *Slaves*, Ayni correspondingly downplayed the other major element of the Uzbek language: Turkic.[76] In a moment of Bolshevik panic about "pan-Turkism," which linked the sedentary Turkic-speakers of Transoxiana and East Turkestan with the Turks of Republican Turkey and the pastoral nomads of the Eurasian heartlands, this ambivalence toward the other Turkic nations of Eurasia insulated *Slaves* from Turkism, the "wrong" kind of internationalism. In *Slaves*. therefore, Kyrgyz and Turkmens are invariably parasites, like Abdurahmon who enslaves the Herati family.[77] Later, "Kazakh" bounty hunters assist in returning escaped slaves, and "Kazakhs" sell arms to the White Army.[78] Tatars fare no better: in one extensive monologue set around the early 1860s, a nameless "Tatar *boi*" defends a potential Russian conquest of Central Asia, arguing that the infrastructure it brings will be good for trade, and that even slaves "emancipated" by the tsar will continue to be profitable to merchants like himself. Ayni does not denounce Kazakhs, Tatars, and Turkmen as such. But insofar as they represent parasitic nomads and class oppressors, Ayni's proletariat excludes them. For Ayni, the proletarian international he represents is a sedentary *Persianate* international.

In contrast to the proletarians who gush forth Persianate verse, in the entire novel, there is only a single scene in which class enemies participate in any way in poetry-making. After the successful raid on Herat, Abdurahmon and Qilich Khalifa hold a feast, where, in full view of their starving slaves, they gorge themselves on meat and drink wine until their bellies are swollen. Meanwhile, a Turkic epic poet (*baxshi*) entertains them with verses lauding their martial prowess. "Where Qilich's men race their horses / The summer pastures (*yaylov*) of Astarabad will turn to desert…Oh bird of Herat, do not fly about, and do not make a sound / Abdurahmon the horseman has come, your life has ended!" Here, the *baxshi* lauds the class enemies as murderers of the songbirds of Herat and despoilers of all cultivated lands, turning even Turkmen grasslands to desert.[79] So pleased are the Turkmen raiders with this "praise" that they reward the *baxshi* with a sheep and a three-year-old slave girl. In contrast to the slaves, who compose lyrics that convey their feelings or portray nature, these class enemies are mere consumers of poetry, just as they are gluttonous devourers of food. And this is no Persianate lyric—it is (from Ayni's perspective) the coarse, heartless epic narrative of Central Asia's nomads, produced not from deeply felt emotion, but for earnings. Ayni's proletariat thus encoded an implicit nomadophobia, which had a longer history in sedentary Transoxanian and Jadid thought, but aligned conveniently with the Soviet agenda, consolidating in the late 1920s to forcibly sedentarize nomads on the steppes of Eurasia.[80]

From the beginning of the novel, women participate equally with men in labor and cultural production alike. In contrast, the class enemy is in general male: the *boys*, mullahs, nomadic raiders, and wealthy capitalists are exploiters of women, and their wives, who often begin as slaves themselves, are identified more with the workers than the oppressors. This changes, however, in Book 5, which covers land reform and collectivization. By the time land reform begins, male class enemies are clearly on their way out. They huddle in dark guest rooms, plotting their revenge, while in the outside world, socialism is reshaping the countryside in ways they cannot control. By contrast, the new collective welcomes their wives and daughters with open arms.

Such a woman is Qutbiya, the daughter of a wealthy peasant, who attracts the affections of Qodir Ergash, the descendant of slaves and a leading activist for the collective farm. Qodir Ergash knows that the more strategic alliance would be a marriage to Fotima, a dutiful Komsomol member. Still, he is unable to resist the magnetic attraction Qutbiya exerts on him. Trusting her declaration of repentance, and lured by her feminine wiles at a secret rendezvous in the dark, Qodir Ergash agrees to marry Qutbiya: "As Qutbiya's thin lips moved toward Qodir and joined with his lips, Qodir gave up his resistance and said to himself with joy, 'I have brought a petit bourgeois [*meshchanka*] woman into socialist construction.'"[81] Tellingly, although the workers in *Slaves* belong emphatically to a Persianate community, here Qodir adapts a word of Russian origin to describe Qutbiya's class status. But this implicit translation should not be taken as a marker of progress. As the remainder of Book 5 reveals, Qutbiya's repentance is insincere. Throughout Book 5, she uses her connection to Qodir to sabotage collectivization in every way possible. Even Qutbiya's name, from an Arabic root meaning "magnetic pole" or "axis," serves to underscore her role as an alternative—and pernicious—point of orientation for Qodir and the working class.[82] Much like in *Mirage*, then, in *Slaves* the class enemy worms its way into socialism through an attractive woman.[83]

Qodir Ergash's sexuality betrays his commitment to the proletariat. Correspondingly, his class enemies express deep anxiety that collectivization will threaten their masculinity. Qutbiya's primary co-conspirator, Sodiq, is a middle peasant whom a *boi* successfully converts to the anti-collectivization conspiracy. As collectivization proceeds, Sodiq divests himself of all his property rather than allowing it to be collectivized, slaughtering chickens and selling his cow. Eventually, Sodiq sees no other way to preserve his property than to join the collective farm under false pretenses, take back control of his property as a collective farmer, and then sabotage it with all his might. In a remarkable passage that was removed from all subsequent editions, Sodiq and his wife discuss the ways that collectivization has upended the gender norms to which they were accustomed. The couple bemoans that women like Fotima are turning less feminine: cutting their hair, becoming tractor drivers and Komsomol leaders. For a moment, Sodiq and his wife speak almost admiringly about the women who cut their hair and come into public: Sodiq's wife even proposes cutting her own hair. Rebuffing her, Sodiq jokes that his wife can cut her hair only on the day he cuts his beard. Then, in a clear moment of sexual innuendo, Sodiq asks his wife to put the children to bed so she can "stroke his beard for a while." Sodiq's wife, in turn, responds with surprise:

> "I feared you would lose your masculinity after you became a collective farmer!" said his wife with a skeptical voice.
>
> "True," said Sodiq, "but my masculinity was under threat (*erligimni yo'qota yozgan edim*) not because I became a collective farm member, but because I lost my property and and got so upset about how badly things were being managed at the collective farm."[84]

The connection Sodiq makes here, among Sodiq's masculinity, his (hetero) sexuality, and his control over private property, strikes at the heart of the novel's narrative logic. Earlier generations of slaves found solace and solidarity in their heterosexual amors, but Qodir's sexuality *betrays* his commitment to the proletariat. Only Sodiq, his class enemy, maintains his masculine sexuality in the face of collectivization.

If we read the novel monologically, Ayni dismisses these anxieties about masculinity. But read contrapuntally, Ayni articulates a certain implicit anxiety about male sexuality, which becomes the proletarian's soft underbelly, a point of vulnerability and an object of unease. The novel ends abruptly, never fully imagining a proletarian Central Asian masculinity. In the concluding scene, Ayni's anxiety about masculinity intersects with a breakdown in Persianate linguistic culture. The novel ends with an emotionally charged confrontation that takes place, significantly, at a Red Teahouse. Qutbiya is unmasked as a class enemy after she falsely tries to frame Qodir as a saboteur, and the Soviet militia enter the Red Teahouse to arrest her co-conspirator. Newly vindicated, Fotima leads the collective farmers in a series of five slogans, all lauding Stalin, and laden with borrowed Russian terminology. "Long live great Stalin, leader of the world proletariat! / Long live the shock-working brigadier and organizer of collective farm construction, our Stalin!"[85]

Her fellow collective farmers join the chant, "shaking the windows of the Red Teahouse." Qodir and Qutbiya, meanwhile, form a dramatic tableau, motionless and speechless:

> Only two people did not move a muscle: One of them, Qutbiya, had fallen on the floor like a corpse; the other was Qodir Ergash, a victor, but like a heroic victor who did not comprehend his own victory, he stood coolly, smiling, with his hands in his pockets.[86]

At the end of the novel, then, at the moment of proletarian victory, Qodir Ergash encounters a block. Fotima inducts herself into the world of Stalin's proletarian international, superseding the Persianate folk lyric with the Stalinist slogan. In this respect, the novel's concluding scenes impose a monological interpretation on the novel, much like Saidiy's snowstorm death does for *The Mirage*. Read backward through Fotima's slogans, all of Qodir Ergash's long lineage—his slave great-grandfather, his sharecropping grandfather, his Red Army father—comes to its fruition in the collective farm. Stalin is a *deus ex machina* in the story of the slaves and their descendants' struggle for emancipation.

And yet, when the class enemies are finally defeated, Ayni leaves his readers in a moment of irresolution: the victory of the proletariat entails a challenge, both to Persianate culture and to Soviet masculinity. The Soviet victory renders Qodir mute. For Qodir Ergash the grandson of slaves, language fails at the very moment that he realizes that his sexuality—his lustful infatuation with Qutbiya—has betrayed him. Fotima's Russian-inflected slogans sit uncomfortably alongside the Persianate folk songs that so long fueled the slaves' fight; and Qodir's immobilization would seem to confirm Sodiq's fear that collectivization entailed emasculation. We need not read *Slaves* in an Aesopian mode to recognize its latent polyphonicity. The novel's conclusion is too neat, too inconsistent with the rest of the text; and it leaves the questions about Soviet proletarian masculinity largely unresolved. As a collection of five barely connected sections all focusing on different characters, *Slaves* barely fits most standard definitions of the novel.[87] While its *siuzhet* may lend itself to a narrative of proletarian victory, a close reading of the text suggest a profound alienation, even an implied self-castration, in the sloganeering Stalinist version of Soviet totality.

If the social contradictions inherent to socialist construction emerged for Qahhor in the form of the evocative realist object, Ayni articulated those contradictions by stretching the boundaries of the novel form: dividing the narrative into five separate sub-plots with distinct temporal and geographical settings and disparate sets of characters; studding the text with poetry; blurring the boundary between fiction and scholarship with his prolific footnotes and archival asides. *Slaves* exemplified the affordances of the novel Bakhtin emphasized most—its omnivorous capacity to absorb the vestiges of older literary and cultural forms—and in so doing, it introduced instability into the totality presumed by the competition prompt. If that prompt presumed the socialist victory to be complete, Ayni's novel-collage indicated that much struggle remained ahead.

Shams's *The Law*

Of all the 1934 prizewinners, Shams followed the novel competition guidelines most scrupulously. The hero of *The Law*, a young factory worker named Sodiq, is proletarian in the most technical sense, and the novel foregrounded precisely what the competition had called for: the fight for "proletarian dictatorship." In Shams's case, this meant the conflict in Kokand from World War I until the Bolshevik victory.[88] As hard as Shams tried to write Kokand and Central Asia into a shared Soviet story of transnational revolution, however, his attempts at historical revisionism fell flat, earning him criticism both for ideological garbling and historical nonsensicality. And yet, inextricably intertwined with the vast historical struggle is Sodiq's more personal struggle: his persistent efforts to find and emancipate his beloved, Nodira, from the clutches of the class enemies that have sullied her reputation. This most superficially ideological novel turned out to rely, not on the principles of class conflict stripped of anti-colonial struggle, but on a logic of masculinity that generated the most potent affective energy in the novel. Qahhor imagined the Soviet public as a bloodless phantom and Ayni as a historic Persianate cosmopolis, but both foregrounded masculinity—and masculine sexuality in particular—as a block to Soviet publicity. In contrast, Shams leaned into hypermasculinity as its bedrock.

On the most straightforward level, *The Law* is a novel of political revolution. It dramatizes the Bolsheviks' fight for supremacy in Shams's native city of Kokand, where local clergy and intelligentsia had put up some of Central Asia's most organized resistance to Soviet power.[89] The novel's action spans from the Central Asian revolt of 1916 and lasts until the Bolshevik victory of 1918 in Kokand. At the time Shams wrote, Party ideologues were rewriting the official story of this entire period, and Shams joined in the revisionist effort. The novel's revisionism begins with the uprising of 1916, which in the mid-1930s was the focus of a major historiographic shift in Central Asia. In 1916, when the tsarist authorities called for a draft of Muslim subjects to the WWI front, it triggered a series of revolts in the cities and steppes of Central Asia, many of which the tsarist army brutally suppressed. Throughout the 1920s, the bulk of Soviet historiography had stressed 1916 as a moment of anti-colonial mobilization, with Central Asian Muslims revolting against Russian settlers and the tsarist authorities that backed them.[90] Beginning in late 1931, the official line changed: 1916 became not a moment of anti-colonial revolt, but of class struggle. New historiography began to obscure the ethno-religious dynamics of the uprising, stressing a narrative of international proletarian solidarity over more uncomfortable colonial hierarchies. In turn, the narrative about 1916 as an internationalist revolutionary movement made it possible to represent the Bolshevik takeover of 1917 as a multinational collaboration rather than a European-led coup. The complex and shifting allegiances of Central Asian Muslims with various European (counter-)revolutionary groups became flattened into binaries between "revolutionaries" and *bosmachi* rebels. Shams's historiographic revision extended also to the Kokand autonomy, the government set up by a multinational group of liberals and moderate socialists that the Red Army defeated in 1918.

Writing in 1933–34, Shams spearheaded this process of historical revisionism in the Uzbek language. Shams's novel can thus be seen as part of a broader tendency toward historiographic revisionism under Stalin.[91] Although the final pages of the novel are now lost, the outcome of this story is clear in advance: by fighting shoulder to shoulder with his fellow proletarians, Sodiq secures the domination of the multinational proletariat over those who would oppress them—a multi-religious, multiethnic coalition of class oppressors, from Central Asian Muslim clerics to tsarist military officers and factory bosses.[92] While Gorky looms large over all three winning competition novels, in Shams's case the influence of Gorky's *Mother* is unmistakable: like Gorky, Shams focuses on a young worker's induction into a worker's struggle.[93] The novel elides the colonial histories from which Soviet domination in Central Asia emerged, and flattens the complex interplay of anti-colonial and class struggle at a moment of historical ferment.

It was this constructed historical narrative of "proletarian struggle" that made Shams's novel technically eligible for the competition prize. But for our purposes, the novel is valuable not primarily because of its obviously tendentious revision of the recent history of Central Asia, nor for its role in "telling October," a phenomenon that is largely familiar to us from other Soviet contexts.[94] What matters, instead, is just how little history this historical novel actually told. When the members of the novel competition jury recommended *The Law* for the third prize in 1934, they did not mention the extended storyline outlining Sodiq's participation in the pro-Bolshevik forces or his activism against the bosses and the clergy. Instead, the jury that commended *The Law* praised Shams's moving presentation of Sodiq's personal relationships: his deceased father, from whose sufferings he "[grew] up to hate the factory bosses"; and Nodira, whose "torture" at the hands of a class enemy brought him to class consciousness.[95] According to the jury, then, *The Law* won the novel prize not for its historical accuracy or its ideological purity, but for its emotional intensity—and, particularly, the emotional intensity of Nodira's story.

From the beginning of the novel, Sodiq's proletarian identity and his masculinity are closely intertwined. When the novel opens, young Sodiq, imprisoned for his role in organizing a rebellion against the WWI draft in Turkestan, helps to orchestrate a prison break and returns stealthily to his hometown. He slips by night into the home of his old work friend, Egamberdi, where he attempts to find out what has transpired during the three months he was away. First, he asks after his ailing father and grandmother, and learns that they both have died without him to support them. Next he asks after the factory and learns that there has been no more "conflict or unrest" (*janjal, to'polon*) since he and his fellow organizers were arrested. Finally, by the light of the moon, Sodiq asks after a girl, Nodira. Egamberdi tells Sodiq that scandalous rumors began to circulate about her soon after Sodiq's departure: "Nodira's really turned bad, she sleeps with young men every night, Nodira needs to be driven from the neighborhood, she's a dirty girl, a thousand curses be upon such young Muslims."[96] Unable to bear the social stigma, Nodira and her mother, Sora xola, have disappeared.[97] Perhaps, Egamberdi conjectures, they fled to a village, where they could hide in anonymity. Just as Sodiq's father and grandmother relied on him for their lives and livelihoods, Nodira relied on Sodiq for her reputation. From the beginning of the novel, then, Sodiq's work as a labor organizer is linked to his effort to maintain the sexual purity—or at least, the reputation for sexual purity—of his chosen beloved. For the remainder of the novel, the struggle to restore Nodira's sexual honor, or *nomus*, becomes a driving force for the plot.

This emphasis was not an idiosyncrasy peculiar to Shams. By the time Shams wrote *The Law*, local understandings of female honor had been in crisis for some time. By the time the Bolsheviks prevailed in Central Asia, it was widely believed among the urban Muslim population that a "respectable" woman did not appear unveiled in public, and socialized primarily in single-gender settings. For some Central Asians, breaching these norms threatened the *nomus*. or honor and respectability, of the woman in question.When Shams wrote *The Law*, then, Central Asians were attempting to negotiate how a woman could participate in the Soviet public while remaining respectable in their families and communities: whether, and how, a woman could retain *nomus* while also participating, unveiled, in socialist construction.[98] When Shams foregrounded Nodira's *nomus* he responded to a debate that was far from resolved in Uzbekistani society.

In describing Shams's fixation on proletarian masculinity over and against other ideological substance, I do not mean to argue that Shams fell back on "traditional" values that he inherited from his cultural or religious background. In fact, arguably, the category of *nomus* itself, as it was mobilized in the modern Islamic world, constituted a reaction to the onslaught of modernity, not a premodern "survival." More recently, a range of scholars, from historians to anthropologists, religious scholars, and philosophers, have demonstrated that the narrative that Muslim women need "saving" or that Islam is inherently oppressive to women was a product of colonial modernity, and in many cases, served to justify imperial intervention.[99] In reaction to these imperial feminist discourses, anti-colonial actors have sometimes adopted resistance to western feminism as a form of resistance to colonial domination.

I thus argue that Shams's struggle with masculinity constitutes a precarious and contingent response to several challenges in imagining the Soviet public in Central Asia. First, the category of the "proletariat" was deeply problematic in a Central Asian context—both because of the distinct economic history of the region when compared to western Europe or European Russia, and because of the uncomfortable fact that most of Central Asia's "proletarians," initially, had been Europeans. Beginning with the Hujum in the late 1920s, official Soviet discourse furnished a readily available and affectively potent narrative about women's helplessness and the (masculinized) Soviet proletariat as a rescuer.[100] Shams does not invent that narrative—he just inscribes a Muslim man like himself into the story.

Still, like *The Mirage* and *Slaves*, *The Law* makes a conscious effort to imagine a proletariat for Uzbekistan. For Shams, Central Asia's proletariat is linked to the European anti-capitalist struggle, with its centers in Germany and the Russian metropole. Of all the competition novels, Shams's hews most closely to Gorky: when Gorky died in 1935, in fact, Shams attested that he had carefully read *Mother* twice, and that he "learned a lot of things from *Mother* when writing *The Law*." Many features of the novel—the young factory worker fighting for liberation; the simple mother figure (Sora xola); the monumental crowd scenes—owe a clear debt to Gorky. Much like Gorky, Shams also takes great pains to show the multinational provenance of the factory workers who fight for Kokand alongside Sodiq. In prison, Sodiq gets his first introduction to the global proletariat through "Meta"—evidently "Mitya or Mitrofan"[101]—a "Russian boy" who had "learned to speak Muslim as smoothly as flowing water."[102] From Meta, Sodiq learns of Lenin, of his work in "Moskop" (Moscow) and "Girman" (Germany).[103] Another fellow-prisoner, Salim the thief, teaches Sodiq how to read and write in Nogay, or Volga Tatar. Sodiq's friends from the Kokand factory are also a multinational bunch, including Yashka and Grishka. Shams's descriptions explicitly racialize some characters: for example, Grishka's "bright blue eyes" are said to "embolden" Sodiq; and Faxri's blond mustache, sculpted nose, and mountain province, Karategin, give him away as a Tajik.[104] The spontaneous internationalism of this proletariat is only underscored by the conspiratorial internationalism of their capitalist enemies: Kokand's wealthy men (*bois*) get help from Austrian medics, British colonialists, Tatar merchants, and Russian capitalists.

Masculinity lies at the heart of the multinational crew's socialist solidarity.[105] In fact, in *The Law*, the proletarians' homosocial bond is solidified by their manly defense of helpless women. Sodiq learns, through witnessing Nodira's mother's public tirades against the rich, that Nodira was forced into prostitution by his wealthy enemy Mirzaqosim.[106] When Sodiq's friends see his despondency about Nodira's disgrace, for example, independently of Sodiq they hatch a secret plan to liberate her from the brothel. Although their effort ultimately fails, it knits the group together in a shared effort to free the oppressed woman. Part III of *The Law* consists almost entirely of the suspenseful story of the Red Army's defense of Sodiq's factory, which Shuroi Islomiya, the ephemeral Ferghana Valley polity that the Bolsheviks eventually overcame, has besieged. The soldiers are all men; within the factory women and children cower. But Sodiq and his "brothers" are defined more by their defense of women than their factory work. In fact, there are no scenes of factory labor in the novel, and in terms of its relevance to the plot, the factory they defend may as well be a medieval fortress. The narrator calls Sodiq's worker prisonmates "brothers," and in the novel, proletarians truly are a band of brothers.[107]

Nodira's story—the only female-oriented storyline in the novel—is not completely devoid of class categories. Her disgrace comes directly at the hand of class enemies, and she is the fatherless daughter of a poor family. However, reflecting how Soviet discourse in Uzbekistan partially displaced class emancipation with gender, Nodira's struggle is presented primarily not as a working-class, but as a woman's plight.[108] Nodira and her mother, Sora xola, are destitute because they lack the protection of a breadwinning father and husband. After her husband's death, Sora turns to gendered forms of labor: she supports herself and Nodira for some time as a washerwoman, but eventually, in order to avoid destitution, she takes on a clandestine lover who helps to support her. After that lover dies, she hopes that a marital alliance between Nodira and Sodiq will secure her and Nodira's future. But when Sodiq goes to prison, Nodira is first aggressively wooed by Sodiq's arch-enemy, the merchant's son, who, rebuffed, offers Nodira money for sex, and, when she refuses, instigates a brutal gang rape against her. Because of Mirzaqosim's machinations, Nodira finally ends up, involuntarily, with her first paid work—in a brothel. Although now a "worker" in the technical sense—but not by Bolshevik standards (not being a factory or farm worker)—she remains first and foremost a woman. Class conflict dominates the historical frame, but gender politics governs Nodira's story.

Shams's linkage between masculinity and proletarian identity emerges in some of the most suspenseful chapters of the novel, in which Sodiq's worker-friends attempt to rescue Nodira from the brothel. When Sodiq's friends come to the brothel, they first encounter her in a state of abject femininity: posing as prospective customers, Sodiq's friends ask the madam to see Nodira, and are told to wait because she already has a customer. The scene emphasizes Nodira's physical appearance: the madam notes that Nodira is one of the two most beautiful women in the brothel, and offers Sodiq's friends a virgin as an equivalent alternative if they prefer not to wait. When Sodiq's friends are finally admitted to Nodira's quarters, her physical attractiveness is just an extension of the sumptuousness of her surroundings: the guest room where she receives Sodiq's friends is adorned with copper dishes, "piles and piles" of rugs, silk mattresses, and musical instruments hung on the walls.[109] Simultaneously orientalized and ornamentalized, Nodira's abject femininity renders her both decorative and passive. In contrast to Nodira, the madam repeatedly uses language that stresses the masculinity of Sodiq's friends: "Make your brothers glad, Nodira! These brothers of yours are some of our city's brave young men!"[110]

After the madam departs, leaving her alone with Sodiq's friends, for a short while Nodira continues to model passive femininity. When they propose an escape, Nodira casts down her eyes and expresses doubt that such a plan could ever succeed. But all that changes when Nodira follows Toshpo'lat's barked command to go with him into the curtained corner of the room (*chimildiq*) reserved for intercourse. Minutes later, not Nodira, but a "very youthful little young man" (*yoshgina bir yigitcha*) emerges with Toshpo'lat from the curtains.[111] As if he has forgotten something, that "young man" returns briefly into the curtains, bringing out a knife and sheath. Nodira enters into the proletarian community through her symbolic transformation into a man. The process culminates with her obtaining of a phallus-knife; and the mechanism of that transformation—the death of her abject femininity—is her symbolic intercourse with the (male) proletarian.

Unfortunately for Sodiq, Nodira's emancipation does not last, and once apprehended by the bourgeois police (*mirshab*), she returns to her abject femininity. Her next form of captivity, however, further underscores the proletariat's masculinity, this time by comparison to its effeminate class enemies. After staying in jail for several days, Nodira is given as a wife to a local official (*mingboshi*) named Sarimsoqxo'ja. The description of Sarimsoqxo'ja emphasizes his apparent virility: he is known for cycling through wives, keeping from three to five wives at any given time; and even beyond his wives, he has a reputation for his womanizing (*xotinbozlik*). But that virility is just an appearance with no substance, for despite all his sexual escapades, Sarimsoqxo'ja has, scandalously, begotten no children.[112] Out of his desire to dispel the gossip about his childlessness, Sarimsoqxo'ja takes Nodira as his wife. Nodira does not oblige him by becoming pregnant, but she does manage to garner special treatment from him by feigning pregnancy symptoms. Sarimsoqxo'ja is only one among several class enemies with questionable masculinity. Throughout the novel, Shams emphasizes the effeminacy of bourgeois characters. As a teenager, for example, Sodiq's cowardly enemy Mirzaqosim loses badly in a fistfight with Sodiq. Once the civil war breaks out, the proletarians bravely fall into formation, while the class enemies, for the most part, enlist ignorant villagers as mercenaries. Even at the brothel, Nodira, in male drag with her phallic knife, is more of a man than the bourgeoisie, who fail to take up arms themselves.

Nowhere is Shams's intense preoccupation with gender politics more clear than in the terms he uses to describe Nodira's struggle—the language not of class conflict, but of gendered respectability. The term *nomus* appears first in the account of Nodira's demise: according to Egamberdi, Sora xola left town because her "nomus" could not bear the destruction of Nodira's reputation.[113] When the wealthy villain, Mirzaqosim, hires a go-between to secure Nodira's sexual services, he openly states, "There are very few people left who would stand on *nomus* in the face of hunger and duress."[114] When Sora xola rejects that go-between, she does so for fear of "*nomus* and the tortures of the day of judgment."[115] Furthermore, around the term *nomus* arises an extensive vocabulary of purity. Nodira is repeatedly said to be "disgraced" (*sharmanda; sharmandayu sharmisor*); the wealthy perpetrators of that disgrace are called "filthy" (*iflos*) and "dogs," epithets that are particularly offensive in Islamic contexts. In conversation with a friend, Sodiq demands "justice" (*insof*) for Nodira, and the friend responds that, by marrying Nodira, he can make her ritually pure (*halol*) again. With reference to Nodira, Shams returns over and over to the Islamicate language of ritual purity.

Shams's use of this vocabulary is particularly striking in light of the corresponding lack of language of class warfare and, more generally, of historical precision. Writing in 1937, Shams's most brutal reviewer, the Turkestani Russian writer Boris Cheprunov, eviscerated Shams for his many "errors."[116] For instance, instead of more technical terms—strike, uprising, demonstration, revolution—Shams consistently used the onomatopoeic Uzbek word *janjal*, meaning "fight" or "uproar." Too often, in Cheprunov's view, Shams avoided terms like "proletarian" or "worker" in favor of the less explicitly Communist term *kambag'al*, or "poor person."[117] According to Cheprunov, Shams confused the February Revolution with the rise of the Shuroi Islomiya, and failed to distinguish between Bolsheviks, Mensheviks, and SR's.[118] In other moments, he noted, Shams made strange distortions of time and space. In one case, a character predicted already in 1916 that Kerenskii would come to power and that Tsar Nicholas II would abdicate the throne—events that did not occur until 1917.[119] Cheprunov treated Shams with unique harshness, but this was not just a matter of Cheprunov's peevishness: a kinder 1937 reviewer, Usmonov, also noted the "vagueness of some historical events and the confusion of one event with another."[120] Meanwhile a member of a writers' brigade that visited from Russia in 1937[121] remarked upon the many factual inaccuracies of Shams's novel, concluding that the novel was "weak from a literary standpoint, politically, and in every way" (*literaturno politicheski i vsiacheski slabyi*).[122] He even claimed that no one actually read the novel before awarding it the prize.[123] For Shams's Soviet critics, the historical inaccuracies were damning indeed. In Shams's defense, of course, the "facts" that Cheprunov took for a given were far from established. In 1933 no rigorous research had yet been conducted on the events of 1917–18 in Turkestan (to this day the period remains something of a scholarly black box), and the official narrative about those years was actively shifting as the official discourse about the Russian Empire shifted from representing it as a violent colonial power to a progressive force with the ascendancy of Russian nationalism.[124]

Under these circumstances, anyone would have struggled to assemble a coherent narrative.

The Law is no history textbook, then. Nor is it a feminist critique of repressive gender norms about *nomus* and respectability. Shams made no attempt to dispense with or call into question the language of *nomus*; instead, he attempted to redefine it to include a poor woman once ensnared by prostitution and a helpless mother who takes on a lover in order to feed her family. These situations do not challenge the discourse of *nomus*. To the contrary, they reinforce it by showing class enemies to be its primary violators. Their primary crime is their violation of helpless women, and, correspondingly, the proletarians' mission is not to overturn, but to reinstate *nomus* as the reigning standard in the face of its bourgeois violators. In other words, for Shams, the primary problem is not the gendered category of *nomus*, but the fact that the bourgeoisie make it impossible for proletarian women to protect it.

It would be simple at this point simply to conclude that *The Law* is not "really" about proletarians at all.[125] It eschews most of the technical language of class conflict in favor of a dense web of vocabulary about ritual purity and sexual respectability. It offers a historical narrative riddled with logical holes and factual errors, while its romantic subplot is so engaging that the competition judges cited it specifically in awarding *The Law* its prize. But this is not a zero-sum situation. Nodira's struggle may be defined primarily by her gender, not her class; but for Sodiq, his class status as a factory worker is so imbricated with his masculinity as to be inseparable from it. Sodiq, unlike Nodira, is both proletarian and lover; his opponents are both class enemies and sexual rivals. For Shams, then, the imagined public is a "proletariat," in the most technical sense. But while the proletariat is only superficially proletarian, it is profoundly, inherently male, and it maps neatly onto fantasies of helpless women, besmirched honor, and manly rescuers.

Cheprunov touched on this issue when he argued that Sodiq's emotions, like those of his fellow workers, were "primitive and savage" (*primitivny. pervobytny*), particularly with reference to Nodira. "What a strange, zoological feeling," said Cheprunov of Sodiq's intense sexual feelings for her. "Sodiq is a man of the moment. He lives only in the moment."[126] If *The Law* was to succeed as a work of Soviet literature, in Cheprunov's view, Sodiq's emotions needed to be reworked—he needed to become, not the spontaneous, hypermasculine hero propelled by his sex drive, but a conscious "positive" hero.

Of the three winning novelists, Shams suffered most during the Terror and its aftermath. At the peak of terror denunciations, his humble origins became a liability. "We pulled Shams up from the lower depths," said one critic, bemoaning the fact that no one had adequately mentored Shams in the process of revising his novel, and consequently, the novel never improved.[127] Shams's humble origins rendered him a valuable literary representative, and at the same time, from the critic's perspective, made him uniquely susceptible to ideological error.

Responding to his critics in March 1937, Shams attributed his "failings" to the rushed time frame in which he had composed *The Law*, and promised to correct his errors if the Writers' Union offered him a paid sabbatical to that end.[128] It is unclear whether Shams ever received the desired sabbatical, but no matter the circumstances, Shams took a pen to his galley proof. In Arabic and Latin scripts, Shams added words, phrases, and extended passages; he scribbled out entire paragraphs and chapters until they were completely illegible; he corrected major errors. By the time he finished, Shams had been excised from the Writers' Union and reinstated, chastened, during the Terror. The novel was never published until 1958, 15 years after Shams's death and five years after Stalin's. To this day, the novel's ending is missing from the published edition, and although Shams expressed an intention to turn *The Law* into the first part of a trilogy, those plans never materialized. Perhaps, had he lived to write Volumes II and III, Shams would have found a way to tame the hyper-masculine "zoological" impulses of his proletarians, to induct Nodira and her sisters into the community of workers. From the vantage point of the late 1930s, Shams's job had been to transform a *janjal* into a revolution, the *kambag'al* into a proletariat. But in 1933, that revolution was still all too nebulous and un-revolutionary. So Shams latched onto the script he found most potent: violated women and masculine rescuers.

Conclusion

When Lukács argued that the socialist novel would veer toward the epic as the contradictions of capitalist society vanished, he articulated an assumption at the heart of the project for novel-writing in the early years of Socialist Realism. The competition prompt called for novels that would articulate an unfragmented totality—a unified struggle of the global working class against feudal survivals and capitalist oppression. In practice, the unacknowledged, intersecting legacies of patriarchy and imperial hierarchy haunted the Socialist Realist novel in Central Asia. Each competition-winning novel attempted to impose a representation of totality—an "epic" frame—on the novel. And yet each novel, in classic Bakhtinian novelistic form, instead accommodates many languages and a great deal of ambivalence, from Ayni's verse-bedecked unconventional five-part novel, to Qahhor's affectively inconsistent Soviet public, to Shams's "zoological" novel of manly derring-do. Precisely as Bakhtin suggested the novel always had done, these novels resisted totality, even undermined it. In Qahhor's case, it was his successful uptake of the norms of nineteenth-century realism that undermined the totalizing vision of Soviet victory. In Ayni's, it was the novel form's capacity to subsume other expressive modes, from the lyric to the archive, that complicated *Slaves*'s drive toward narrative closure. Meanwhile, Shams's dutiful imitation of Gorky's model novel did little to help him achieve a wholistic vision of Soviet totality. By the time the selection committee announced the novel competition results, the caption to the cartoon, that "the one who jumps in time and keeps the tempo will be first," carried an unintended irony: there *was* no first-place winner.

Socialism Mediated: The Making of Soviet Culture in Central Asia. Claire Roosien, Oxford University Press.
 DOI: 10.1093/9780198971153.003.0005

4
Songs

Introduction

This chapter is about music, but by way of introduction, I begin not with a song, but with a poem. In 1932, a seventeen-year-old girl named Zulfiya published one of her first poems in *New Way*, the official Uzbek women's journal. Its title, "Her Every Movement Sets the Tempo," did not just forecast the contents of the poem: it resonated with the other contents of the journal, and indeed, of official Soviet discourse of the time in every national language and every mass medium.[1] During the first two Five-Year Plans, the word "tempo" appeared in the headlines of *Pravda* and *Pravda of the East*; it filled the front pages of *Red Uzbekistan* and, in *New Way*, it organized the dull articles that appeared at the beginning of the issue, encouraging a "Bolshevik tempo" in silk-weaving or cotton-picking or nursery-building. A few pages before Zulfiya's poem, an article called for "Bolshevik tempo" in grain production during the critical summer growing season. With "tempo" in the title of her poem, Zulfiya confirmed its timeliness for current events, its relevance to the all-out effort for fulfilling the Plan.

In the poem, Zulfiya applies tempo across multiple scales. Shrinking the massive industrial scale of the Pravda headlines, Zulfiya maps Bolshevik tempos onto an individual woman's body. The poem's heroine, a textile factory worker named Marhamat, works to thread and place bobbins on a weaving machine. As she works, she follows Bolshevik time-discipline by working in shifts (*smena*), but even on the most momentary level, the motions of her body mark an insistent beat, "like a wave," as if rising and falling rhythmically. Indeed, the title might more accurately be translated "Her Every Movement *Is* a Tempo," as if Marhamat has synchronized her very body with the movements of machinery. The machines mirror her movements in turn, crying out "Give me work!" and begging for more thread by "opening their embraces wide."

If the poem articulates a cyborg-like synchrony between machine-woman and anthro-machine, it also conveys a sense of lateral connection between women workers. The poem is written in the first person, as if another factory girl is praising Marhamat. The first stanza, which is nearly identical to the last, reads thus:

> Her every movement sets the tempo,
> That's the look within her eyes.
> She, that bright girl, Marhamat,
> Is a shock-worker just like me.

Marhamat's rhythm links her body to the other factory workers. Zulfiya emphasizes this lateral connection as Marhamat operates the machines: "She locks eyes with a girl / the movement like a wave." The final line stresses Marhamat and her colleagues' state of emotional arousal: the Uzbek word "to be agitated" (*to'lqinlanmoq*) derives from the word for "wave," *to'lqin*. At the same time, the language of a wave creates an impression of a certain rhythmicity and regularity to Marhamat's movement. It also conveys a sense of lateral synchrony: Marhamat does not act alone; she is merely the crest in a wave of other women like her. Marhamat's tempo organizes the public of working women and in turn, inducts them into the public of all those working to fulfill the "industrial-financial plan" (*prom-fin plan*).

Bolshevik tempo also organizes Zulfiya's poetic meter. With minor exceptions, the poem follows an insistent folk meter, alternating lines of seven and five syllables. The poem reflects the turn away from Persianate poetic meter (*aruz*), now widely condemned as elitist and obscure, and to a folk meter, *barmoq*, derived from oral poetry. Its name, *barmoq* (lit. "finger"), reflects its simplicity: the syllabic meter consists of a fixed number of syllables in each line that can be counted on the reader or reciter's fingers. Just as Marhamat's body participates in a Bolshevik tempo, Zulfiya's verse mimics that Bolshevik rhythm, keeping time with the regular beat of the weaving machines.

This poem conveys the importance of *tempo* as an organizing principle for the socialist public in Central Asia, linking practices of bodily cultivation, time-discipline, labor practices, and cultural production. For Zulfiya and her comrades, the meters of poetic and musical form were intrinsically connected to the rhythms of production. To lose the tempo was no less than to interrupt the flow of socialist construction. Music, like poetry, mobilized the masses as a productive public.

The discourse about musical form articulated a much broader tension between "national form" and the temporality of socialist modernity.[2] In his paradigm-shifting speech at the 1932 Fifth Plenum of the Central Committee of the Communist Party of Uzbekistan, Akmal Ikromov represented the entire project of socialist culture in Central Asia in terms of tempos. He began by complaining: "Our cultural construction still lags behind the accelerating tempos of socialist construction and the growing demands of the laboring masses,"[3] and concluded that the most urgent task facing socialist culture in Uzbekistan was to "speed up the tempos of cultural construction during the second Five-Year Plan"—as if poems and novels were so many factory-made widgets. Ikromov articulated a temporal disjuncture between the temporality of socialist construction and "our" (Uzbekistan's) cultural construction. Tempo informed Ikromov's representation of cultural construction on a broad scale, but it was all the more relevant to music.

> Today, even a rank-and-file collective farmer begins to recognize that the old Uzbek music does not satisfy him. Uzbek music was created many years ago, when the Uzbek people and Uzbek laborers carried a double burden: the yoke of the khans and beks and the yoke of tsarist imperialism. Precisely for this reason the main motif of Uzbek music is weeping, tears, and woe. *These motifs do not meet the demands of the day.* It is dull to listen to such music.[4]

An editorial cartoon published in Uzbekistan's flagship satirical journal made clear precisely what Ikromov was referring to: the supposedly lachrymose melodies of the *maqom*, the suite of songs that had dominated Transoxanian classical music (Plate 6). While the performers were singing the slow, mournful melody of the famous "Iraq" piece from the maqom, the cartoon made it clear that the new Soviet public demanded music in keeping with the times. Another leading politician, Fayzulla Xo'jayev echoed Ikromov, arguing that too much Uzbek Soviet music couched important ideological messages in "old, mournful Uzbek motifs."[5] Ikromov, like Xo'jayev, walked a fine line. On the one hand, like countless cultural mediators across the Soviet Union, he argued that much of the music of the past was intolerable for the new socialist society. On the other hand, Ikromov insisted it would be a "left-deviationist" (*levatskaia*) error to reject "old" Uzbek music entirely. Ikromov articulated a tension in the slogan that music needed to be national in form, socialist in content. Insofar as music was national, it maintained continuity with history. Insofar as it was socialist, it needed to slough off the old, slow, sad rhythms of the past. National form did not exist for its own sake; it needed to be synchronized with socialist rhythms.

This chapter considers how cultural mediators transformed music into a medium of Soviet state publicity in Central Asia. At a moment when much of

Central Asia's musical heritage was being transformed beyond recognition, Uzbekistan's mediators used popular song (*ashula*) to create the synchronicity between proletarian tempo and national form that Ikromov desired. In its modularity, its mass reproducibility, and its capacity to facilitate Bolshevik rhythms and consequently, Bolshevik moods, the Uzbek popular song came into its own over the course of the 1930s. Derived from folk music but also distinct from it, the mass song was more than just a musical form: it was a medium of mass publicity carrying with it a whole host of new social practices and cultural imaginaries. A well-crafted popular song was supposed to help ordinary Central Asians to imagine themselves as part of a shared public of listeners, dancers and performers, and also to engage in that public on an embodied, affective level: not merely to *assent* to socialist construction, but also to step in time with its beat.

This dynamic was not specific to Central Asia. The Central Asian project for mass song took shape within a broader all-Soviet program to promote amateur music and Soviet "folk" music.[6] Music was an integral part of Soviet mass festivals from the very earliest years of the revolution, and popular songs rang out over the ritualized mass festivals of the Stalin era, whether in Moscow or Tashkent.[7] Musicians and performers throughout the Soviet Union understood music to be a critical tool for engaging the masses in socialist construction. The story I tell is thus not exclusive to Central Asia. Still, to this day scholars of mass and popular culture have focused on a generalized "Soviet" people, with an implicit presumption of Russianness.[8] Furthermore, while studies have examined art music such as the opera or metropolitan institutions like the musical theater, they have not considered popular musical forms so attentively. Music is often an afterthought in research on broader cultural phenomena, such as mass festivals and popular mobilization. Much could be said about these songs from a musicological perspective, but my focus here is distinct. This chapter asks what happened when all-Soviet systems of mass publicity confronted the problem of cultural difference, including the musical form and social performance practices that came along with it.

The story I tell is also not exclusive to the Soviet Union. Elsewhere in the Islamic world, modernizing states were turning to rearranged "folk" songs as a device for cultivating new political imaginaries. We might linger on an example from the People's Houses of Republican Turkey, where activists stressed choral performance as an essential device for turning peasants into Turks. One Turkish activist named Hamit Zübeyr argued that choral music, organized at People's Houses and People's Rooms, could create a unified

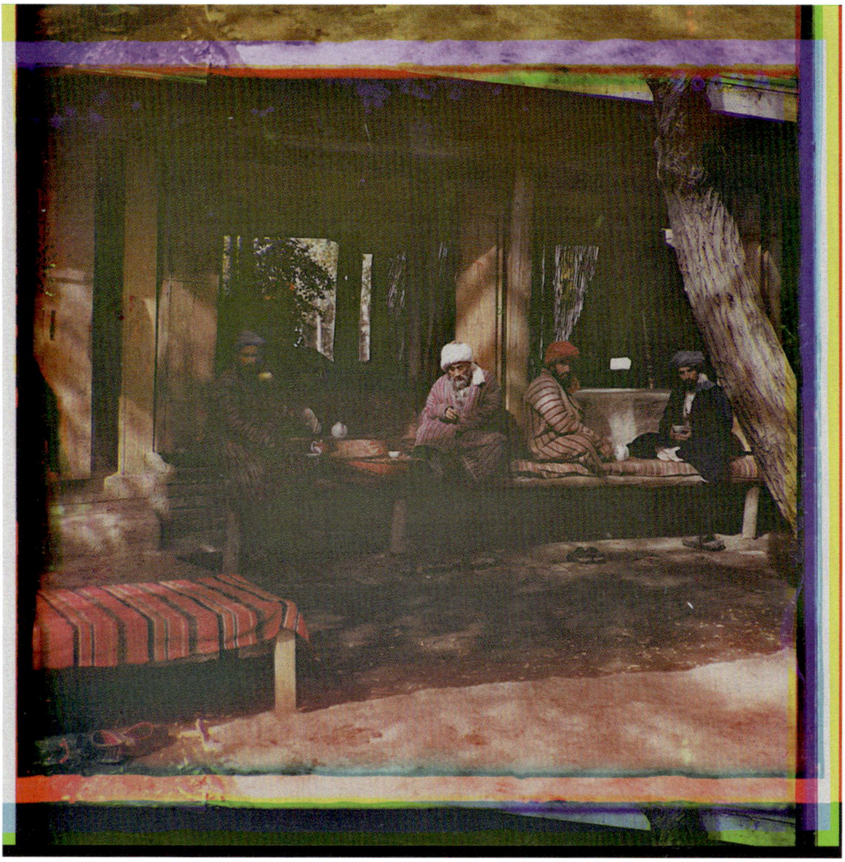

Plate 1 Pre-revolutionary teahouse in Samarkand, Library of Congress, Prints and Photographs division, Prokudin-Gorskii Collection, LC-P87- 8002A.

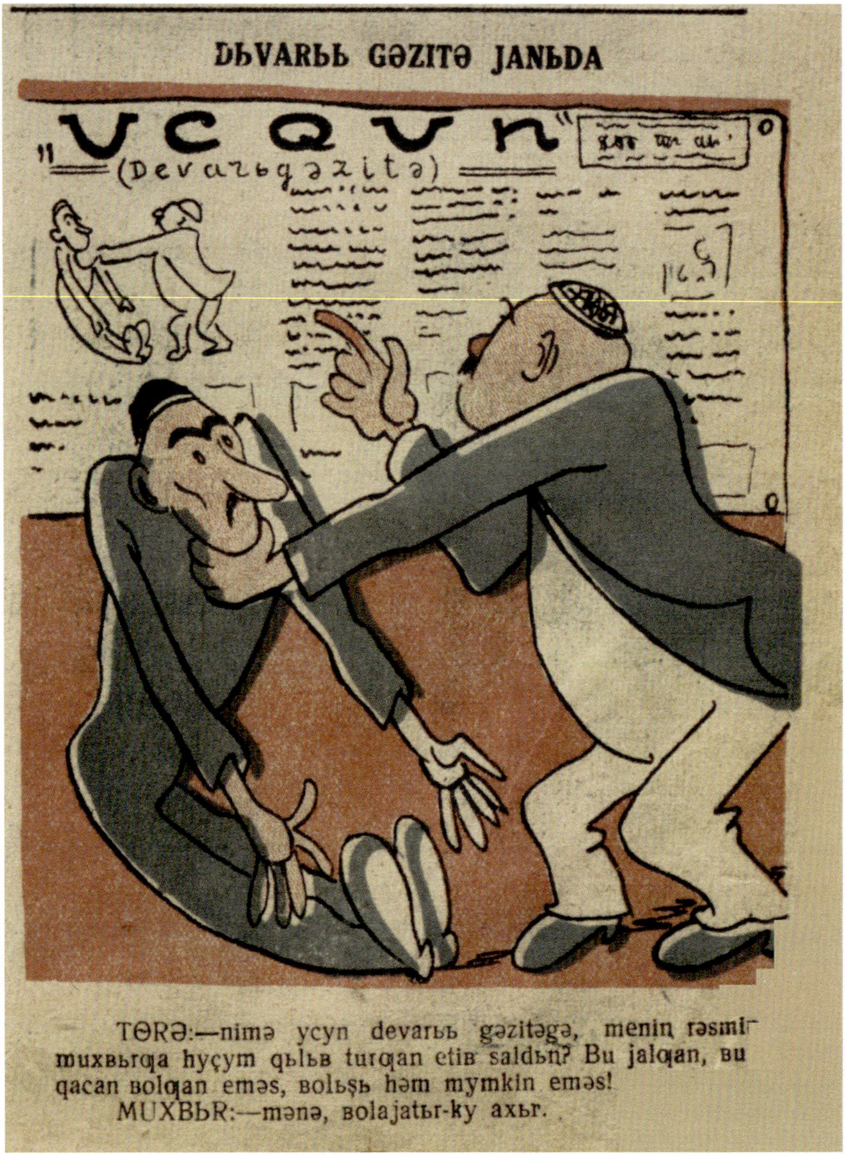
DƄVARƄƄ GƏZITƏ JANƄDA
"UCQUN"
(Devarƅgəzitə)
TƟRƏ:—nimə ycyn devarƅƅ gəzitəgə, meniꞑ rəsmi muxʙƅrƣa hyçym qƅlƅʙ turƣan etiʙ saldƅꞑ? Bu jalƣan, ʙu qacan ʙolƣan eməs, ʙolƅşƅ həm mymkin eməs!
MUXBƄR:—mənə, ʙolajatƅr-ky axƅr.

Plate 2 Editorial cartoon, "At the Wall Newspaper," uncredited, *Mushtum*, no. 9 (1931), 5.

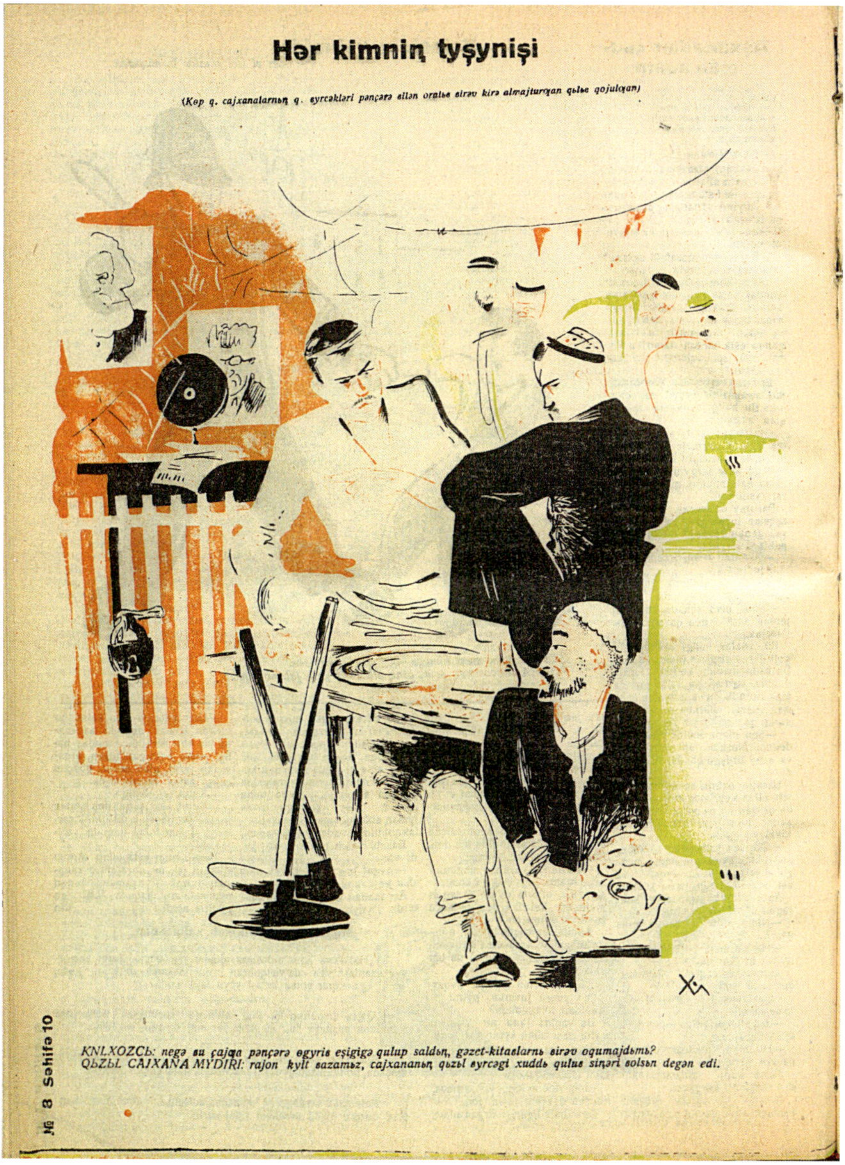
Hər kimnin tyşynişi
(Kəp q. cajxanalarnьŋ q. ьyrcəkləri pənçərə ьilən oralьь ьirəv kirə almajturqan qьlьь qojulqan)
KNLXOZCЬ: negə ьu çajqa pənçərə ьgyriь eşigigə qulup saldьŋ, gəzet-kitaьlarnь ьirəv oqumajdьmь?
QЬZЬL CAIXANA MYDIRI: rajon kylt ьazamьz, cajxananьŋ qьzьl ьyrcəgi xuddь quluь siŋəri ьolsьn degən edi.
№ 8 Səhifə 10

Plate 3 Editorial cartoon, "What Everyone Thinks," uncredited, *Mushtum*, no. 8 (1933), 10.

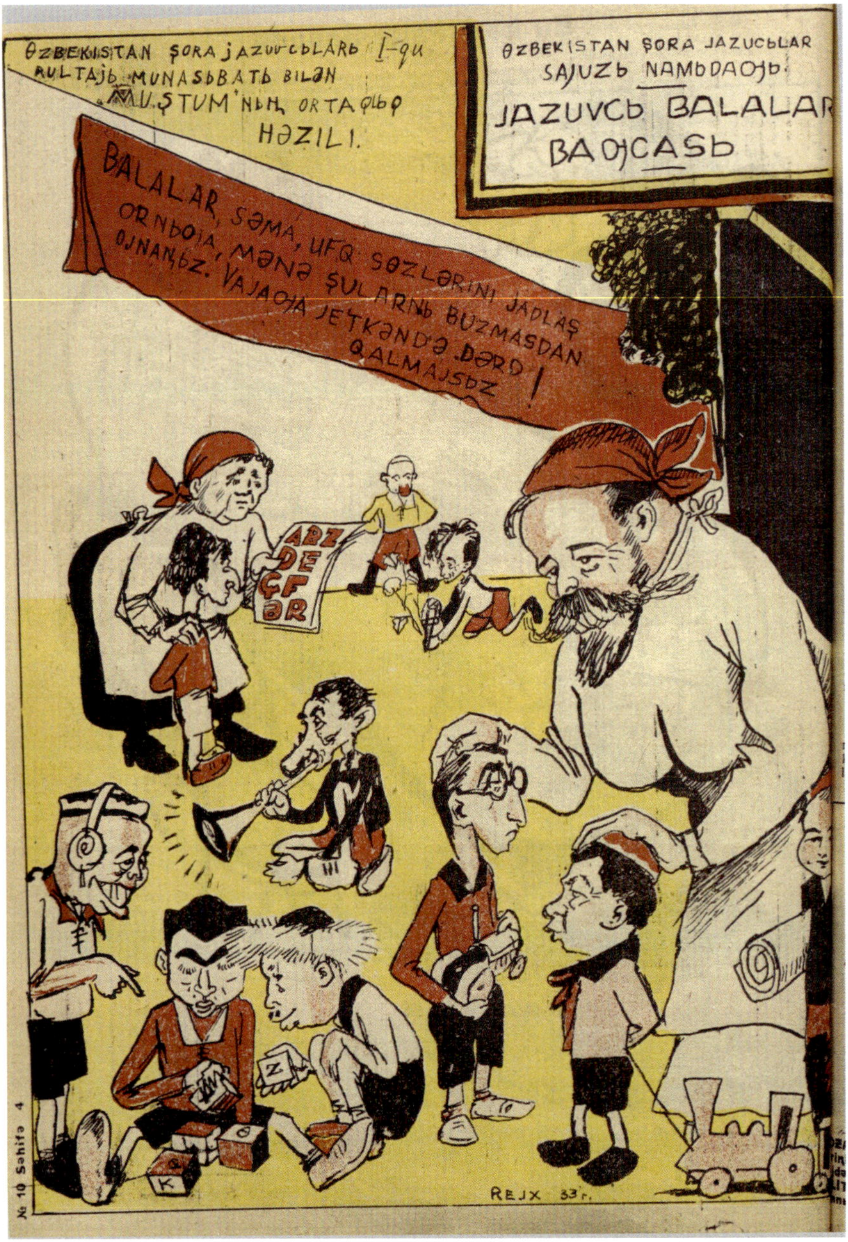
ƟZBEKISTAN ŞORA JAZUVCЬLARЬ I-qu RULTAJЬ MUNASЬBATЬ BILƏN MUŞTUM'NЬꞐ ORTAƢЬƢ HƏZILI.
ƟZBEKISTAN ŞORA JAZUCЬLAR SAJUZЬ NAMЬDAƢЬ:
JAZUVCЬ BALALAR BAƢCASЬ
BALALAR, SƏMA, UFQ SƟZLƏRINI JADLAŞ ORNЬƢA, MƏNƏ ŞULARNЬ BUZMASDAN OJNANЬZ. VAJAƢA JETKƏNDƏ DƏRD QALMAJSЬZ!
ABZ DE ÇF ƏR
Z
Ɵ
K
REJX 33 г.
№ 10 Sahifə 4

Plate 4 Editorial cartoon, "A Friendly Jest in Honor of the First Congress of Soviet Writers of Uzbekistan," *Mushtum*, no. 10 (1933), 4.

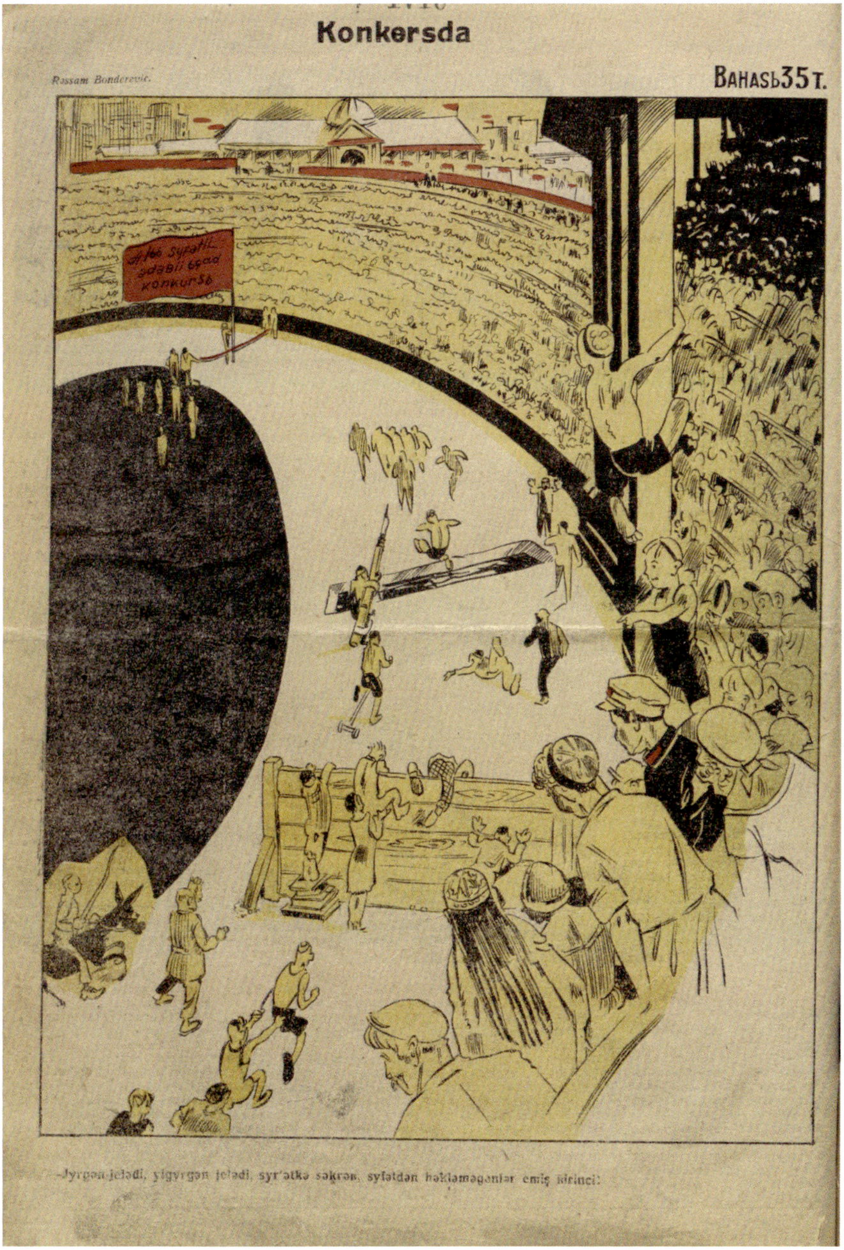
Konkersda
Rassam Bonderevic.
BAHASЬ35T.
–Jyrgən jeladi, yigvrgən jeladi, syr'atkə səkrəв, syfətdən həkləməgənlər emiş kirinci!

Plate 5 Editorial cartoon, "At the Competition," *Mushtum*, no. 16 (1933), back cover.

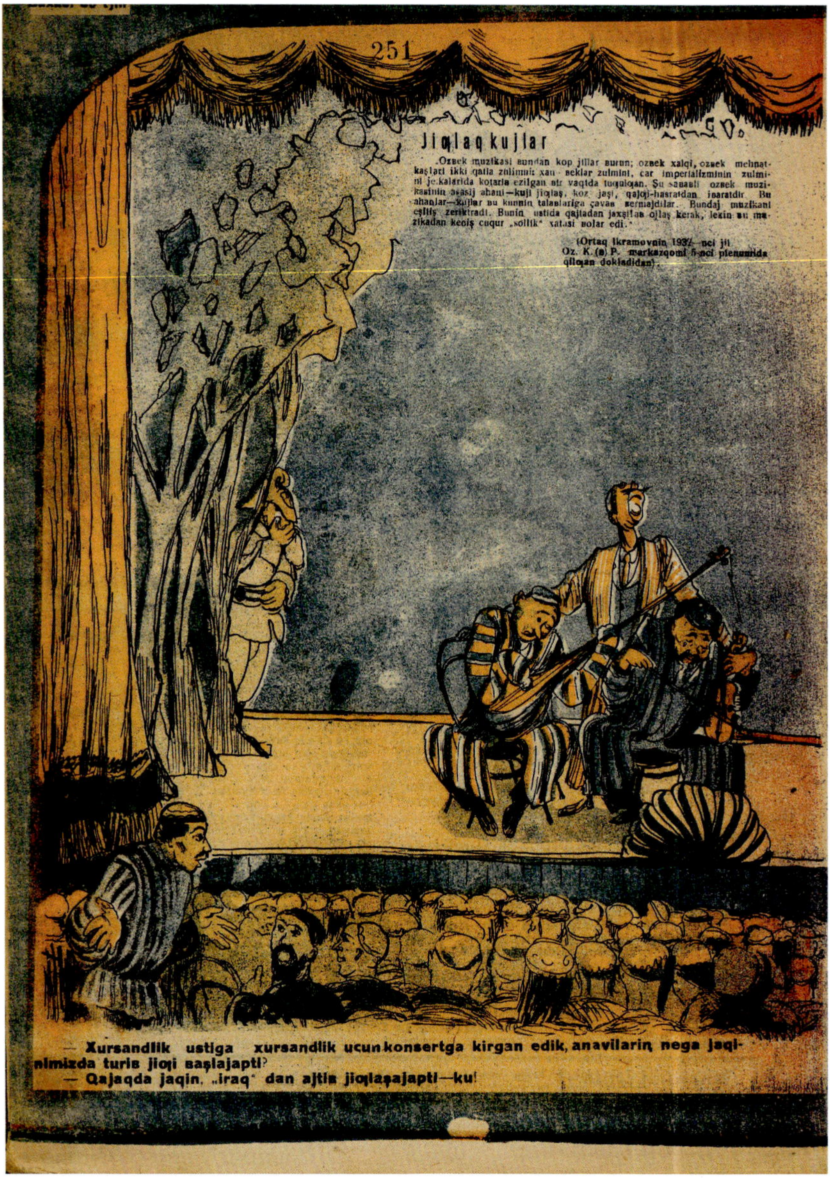
251
Jiqlaq kujlar
„Ozʙek muzikasi ʙundan kop jillar ʙurun; ozʙek xalqi, ozʙek mehnatkaşlari ikki qatla zulimni: xan · ʙeklar zulmini, car imperializminin zulmini jelkalarida kotarib ezilgan ʙir vaqtda tuqulqan. Şu saʙaʙli ozʙek muzikasinin asasij ahani—kuji jiqlaş, koz jaşi, qajqi-hasratdan iʙaratdir. Bu ahanlar—kujlar ʙu kunnin talaʙlariga çavaʙ ʙermajdilar. Bundaj muzikani eşitiş zeriktradi. Bunin ustida qajtadan jaxşilaʙ ojlaş kerak, lekin ʙu muzikadan keciş cuqur „sollik“ xatasi ʙolar edi.“
(Ortaq Ikramovnin 1937—nci jil
Oz. K. (ʙ) P. markazqomi 5-nci plenumida qilqan dokladidan).
— Xursandlik ustiga xursandlik ucun konsertga kirgan edik, anavilarin nega jaqinimizda turiʙ jiqi ʙaşlajapti?
— Qajaqda jaqin, „iraq“ dan ajtiʙ jiqlaşajapti—ku!

Plate 6 Editorial cartoon, "Weepy Songs," *Mushtum*, no. 2 (1936), back cover.

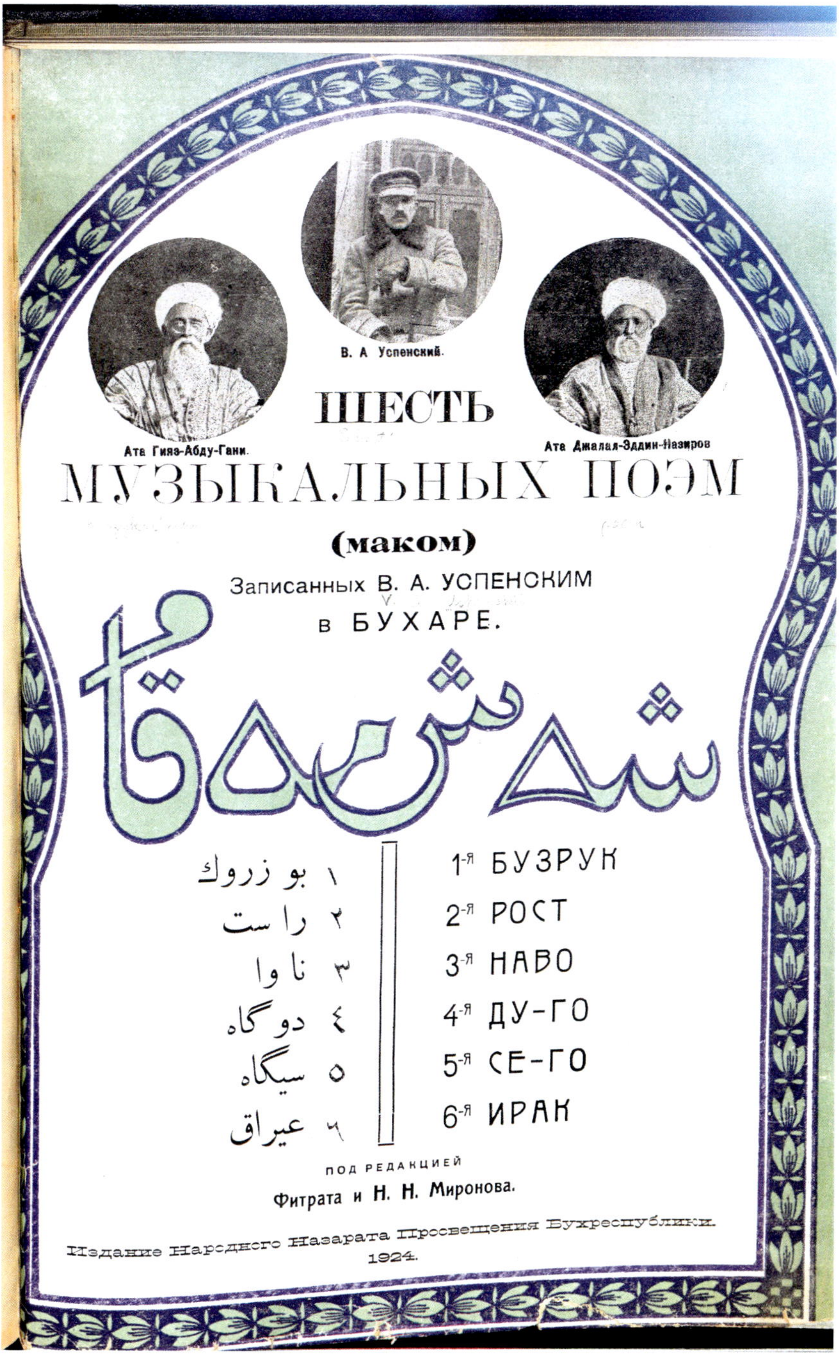

Plate 7 Front cover of Fitrat and Uspenskii's *Shest' muzykal'nykh poem* (Bukhara: Izdanie narodnogo nazarata prosvescheniia Bukhrespubliki, 1924).

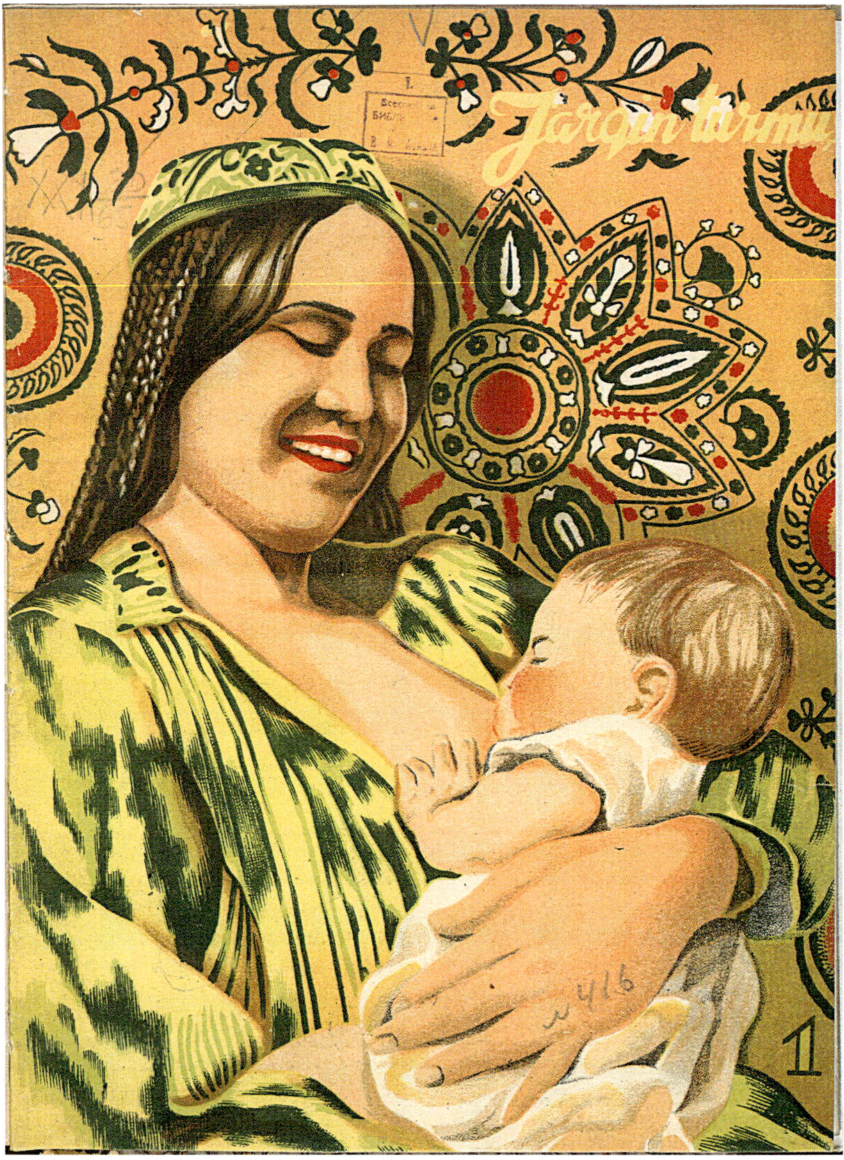

Plate 8 Women's magazine cover showing Uzbek woman wearing a silk or semi-silk dress, *Yorqin Turmush,* no. 1 (1937), front cover.

"social body and nation" (*ictimai vücüt ve millet*) out of a country divided along lines of "dialect, creed, and culture."[9] In choral singing, he continued, "the individual melts away in the group and loses himself." For Zübeyr, however, the ideological *content* of such music mattered little: he analyzed Soviet and Fascist musical mobilization neutrally and in parallel.

On the broadest level, however, both states understood participatory music as a tool for state publicity. Music offered many affordances not present in more staid and academic mediums like the novel. Illiterate or semi-literate populations could access music alongside the highly educated, and music capitalized on skills and practices with which even rural citizens were already familiar. Music has always produced collective effervescence in the moment, but in the age of mass publicity, modern states channeled that energy toward imagined communities beyond the face-to-face: the community of proletarians, the nation. In the new mode of musical mass publicity, an individual concert, festival, or performance facilitated both a sense of local belonging and broader political affect. Music could rouse soldiers to abject self-sacrifice and motivate workers for backbreaking labor. More broadly, it facilitated a sense of shared political participation even in the absence of mechanisms for democratic engagement. Amplified through the radio, it reached a far broader geographical span than ever before.

For music to work as a medium of state publicity, both musical form and the social practices around music needed to change. The chapter thus begins with a brief discussion of musical performance practices before the Soviet period and an analysis of how, during the 1920s, former Jadids collaborated with an enthusiastic cohort of European musicologists, working to imagine a musical modernity for the Uzbek nation by creating a body of national songs. Then, I turn to several musical mediators, examining how they remade Central Asian song over the course of the 1920s and 1930s. I consider their participation in the musical-cultural Olympiad of 1934 to illustrate the profoundly transformed social setting and reconstituted repertoires of socialist music for a mass public.

The "Music of the Past"

The year is 1913. On a summer evening, a small group of musicians form a circle in the courtyard of one of the palaces of the Bukharan emir. Two men sit playing long-necked stringed instruments—a *tanbur* and a *soz*—and another holds a round drum, a *doira*, with a sheepskin stretched over the rim, jingling bits of metal adding to the percussive rhythm. As the instrumentalists play an extended prologue, the singer closes his eyes, feeling the cool of the evening descend. He begins to sing, the melisma emerging fluidly from his throat. The modes of the *maqom* suites are as familiar to him as the tongue he speaks with his children; like a language, he improvises the melodic figures as he sings, performing the mode in a way that is both completely familiar and entirely unrepeatable. The texts he sings derive from classical Persianate poetry, and the *aruz* meter of the classical poem he sings is intimately linked to the meter of the melody. As he completes his opening phrase, the assembled audience—the emir and several honored guests—nod in unaffected pleasure.[10]

Not far from the palace, at the market near the *lab-i hauz*, the pool at the center of the city, an adolescent boy performer (*bacha*) begins his evening performance (Figure 4.1). He wears a bright silk robe, jangling jewelry, and an embroidered skullcap. Like the courtly musicians, he has never relied on written musical scores for his performances. Instead, from his mentors he has

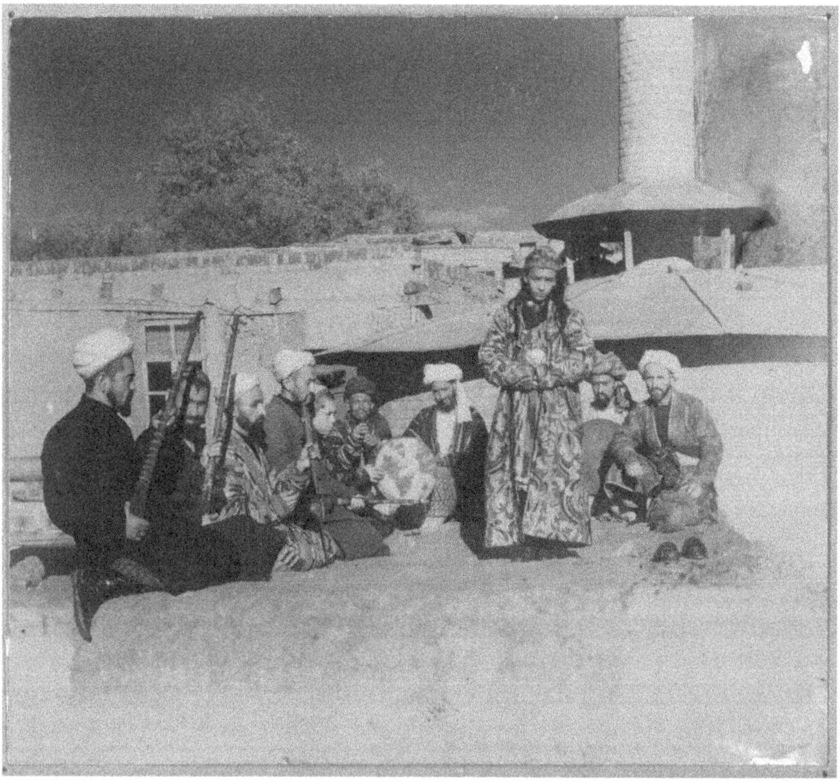

Figure 4.1 Bacha's dance, Library of Congress, Prints and Photographs division, Prokudin-Gorskii Collection, LC-DIG-prok-02309.

memorized a vast repertoire of popular songs: some evoke Sufi mysticism, while others have a bawdy subtext. On major market days, popular singers will come to the market square to accompany entertainers: tightrope walkers, puppeteers.

Women perform music too. The *dutar*, a two-stringed lute, is particularly associated with women; some members of the emir's household perform for him and his guests. Tonight, in a walled courtyard in the Ferghana Valley, a Tajik family is celebrating a wedding. A curtain separates the women from the view of their male counterparts, freeing them to sing, play, and dance uninhibited. Tonight, a group of *sozandas*, female wedding performers, sings a festive song: one virtuosic singer chants brief, two-line verses while a group of her fellow performers respond with a repeated refrain.[11]

These are just a few of the many ways people make music in Central Asia before the Bolsheviks. I have not begun to touch upon nomadic musical traditions, or the generic variety that obtained among all these various performers. Nor have I begun to address the forms of rhythmic and melodic performance that Central Asians do not consider music at all: the call to prayer that resounds over city skylines at dawn and dusk; incantations to heal the sick, and recitations to mourn those who die. In 1913, when the emir entertains his guests and the *bacha* his patrons, it is hard to imagine how much the soundscape of Central Asia will change within twenty years.

Music was always political. For influential men in Central Asia, cultural patronage had long been a way of exhibiting one's wealth, good taste, and clout. Beginning in the late medieval era, stories abound of medieval Central Asian courts poaching poets, miniaturists, and musicians from other courts as a way of jockeying for power in times of political competition.[12] This basic structure held true into the late Russian imperial period. In Khiva, Muhammad Rahim Khan patronized virtuosic *maqom* performance as a way to claim cultural authority when the Russian imperial order weakened his political and military power.[13] Cultural patronage by powerful men bankrolled the work of professional musicians in Transoxiana.[14] The last Bukharan Emir, Alim Khan, was known for impressing his visitors with performances by local Jewish musicians and dancers at his court when entertaining visitors. Sometimes, according to the grandson of one such performer, the emir would invite several small groups of performers to take turns performing the same piece, creating a "sort of competition."[15] According to one 1934 account based on an interview with a former court musician, the Bukharan Emir also sponsored an orchestra consisting of seventy to eighty Uzbek instruments, as well as an orchestra comprising exclusively European wind instruments, which was managed by a European staff member.[16] All of these musicians were well provided for by the Emir in return for an agreement that they would perform exclusively at his court.[17]

When Ikramov condemned the music of the past, the main object of his critique was the *maqom* in which many courtly musicians specialized.[18] Although primarily a "classical" tradition, the *maqom* became an oft-referenced foil to the popular repertoire that Soviet-era musicians were building. The *maqom* began as a collection of melodic modes, but by the early nineteenth century the term had come to refer to a "suite of musical pieces sequentially organized by melodic mode, metrical pattern…and rhythm."[19] Different sedentary regions of Central Asia developed different versions of the *maqom;* the territory that became Uzbekistan had three primary versions of *maqom*, associated with the courtly cities of Bukhara, Khiva, and Kokand.[20] Given its courtly associations, then, it makes sense that the Bolsheviks condemned it.

To find more popular entertainments, one could begin with the teahouse. Teahouse owners competed for customers by seeking out the best musical performers for the entertainment of their guests.[21] Musical sets could include both "classical" music (presumably *maqom*) and popular song, which was often accompanied by other performances, such as the entertainment of a *qiziqchi*, a local clown or comedian. Dancing boys provided the main entertainment at teahouses.[22] Both dancing boys and popular singers were organized into a guild (*g'olibxona*), while another guild, the *mehtorlik*, organized the activities of some musical performers as well as acrobats.[23] Well-off men sometimes hosted popular entertainment (*tomosha*) in their homes, and neighborhoods often had their own musical ensembles, comprised of local artisans, who performed on holidays and other special occasions.[24]

Among the genres of popular music, the *ashula* and the *qo'shiq* are the clearest antecedents for Soviet popular songs. The terms are defined differently by different musicologists. According to nineteenth-century ethnographer Avgust Eikhgorn, *ashula* described a range of lively dancing songs that were not dedicated to a specific event, such as a wedding.[25] He collected a variety of such *ashula*, most of whose lyrics comprised impressionistic verses on love and nature themes. Soviet scholar Beliaev, in turn, described the ashula as "songs in large two-part form,"[26] distinguishing it from the "small two-part form" of the *qo'shiq*. Later scholars distinguish the two genres based on their use of folk *barmoq (qo'shiq)* or classical *aruz* meter (the *ashula*).[27] Regardless of their generic distinction, the social setting for the songs was similar: both were popular songs for general entertainment outside the realm of ritual practice. In contemporary Uzbek, the two terms are synonymous outside the narrow circle of specialists. Indeed, it is arguably in the context of

Soviet mass publicity that the generic divisions between song types began to blur. It is these song genres—the *qo'shiq* and the *ashula*—that the great popularizers of the 1930s would adopt as Soviet songs.

Whether in courtly, religious, or commercial contexts, in the pre-Soviet period, musical production and performance occurred exclusively in face-to-face settings, linking people through relationships of kinship and patronage. This was true also of musical education. In order to learn to perform the *maqom*, for example, an aspiring musician apprenticed himself as a student, *shogird*, to a master musician, or *usto*. Through years of in-person training, over time, the young musician learned to perform the various *maqom* modes, and eventually, gained the experience to become training his own students. The *maqom* was thus transmitted orally, and professional musicians tracked their lineage in a long hierarchy of teachers and students, fathers and sons. Similarly, popular musicians, such as *bachas*, learned their performance practice by apprenticing themselves to more experienced performers.

The extent to which Central Asians understood music as a face-to-face phenomenon can be illustrated by two exceptions that prove the rule. Scholar Theodore Levin relates that in the latter years of Russian imperial rule, one Bukharan Jewish musician in the service of the Emir, Leviche Babakhanov, gained renown throughout the Russian Empire for his beautiful singing voice. A gramophone company in Riga, Latvia heard of him, solicited a letter of permission from the tsar, and sent a representative to Bukhara to record Babakhanov's performance of the *maqom*. Until that point, Babakhanov had permission to perform exclusively for the Emir. According to Babakhanov's grandson, the emir told him, "If they record you, then anyone will be able to hear you and you will be lower than everything; your music won't have any weight."[28] Unable to resist a letter from the tsar, however, the Emir granted permission for the recording to be made.[29] Nevertheless, his reticence to allow his star performer to be recorded demonstrates that for the Emir and his circle, music was not a mass medium, but an exclusive and intimate performance practice.

The second illustration has to do with notation. When the *maqom* was written down, as it had been occasionally since around the twelfth century, this usually involved simply transcribing its texts with commentary including the name of the melody to which the text could be performed. The melodies themselves, however, were not transcribed; it was assumed that the performer knew them by heart. These early "transcriptions" of the *maqom* were mere "knots [in a string] for the memory," intended to be auxiliary to the in-person hierarchy of master and apprentice.[30] In the late nineteenth century, one attempt was made in Khorezm to fixate not only the names of *maqom* melodies, but the melodies themselves. According to Otanazar Matyakubov, these attempts at notation grew out of a small circle (*dasta*) of *maqom* performers, all connected with the court of Muhammad Rahim Bahadur Khan. This circle worked intensely together and developed aspirations to transcribe a canon from which to develop a "new phase in the maqoms."[31] Accordingly, for their own use they devised a new form of notation specifically for the *tanbur*. Using this notation, they produced manuscripts of the *maqom*, eight of which survive to this day.[32] The notation thus represented an effort to create a small number of canonical copies of the *maqom* that the musicians could use in their own efforts to reshape their performance practice. However, they produced only hand-written copies, intended for use by musicians trained in the traditional hierarchies and in court circles exclusively. At this stage, notation did not enable music to address a public of strangers, but embodied, local communities of practitioners.

National Songs for the National Public

The Soviet state did not invent the effort to reform Central Asian performance practice. Indeed, the men who would become leaders in Soviet popular performance, Hamza (1899–1929) and his comrade Qori-Yoqubov (1896–1957), are better seen as part of a broader environment of Jadid and Islamic performance from well before 1917. Some readers will remember Hamza from Chapter 1 as the young activist who was murdered after attempting to repurpose a local shrine for a Red Teahouse. Such was his demise, but before he became a Soviet activist, Hamza was like most Jadids an avid newspaperman and an eager advocate of new-method education, opening schools in four cities during his early twenties. The records of Hamza and Qori-Yoqubov's activities, particularly in the early years after 1917, are notoriously spotty. The extent to which Qori-Yoqubov and Hamza supported the anti-Soviet Sho'royi Islom in Kokand, for example, is unclear in the absence of extensive archival documentation, though there is some evidence that Qori-Yoqubov worked as a courier and watchman for the Sho'royi Islom in 1917.[33] There are sufficient archival hints, however, that suggest that the transition from Jadid reformer to Soviet activist was not as smooth in either case as the Soviet-era biographers would have it. To the extent it is possible, then, I have collated published materials with the available archival materials, including a rich collection of oral history interviews with Central Asian musicians and performers conducted during the relative openness of the Thaw years of 1956–57.

Hamza and his fellow Jadids sought to transform Central Asia's musical culture in two main ways.[34] First, they began to shift the social setting for musical performance. Jadids introduced European-style theater to Central Asia, first by hosting performance troupes from Tatarstan and Azerbaijan, and then by producing their own plays, which often included songs. Jadid societies held "musical soirees or benefit concerts," which could include theatrical and musical performances.[35] Independent of courtly or religious institutions, such events heralded a new kind of associational life in Central Asia. In developing a public performance culture, Jadids created opportunities for a new kind of relation among strangers. Rather than addressing friends, family, patrons or clients, the Jadid theater created a space for otherwise unrelated people to come together around performance.[36] Alongside the theater, music thus became a focal point in the Jadid milieu.

More importantly, perhaps, Jadids pioneered the use of "folk" genres for popular enlightenment. Hamza was among the most avid proponents of song-as-enlightenment, pioneering the use of reworked folk songs for popular entertainment and enlightenment. Between 1915 and 1917, Hamza published a five-volume collection entitled *National Poems for National Songs* (*ashula*). The collection did not include musical notation: Hamza assumed the users of the collection knew the melodies already, and indeed, some of his early collaborators claimed he did not know musical notation anyway.[37] Instead, Hamza transformed the lyrics of folk songs—with their frivolous love themes, their superstitious subtexts—into anthems of progress. For example, the first song in the collection is based on a religious pilgrimage song about a much-beloved shrine in O'sh. Like many Jadids, Hamza was an outspoken critic of shrine pilgrimage. He converts the song's undesirable lyrics to a war anthem on behalf of both the Turkestani nation and the tsar: "Long live the nation (*millat*), long live our great king (*shahanshoh*)...Level Hungary to the ground /...break the land of Germany."[38] In the context of the tsarist war mobilization and the anti-colonial revolt it inspired, the anthem conveys Hamza's allegiance to the tsar in a fraught political moment. It also makes a space for a modern Turkestani nation within the tsarist order. Other songs replace expressions of fidelity to community elders (*to'ralar*) with national pride and a cult of youth. "We wish you peace, we wish you good health / Ah, dear elders, oh God (Allah)!" becomes "Unite, Turkestan! / Long live the youth of our nation (*millat*)."[39]

Already in this transitional moment, Hamza articulated a striking optimism about the power of popular song to inculcate "enlightenment." Hamza's logic about songs paralleled the logic behind the Red Teahouse: they were popular already, so why not put them to good use? By circulating these songs among the common people (*avom*), Hamza hoped to bring them over to his side; by exposing them to his verses in song form, he hoped to attract them, little by little, to higher-prestige cultural forms like written literature.[40] Indeed, many of the early members of Hamza's performance groups harked from popular performance traditions. Many Turkestanis would never read Hamza's poetry, but he hoped that hearing it sung by a *sozanda* might have the same salutary social effect. Others might not have attended an agitational speech, but an agitational speech preceded or followed by a rousing song and dance performance could always draw a crowd.

Popular and Professional

Summer 1919. A crowd gathers on Old Juva Square in Tashkent, waiting on a troupe of musicians from Ferghana to arrive. Suddenly the crowd murmurs: an open trolley is pulling into the square, carrying a group of musicians. Some hold wind instruments and hand drums, while others prepare to sing. As the trolley enters the square, a stately performer rises and begins to sing a new Hamza song in Uzbek, "Oh, Workers!"[41]

> Oh, workers!
> Oppressed laborers!
> Down with the tyrant *bois*!
> Don't let freedom slip from your hands,
> Long live hired servants![42]

The song is an *ashula*, but it differs profoundly from the "frivolous" *ashulas* Eikhgorn collected in the nineteenth century. The song may entertain—this crowd certainly enjoys the performance—but for the troupe director, Hamza, and for the performer, Muhiddin Qori-Yoqubov, this *ashula* is dead serious. Later that year, Qori-Yoqubov would carry a rifle as he toured the Transcaspian front boosting the Red Army's morale.[43] For now, the song is as good as a weapon. Over the course of August and September 1919, Qori-Yoqubov will perform in the theaters and squares of Tashkent. In one performance, he plays the role of a hired servant in a play by Hamza. After his master brutally beats him, the servant lifts himself off the ground on his elbows and quietly begins to sing the song from Old Juva Square, gradually gaining in volume until he laboriously leaps up and sings triumphantly to the end: "Down with the tyrant *bois!* Don't let freedom slip from your hands."[44]

Hamza's collaborator, Muhiddin Qori-Yoqubov, shared many components of Hamza's biography (Figure 4.2). Qori-Yoqubov's musical-theatrical agenda took shape in dialogue with multiple popularizing traditions: Islamic religious practice, the Jadid nationalizing project, and the avant-garde agenda for proletarian massification. Born, like Hamza, in the Ferghana Valley, Qori-Yoqubov was the son of a scribe and teacher who died in 1898, apparently while participating in the anti-imperial uprising led by Dukchi Eshon (Muhammad Ali Madali).[45] Raised by his stepfather, a plasterer, Qori-Yoqubov trained as a Qur'an reciter (*qori*)—hence his surname. He quickly became known for his melodic voice, both in folk song and religious performance. According to his Soviet biographers, in 1916 he founded an "orchestra" of wind instruments in Ferghana, incorporating both European and Central Asian instruments. Until 1917, however, Qori-Yoqubov merely moonlighted as a musician, working in a variety of hired positions in Andijan and Ferghana. The upheaval of 1917 made him a professional. Beginning in 1918, Qori-Yoqubov participated in a shifting assortment of performance troupes in the Ferghana Valley, including the "Muslim Youth Drama Troupe" and the "Karl Marx Troupe," which performed for Red Army troops in Transcaucasia and Central Asia, respectively. By 1921, he was directing a troupe of his own, performing primarily the songs and plays of Hamza.[46] Over the course of his career, Qori-Yoqubov cultivated an image as both a national virtuoso (the "Uzbek Chaliapin") and a diehard revolutionary. It is perhaps suspiciously fitting that Qori-Yoqubov claimed he was born on May Day in 1896.

If Qori-Yoqubov was Uzbekistan's native son, his first wife Tamara Khanum (1906–91) was its adopted daughter (Figure 4.3).[47] A charismatic young dancer, choreographer, and organizer of Armenian descent, Tamara Khanum had grown up in the Ferghana Valley after her father was exiled from the Caucasus because of his participation in a factory strike. The young Tamara's upbringing was decidedly multinational: Tamara Khanum's grandmother took her to an Orthodox Christian church, and she attended a school for the children of railway workers, who at the time were mostly European. Tamara joined her Muslim neighbors at play and at celebration, and learned Central Asian performance both from her father (who played the *tar*) and her neighbors. As a young teenager, she became the devoted protégée of the renowned percussionist, Usto Olim Komilov; and of a dancer named Yusuf Qiziq Shakarjonov. In the early post-revolutionary years, Tamara Khanum was one of very few skilled local woman musicians who were also willing to perform for a mixed audience on stage. Deeply immersed in Muslim performance traditions but lacking the gendered taboos of many of her Uzbek colleagues,

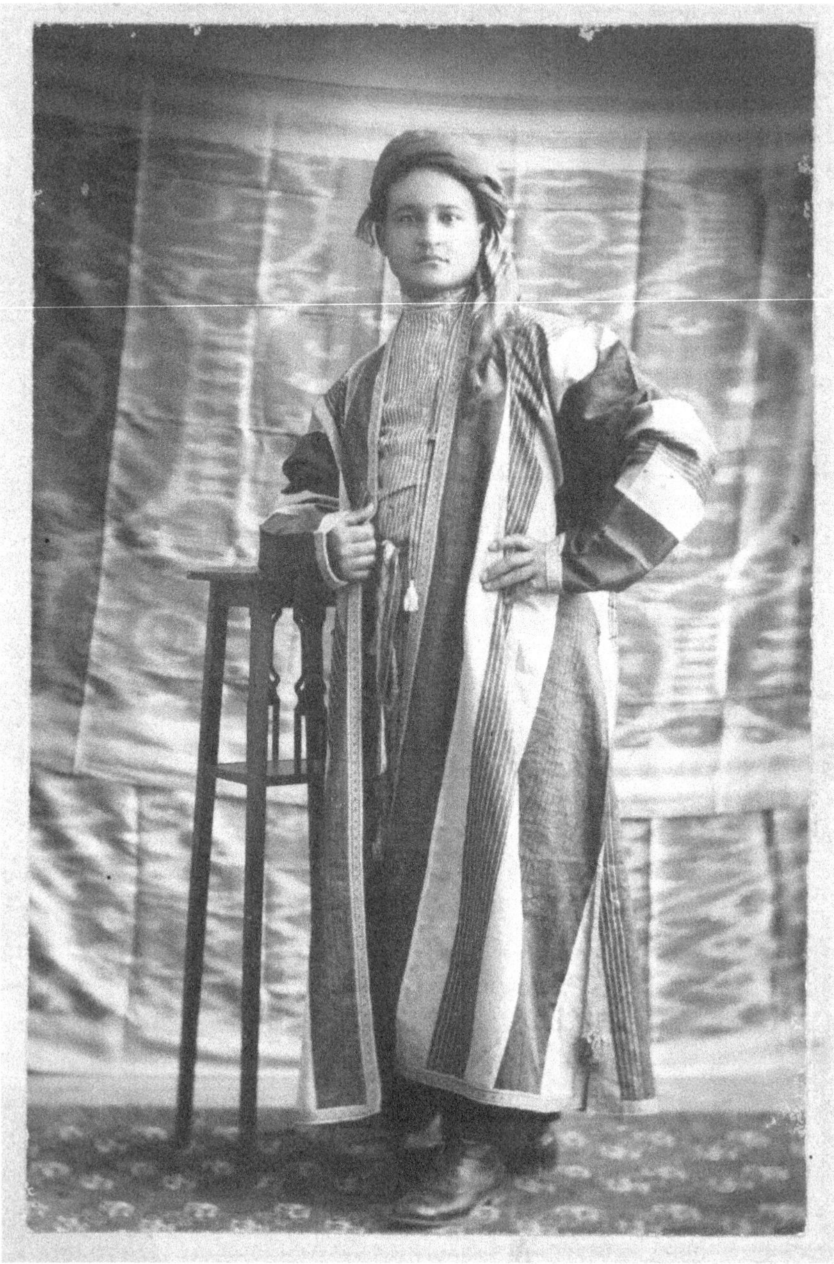

Figure 4.2 Muhiddin Qori-Yoqubov in his youth (1910s or 1920s), courtesy of Turkestan Archive.

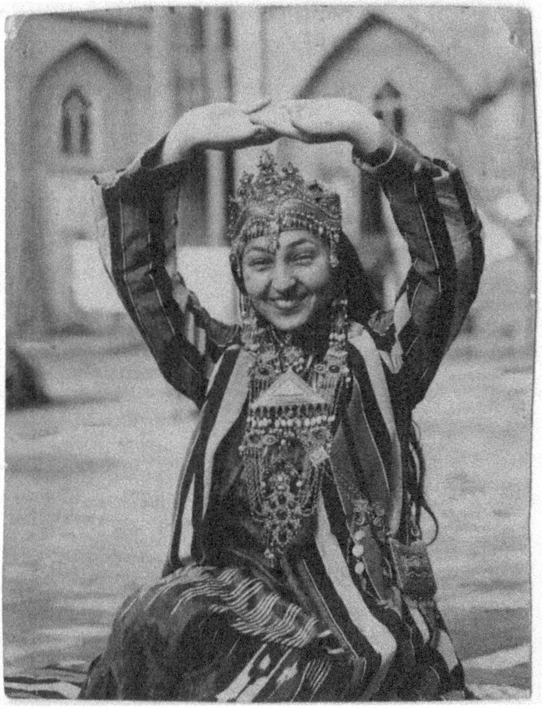

Figure 4.3 Tamara Khanum, uncredited photo, courtesy of estate of Langston Hughes and Beinecke Rare Book and Manuscript Library.

Tamara Khanum filled an important gap in early Soviet Uzbek performance culture.[48] In 1923, she joined Qori-Yoqubov's performance ensemble and soon married him. The pair eventually split amicably, but their union resulted in two daughters, the first of whom, Vanzetta, they tellingly named after Sacco's Italian anarchist partner, Bartolomeo Vanzetti. Like Qori-Yoqubov, Tamara Khanum became known for her remarkable charisma as a performer, charming international visitors like Langston Hughes, and wooing global audiences from Paris in 1925 to Delhi in 1958.

Jadid Music, Soviet Music

Qori-Yoqubov and Tamara Khanum developed their revolutionary Central Asian performance practice in the early years after 1917, but that project did not supplant the Jadids' nationalizing effort. Hamza was one among many Jadids who considered music a critical medium for organizing and modernizing a national public, and the early Soviet–Jadid conjuncture gave new institutional support to some of their efforts. Among the leading movers and shakers in Uzbek culture of the early 1920s, polymath Abdurrauf Fitrat laid the groundwork for Ikromov's revaluation of Uzbek "national" culture.[49] Two major projects expressed Fitrat's vision for Uzbek music: Fitrat's 1926 treatise *Uzbek Classical Music and Its History*, which laid out a vision for the future of Uzbek music; and a transcription of the Bukharan maqoms using European notation that he commissioned from Russian scholar V. A. Uspenskii in 1924 (Plate 7).[50]

Taken together, the two projects offered a new vision for Central Asian music. First, they rendered Transoxania's multi-lingual, transregional musical culture an Uzbek *national* project. As Alexander Djumaev has shown, Fitrat repeatedly declined to publish the texts that accompanied the *maqom* melodies transcribed by Uspenskii. The sole surviving copy of the texts, preserved only in handwritten form in two school exercise books, indicates that the vast majority of the *maqom* transcribed by Uspenskii were originally performed not in Turkic/Uzbek, but in Tajik/Persian; not by people of Muslim heritage, but primarily by Jews.[51] Djumaev concludes, "there was a deliberate act on Fitrat's side to replace the *shashmaqom*'s original texts with other texts."[52] *Uzbek Classical Music* acknowledged the links between Transoxania and the rest of the Islamic world, but also insistently reified a distinctly Turkic-speaking "Uzbek" nation going back at least to the fifteenth century.

Regional diversity, as well as linguistic heterogeneity, troubled Fitrat's notion of a unitary national music. In 1928, Fitrat complained that musicians in different cities performed the same song in different ways: "The same song [*kuy*] is performed differently in Khiva, Bukhara, Ferghana, and Tashkent."[53] In other words: the various cities that were supposed to be part of one nation in fact exhibited regional variation. The variation made sense before 1917, when Khiva and Bukhara had been the capitals of rival khanates, while Ferghana and Tashkent had been administrative centers of Russian Turkestan. For Fitrat, however, all four cities now represented the unified Uzbek nation, and accordingly, it was imperative to regularize musical performance in each city. Nationalization entailed standardization.

To that end, Abdurrauf Fitrat decided that educating young musicians was a prime imperative. If Jadids had emphasized "new method" literacy education, focused on reading rather than memorization, so Fitrat's musical education project stressed formal training and music literacy over oral performance practice. In 1921, Fitrat organized the School for Oriental Music in Bukhara, whose instructors included former court musicians; in 1927 it was renamed the Eastern Musical Tekhnikum.[54] He participated in a short-lived effort to organize an Uzbek opera studio in Moscow in the mid-1920s.[55] During the 1920s, conservatories, later renamed tekhnikums, also opened in Bukhara, Samarkand, Ferghana, and the old and new cities of Tashkent.[56] In 1928, with Fitrat's support, a "Research Institute for Uzbek Music" opened in Samarkand under the direction of Russian composer and Orientalist, Nikolai Mironov.[57] The People's Commissariat of Enlightenment, Fitrat argued, needed to develop a standard program for musical instruction at all these institutions. The new curriculum was to include transcriptions of songs. Even Khorezmian notation, which had received a renewed traction among those sympathetic to the Jadids, would suffice if need be.[58] In theory, these new educational institutions were to replace the social networks in which music had previously been transmitted and performed, from courtly circles to Sufi *khanaqas* and *qalandar-khanas*.[59] The meaning of professional musicianship changed dramatically in this moment. *Maqom* performers were channeled into the new *tekhnikums* and research institutes, while "popular" musicians from the *mehtorlik* now became members of a Professional Union of Art Workers (RABIS).[60]

Fitrat was not entirely bereft of concern for the "masses" or their revolution. In his volume on Uzbek "classical" music, for example, Fitrat opened with a disclaimer about the limits of his research. According to Fitrat, Uzbek poetic meter could be divided into *aruz* meter and *barmoq*, or "folk" (*el*) meter.[61] Likewise, he argued, musical form could be divided into "formal songs" (*usul vaznidagi kuylar*) and "songs without form" (*usulsiz kuylar*). The "formless" songs, like *barmoq* meter, were a "folk" form of music. Despite the term he coined for them, Fitrat argued that these songs were no more "without form" than *barmoq* poetry was "without meter." Fitrat did not entirely dismiss the folk songs, which in his words boasted a "fiery cadence, full of flame," but he concluded that he did not have the resources to do them justice, and restricted himself thenceforth to the "formal" tradition.

Fitrat also laid the groundwork for Ikromov's insistence that musical form mattered for socialist construction as much as, if not more than, lyrics. In his 1928 article on music, Fitrat argued that some *maqom* modes—namely, *navo* and *iroq*—might be appropriate for feasts and festivals (*to'y* and *ziyofat*), but did not convey the right mood for revolution. In order to create a revolutionary music, Fitrat proposed identifying classical rhythms and melodies that conveyed the appropriate mood, as well as gathering folk songs for that purpose. Before the Revolution, Fitrat claimed, the yoke of the elite "khans and beks" had dried up Central Asian music "at its root." Meanwhile, "progressive" (*taraqqiyparvar*) individuals had unfairly shunned their own national music, claiming that "the tanbur and dutar were condemned to death just like the hookah (*chilim*) and opium pipe (*nosqovoq*)."[62] Now that the Revolution had freed Central Asia from the backward despots that had once ruled it, Uzbek culture could become modern while also remaining true to its national roots.

In 1929, Fitrat was denounced and marginalized in a massive purge of "bourgeois nationalists" that swept the entire Soviet Union. In a programmatic article in cultural journal *Alanga* (*The Flame*), one Muhitdinov excoriated a nebulous category of "nationalists" because they "idealized the khans' age," and because of their attachment to national melodies "left over from the age of Chingiz Khan and Timur."[63] So attached were they to these "bourgeois nationalist" musics, they did not bother to gather "contemporary songs from the everyday life of working Uzbek farmers."[64] Muhitdinov's attack was suffused with conspiracy theory, and it is difficult to identify any individual active in the 1920s who actually espoused all these views, at least in public. But the article made it clear that Jadids like Fitrat were the intended target. After years of ostracism, Fitrat was shot by a firing squad during the peak of the Great Terror in 1938.

Fitrat may have disappeared from public life, but his ideas had long repercussions for the Soviet project of musical modernity. When Ikromov insisted that there was much to redeem in historic Uzbek musical traditions, he channeled Fitrat's defense of Uzbek music history; when he complained that certain modes conveyed an inappropriately mournful "mood" for organizing the masses, he resurrected Fitrat's ideas about the uneven utility of various *maqom* modes. For the first time, under the tutelage of the Jadids, a musical performance tradition that was multilingual, improvisatory, and transmitted through face-to-face networks, became a medium for the (national) public, rooted in state-sponsored institutions, oriented toward popular "enlightenment," and reliant on the print media and recording technology for distribution.

If Fitrat prioritized urban professional performance, Qori-Yoqubov gained a reputation both as a professional as a popularizer. Qori-Yoqubov's passion for "mass"-facing music is especially remarkable given that by the mid-1920s he had already made his name on the most renowned stages of Tashkent, Moscow and Paris. In spring 1922, at his own initiative, he traveled to Moscow, where he studied with renowned avant-garde theater director Vsevolod Meyerhold, then director of amateur arts at the Communist University for the Toilers of the East. In 1923, People's Commissar for Education Anatoly

Lunacharskii reportedly recommended he travel to Italy to study opera there, but the plans failed because he was unable to secure an Italian visa. Qori-Yoqubov nevertheless got his opportunity to visit Western Europe in 1925, when he and Tamara Khanum spent several months in Paris to represent the Soviet Union at the World's Fair, arriving in the city, fittingly, on Bastille Day. According to Tamara Khanum, the couple attracted crowds wherever they went: Qori-Yoqubov made himself immediately recognizable by donning a Bukharan robe (*khalat*) over his tuxedo, while long lines of people waited after their concerts to try on Tamara Khanum's stage costume, including her colorful *atlas* robe and gold slippers.[65] In response to popular demand, the couple extended their tour beyond the four performances that had been originally scheduled.

Upon returning to Uzbekistan, Qori-Yoqubov founded a series of popularizing counterparts to the more professionally oriented musical institutions led by Fitrat. The Uzbek Ethnographic Music Ensemble he founded in 1926 gathered over 500 folk songs with a view toward adapting them for the stage, and the ensemble was soon reorganized as the Musical Theater of Uzbekistan (1929), laying the foundations for what in 1939 would become the Opera-Ballet Theater of Tashkent. For this reason Qori-Yoqubov is frequently remembered as a founding father of the Tashkent theater scene.

In the 1920s and 1930s, however, Qori-Yoqubov devoted much of his effort to bringing music to the provincial towns and village squares of Uzbekistan. The Ethnographic Ensemble brought together singers, dancers, and musicians from around the country for massively popular performances. Costume designer Begimxon Kamilova remembered that at her first concert in 1928, there were far too few tickets to meet demand and the police had to be called to restore order.[66] The group toured around Uzbekistan and, eventually, the entire Soviet Union, attracting adoring audiences everywhere they went. Like Hamza's, Qori-Yoqubov's work was bidirectional: it collected folk material from among the "people," but it also repackaged that material and brought it back to those same people in formats—the stage play, the theater concert—that may not have been familiar to them.

Popular as it was, the ethnographic ensemble was not without its detractors. In March 1927, one Komil Aliyev published a harsh critique of Qori-Yoqubov and his ensemble in paper of record *Red Uzbekistan*. In emphatic bold print, Aliyev accused the ethnographic ensemble of "arousing lewd feelings and promoting disrespect for the fine arts among the people (*xalq*)."[67] The ensemble, Aliyev argued, had capitalized on the appeal of Russian performer Elena Iupatova, who "ruined the morals" (*ahloqini buzdi*) of young and old alike; some performances, he claimed, were completely inappropriate for the children who attended.[68] The raucous performances were profiteering off the common people, who spent outrageous sums of money on tickets, and the ensemble's "festivals" (*bazm*) merely repackaged the decadent performances that had once been sponsored by the merchants and wealthy men (*boy*) of yore. It is unclear precisely what the ensemble was performing in these early years of its existence, but Aliyev's critiques of the Ensemble reflected widespread NEP-era suspicion about private profit and sexual degeneracy. He also likely tapped into a general anxiety about women's stage performance as "uncultured" and sexually provocative, an anxiety that religious conservatives and Communist hardliners shared.[69]

The following day, another writer, M. Rasul, responded in defense of the troupe.[70] To be sure, he admitted, not all the troupe's oral materials "serve our ideology." But it was not for no reason that the central election commission thanked Qori-Yoqubov for attracting 35,000 farmers (*dehqon*) to elections. According to Rasul, Uzbekistan's "people" tended to prefer musical concerts to stage plays. By organizing musicians of the old world, who had "spent their entire lives completely unknown in private festivities and performances (*bazm va sahna*)," Qori-Yoqubov had done a great service to the Soviet performing arts in Uzbekistan.

The debates surrounding the Ethnographic Ensemble reflected both the power and the pitfalls of music as a tool for mass mobilization. Musical performance was by far the most popular medium of Soviet mass culture in Central Asia, and could attract crowds to initiatives they would otherwise find uninteresting or unattractive—whether elections to the Soviet or collectivization. But music also had the potential to foment other, less tractable feelings: erotic arousal, carnivalesque frenzy.

Music and the Mass Public

On a Sunday in mid-June 1934, the Central Asian Bureau of the Komsomol held opening ceremonies for the first Central Asian Musical-Artistic Olympiad. Newspapers reported that 40,000 people attended the opening festivities in Tashkent's Dinamo Stadium and in the adjacent Gorky Park.[71] The competitors, all amateur musicians and dancers, had triumphed in local and regional olympiads held around the republics of Kyrgyzstan, Tajikistan, Turkmenistan, and Uzbekistan. As the ceremony progressed, hundreds of performers filed in to the accompaniment of a band. They listened to rousing speeches from Party officials, including Comrade Oxunboboyev, then Chair of the Executive Committee of the Communist Party of Uzbekistan; and Shapurji Saklatvala, a visiting leader of the British Communist Party and former British MP. The evening's festivities concluded with a fireworks display. Over the course of four days, the contestants performed for the people of Tashkent at parks and theaters around the city, and on the last day, a lucky few were awarded prizes and the privilege of competing at the upcoming amateur music Olympiad in Moscow.

The Olympiad is a telling example of a new mode of musical mass publicity in 1930s Central Asia. In some ways, the Olympiad apotheosized the Jadid project for national modernity in music. It emphasized transcription and education beyond the face-to-face; it mobilized folk songs on behalf of a state-sponsored "enlightenment" project, much like that of the Red Teahouses. But from the perspective of musical performance as it had been practiced in Central Asia before, from the *ustod-shogird* norms of transmitting the *maqom*, to Fitrat's music for the modern national public, the Olympiad represented a major departure. Both repertoire and performance practices facilitated an imaginary of a universal proletarian public—from the collective farm circle to the Moscow orchestra. Young people would learn to play and sing at popular music circles at Red Teahouses, factories, and schools, using factory-made instruments and printed musical scores. The new musical culture would be of the "masses" and for the "masses." Some early projects were decisively avant-garde: the "Blue Blouses" (*Sinie Bluzy*), led by dancer Ali Ibrahimov "Ardobus" from 1931 to 1933, organized performances starring Young Pioneers who shouted slogans while wearing blue blouses and shorts, and ending with a human pyramid.[72] The Olympiad represented the triumph of another model—one that appropriated folk performance traditions in a Soviet mode.

When the Komsomol announced its plans for the Olympiad, it appointed a steering committee of twenty-two members, among whom the main movers and shakers were the two stalwarts, Muhiddin Qori-Yoqubov and Tamara Khanum.[73] Qori-Yoqubov and Tamara Khanum were the perfect pair for the job, carrying both national and revolutionary credentials. The Olympiad of 1934 was their opportunity not to bring Central Asian music to the world but to bring their refashioned vision of Central Asian music—and musical literacy—to the "masses."

Haphazard as the preparations may have been, the Olympiad opened with a bang, and the periodical press went to work to emphasize its significance.[74] On the opening day of the Olympiad, for example, an article published in

Yosh Leninchi began with a familiar thesis from Ikromov: the arts had once been a "weapon of exploitation" by the *bois*, the *beks*, and the bourgeoisie. Now, the dictatorship of the proletariat ensured the creation of a culture for the masses, one that would be "national in form, socialist in content." The article pointed out multiple axes of "massness" that were now included in cultural production: there were many "Uzbek, Tajik, and Turkmen girls, once imprisoned in four walls and deprived of the outside world." In addition to women, the article claimed, the Olympiad had brought in people from far-off rural corners of the region: "Here are Andijan, Yangi Qo'rg'on, Kokand, and many others. Here is Jarqo'rg'on province, far away from culture and the centers of scholarship."[75] The Russian-language newspaper *Komsomolets Vostoka* echoed these claims, adding to them a florid triumphalism about the Olympiad as a statement to the other nations of the "East." One article from the Olympiad's opening day claimed that, in contrast to the cultural riches available to Soviet Central Asia's masses, Persia had but two national theaters, and Afghanistan had only one.[76] Both in execution and representation, the Olympiad addressed a transregional, transnational, multi-gender, multi-ethnic proletarian public.

In discussing young performers from distant rural regions, the press coverage implicitly referred to the music and choral circles the Party and Komsomol had begun organizing around the republic of Uzbekistan. Schools, factories, collective farms, and other workplaces began hosting music circles already in the 1920s, although Red Teahouses conducted amateur music work on the largest scale. If the limited available statistics on Red Teahouses can be taken as representative, musical and choral circles were the most common type of circle they sponsored in 1930s Uzbekistan, outstripped only by basic literacy training circles. Music circles also far outstripped literary, visual art, physical culture, anti-religious, drama, and other types of "enrichment" activities that Red Teahouses were encouraged to organize.[77] The Olympiad reflected the youthfulness of circle musicians: over 80% of Olympiad participants were under twenty-four years old.[78]

The activities undertaken during the four days of the Olympiad further underscored this dynamic. On June 18 and 19, amateur groups performed at a variety of institutions around Tashkent: Gorky Park, Kafanov Club, Hamza theater, and a variety of factories; many performances were also broadcasted on the radio.[79] Audiences at the competition performances added up to as many as 8000.[80] A group of young Uzbek women impressed the audience with their skills on the *doira* tambourine and *dutar*, a group of Baluchi collective farmers from Turkmenistan put on a striking dance with sticks, and the Tashkent Profintern, comprising performers primarily of European background, was commended for its skillful use of "topical" material. Welders played the *dutar*, and collective farmers exhibited their talent for singing.[81] A young Ashkhabad prodigy named Nuri-Sari performed virtuosically on the *kamancheh*, a stringed instrument played with a bow. Meanwhile, two of his comrades, both of whom had been admitted to the music tekhnikum after beginning their careers on collective farms, performed exceptionally well on both European and "national" instruments.[82]

In each case, the performers did not only represent their individual performative talents; they stood in for the achievements of many others like them.[83] Photographs of Olympiad participants duly included women and men from a variety of national backgrounds, even if that required creating a photographic montage. The *dutar*-playing Uzbek women exemplified the new freedoms granted by the Party to women like them throughout Central Asia. Performers from collective farms represented the opportunities for self-improvement now available to rural "workers." Non-Europeans' and non-titular minorities' inclusion on a (purportedly) equal footing alongside Europeans served as evidence that Great Russian chauvinism was now a thing of the past. Uzbekistan's children stood in for the workers of the entire "East." Saklatvala, who was present at the Frunze team's performance, was so impressed that he requested an interpreter to convey his regard: "[Nuri-Sari's] playing reminded me of home. I think the hour will soon come when the children of India's workers will also be able to display their gifts and talents on the stage."[84] Both the Olympiad pageantry and the press coverage foregrounded the women, youth, workers, and collective farmers as representatives of a mass public. With its carefully conceived program, its wide-ranging media coverage, and its intentional use of (inter-)national forms, the Olympiad invited not just the in-person participants, but the entire mediatized public around Central Asia, to imagine themselves as part of a Central Asian, all-Soviet, and global proletarian public.

It should be stressed that the Olympiad's actually existing social dynamics did not correspond to these normative expectations. The gender balance was dramatically skewed, with male participants outnumbering female ones by a factor of nearly 6 (Chart 4.1).[85] Many of the female participants seem to have been prepubescent girls: Tamara Khanum notwithstanding, the strong cultural restrictions and real bodily danger facing adult women performers likely served as a deterrent. More than one woman performer had been murdered over the early Soviet years, and Qori-Yoqubov had struggled mightily to attract women performers to his ensembles.[86]

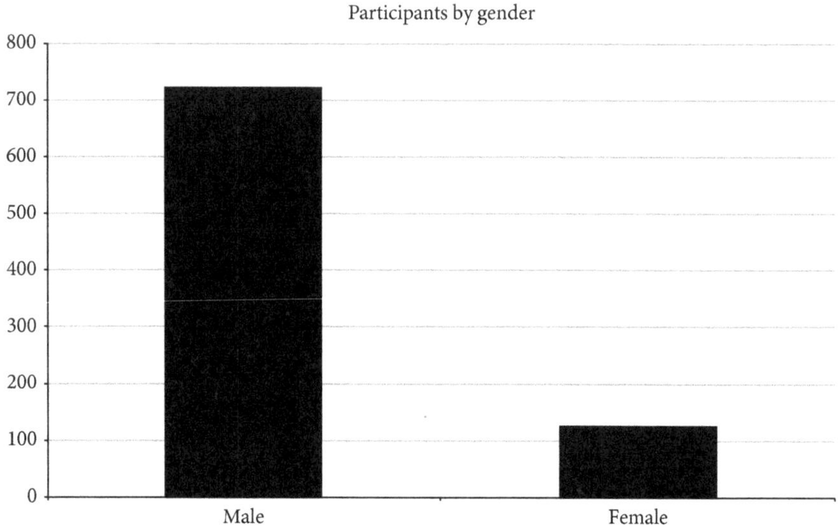

Chart 4.1 Olympiad participants by gender; statistics from RGASPI F. M-63, op. 1, d. 260, l. 35.

Russians and other Europeans were overrepresented both at the regional qualifying Olympiads and at the all-Central Asian festivities; Russians comprised over 40% of the participants in Tashkent. The event also skewed urban. Of 849 total participants in the all-Central Asian Olympiad, a mere 283 had never visited Tashkent. If the statistics about qualifying events are any indication, urbanites far outnumbered the collective farmers in attendance.[87]

The national makeup of the Olympiad also revealed a more complicated picture than the multinational mixing represented in photographs. Although Russians represented a small minority of the overall Central Asian population, they comprised over 40% of the Olympiad's participants (Chart 4.2).[88] In other significant feeder cities as well, Europeans dominated the statistics. At the qualifying Olympiad in Kokand, for example, there were 235 urban participants. Of these, only ninety-five were Uzbeks; the remainder comprised Europeans (120 competitors) and local Jews (twenty competitors).[89] The overrepresentation of Europeans also reflects the fact that, while musicians and musicologists from Fitrat's circle had taken a beating in the "bourgeois nationalist" purges of the late 1920s, Russian musical institutions continued their activities largely unassailed.[90] Russian groups thus benefited from the expertise of experienced performers, while members of local nationalities were reduced to relying on the dregs of decimated cadres. Finally, there are some indications that Russians' antipathy or indifference toward the

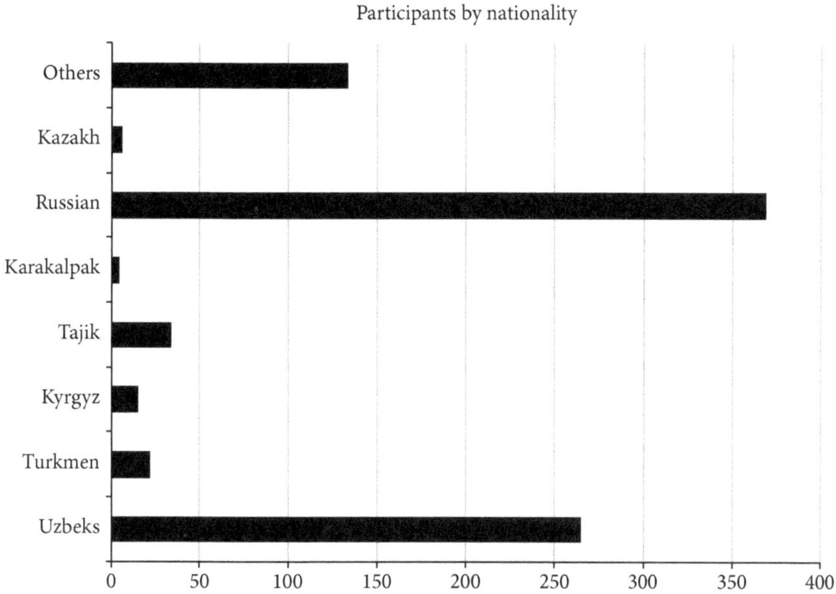

Chart 4.2 Olympiad participants by nationality, statistics from RGASPI F. M-63, op. 1, d. 260, l. 35.

non-Russians around them prevented more active ethnic mixing. For example, a May 1934 inspection of Tashkent's amateur musical institutions reported that Uzbeks were severely underrepresented in two of Tashkent's most active institutions. The Kafanov Club, which served the workers of the Tashkent Hydroelectric Station (*Tashges*), was revealed to include only thirteen Uzbeks out of a total of ninety-five participants in amateur music programs.[91] To make matters worse, although Uzbeks comprised 70% of Tashges's workers, only two of these Uzbeks actually worked at Tashges—the other eleven had been invited from outside. In the Tashkent typographers' club, likewise, only Russian-language amateur groups were active; no apparent efforts had been made to integrate non-European populations into their activities. Generally, the de facto assumption seems to be that "national" ensembles included only local nationalities, while ensembles performing European music incorporated non-Europeans as a minority.

Despite the rhetoric about bringing culture to Uzbekistan's masses for the first time, in fact the Olympiad organizers had no choice but to rely on older cultural forces. Like so many Stalin-era projects, the Olympiad called for massive organizational work in a short period of time. A large proportion of the Olympiad participants began participating in music circles less than six months before the event (Chart 4.3). After those who began participating

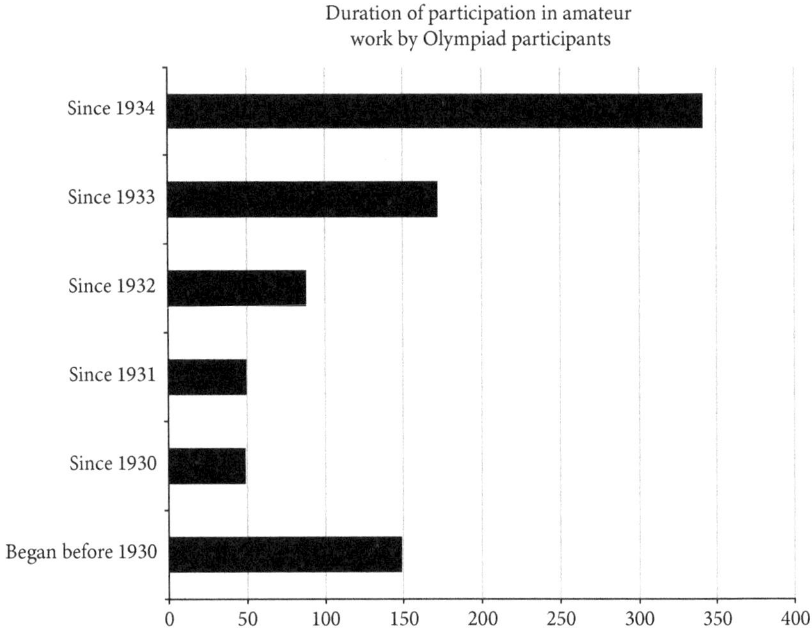

Chart 4.3 Duration of participation in amateur work by Olympiad participants, statistics from RGASPI F. M-63, op. 1, d. 260, l. 35.

in amateur music during the six-month runup to the Olympiad, the most numerous group comprised youth who had begun participating before 1930—well before Soviet amateur music systems were set up.

Under the circumstances, participants with pre-existing musical experience outside the new-found amateur circles had a clear advantage. And where did that experience come from? The older networks of musical instruction which had been so important for Qori-Yoqubov's early ensembles, but whose influence the Olympiad organizers rendered invisible. As Ikromov had insisted, former court musicians had an important role to play in developing Soviet musical culture. One such court musician, Ota Jalol Nosirov, was the source for Uspenskii's transcription of the *maqom*.[92] Another court musician, Hoji Abdurahmon, purportedly fled the Emir for Istanbul by way of Afghanistan and India, returning only in the Soviet period. He then became an instructor of the *tanbur* at the Musical Research Institute in Samarkand.[93] In 1930, *Alanga* even published an extensive article about historic lineages in Uzbek music, based on interviews with multiple musicians from Tashkent, Kokand, Marg'ilon, and Andijon. The author, G'ulom Zafariy, evaluated Central Asian political dynasties based on their attitudes toward music, representing Timur and his descendants, along with Ali Shir Nava'i, as "defenders" of music against the onslaughts of Islam.[94] Zafariy, both citing and building on Fitrat, took pains to argue that Uzbek music was not derivative of Iranian or Arab music. A full-page map representing the personal networks of music instruction in seven of Uzbekistan's cities accompanied Zafariy's article (Figure 4.4).

While the Timurids and their Jadid boosters vanished from the record by the mid-1930s, the traditional networks of musical transmission did not. For example, Nuri-Sari, a Frunze boy who impressed audiences with his virtuosic *kamancheh* performance, turned out to be the son of a *baxshi*.[95] In his research on Central Asian music, Theodore Levin offers further examples of musicians who brought prior expertise to amateur music circles and thence to official musical culture. For example, renowned *dutar* player Turgun Alimatov learned to play first at (black) teahouses in the 1920s.[96] Only after the government repressed these teahouse musicians did he join the amateur music circle at his school. Another musician interviewed by Levin, Ma'ruf Xoja, reported that he first began singing and playing the *tanbur* after hearing an older musician perform at a funeral in his community.[97] From that musician's students, Ma'ruf Xo'ja obtained recordings of his performances and modeled his performance style on the recordings. One year after Ma'ruf Xo'ja began playing the *tanbur*, he joined an amateur music circle run by the silk factory where he worked.[98] And Flora Roberts has shown that beginning in the 1930s, collective farm orchestras became refuges for renowned performers of the *maqom* who were no longer welcome in cities. Under the auspices of new institutions for amateur music, they ended up creating relationships of patronage with collective farm directors that resembled the patronage relationships at a Central Asian court fifty years before.[99]

Repertoire for the "Masses"

Despite the mismatches between aspiration and reality, the Olympiad laid claim to a new vision for music in Central Asia. Making Transoxanian music a medium for the masses entailed significant changes not just in performance practice, but also in musical instruments and repertoire.[100]

We might begin with the instruments themselves, whose very timbre was seen as an expression of the mournful and oppressive past. Leading musicologist Viktor Beliaev argued that certain instruments produced a "wailing" tone deriving from false religious narratives about the "vanity of human life."[101] These instruments needed to be reformed—whether with respect to

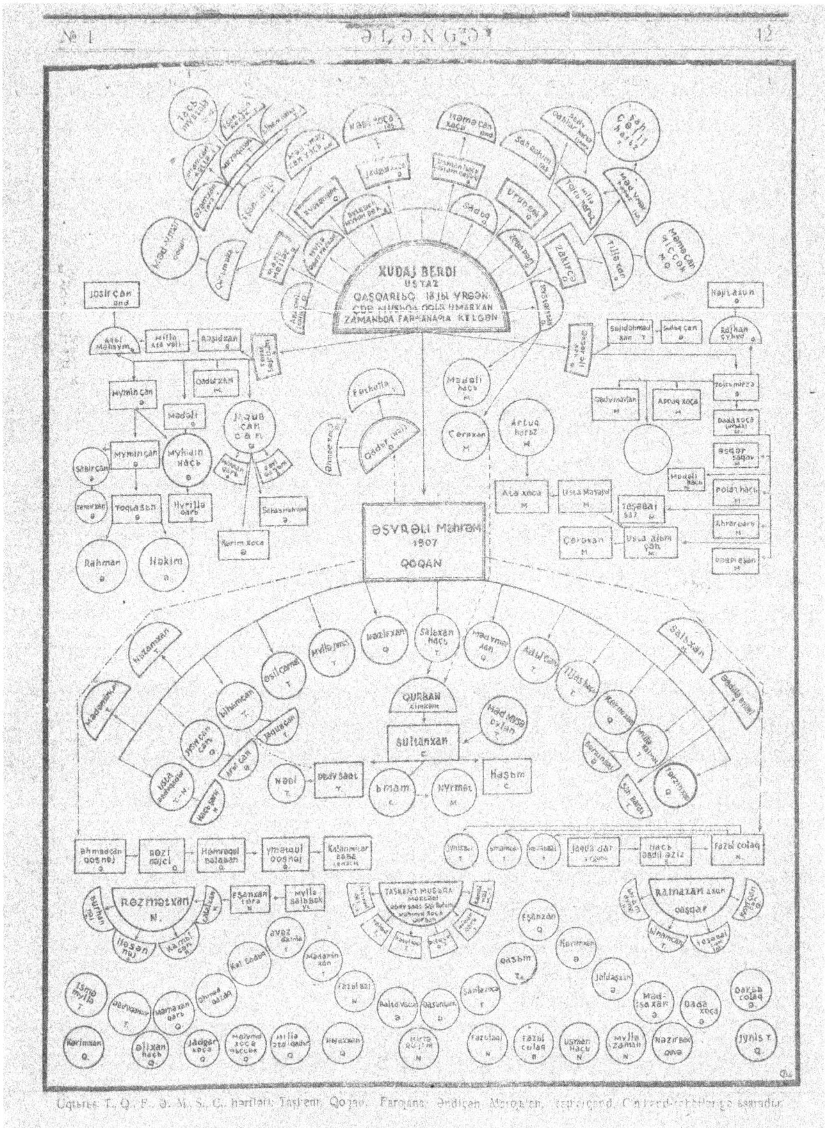

Figure 4.4 Diagram of musicians' networks in the cities of Kokand, Tashkent, Samarkand, Marg'ilon, Ferghana, and Shymkent, including Yunus Rajabiy and others and extending back to the eighteenth century, G'ulom Zafariy, *Alanga*, no. 1 (1930), 42.

performance technique, as in the case of the *nai* flute; or with respect to the physical form of the instrument, as in the case of most stringed instruments. Instruments that had been made for small, improvisatory ensembles in a teahouse or court needed to be updated for the concert hall and the mass festival. Master instrument makers began experimenting with new materials, construction techniques, and instrument types. They created instruments of different sizes to maximize resonance and to facilitate ensemble performance. For example, harmonized music could be played by three different sizes of the traditional Uzbek bowed instrument, the g'ijjak: a treble, tenor, and bass, corresponding roughly to a violin, viola, and bass.[102] To produce the large number of instruments required by the new mass ensembles, a factory opened in Tashkent.[103] Plans were made to open a large, all-Soviet factory in Chuvashia that could produce national instruments for all the republics, prioritizing affordability, volume, ease of use, and facility with western scales.[104] Musicologists like Beliaev even recommended repositioning the frets on fretted instruments like the *tanbur*, so their scales would align with so-called "universal" European scales.[105] In theory (although almost certainly never in practice), a reconstructed Soviet *tanbur* would be loud enough and tuned appropriately so it could play with any ensemble in Uzbekistan and even with an orchestra in Moscow. Other Central Asian instruments were naturally well-suited to socialist construction: Beliaev believed the massive Uzbek *surnai* "surpassed the European oboe and the English horn both in the volume of its sound and the uniqueness of its timbre." He even suggested incorporating the *surnai* into European orchestras.[106]

In addition to instruments, the Olympiad forced many leading figures to consider musical repertoire more seriously. Projects to produce a new repertoire had begun before the Olympiad but had yet to come to full fruition. An official report after the Olympiad lamented that the vast majority of Olympiad participants performed pieces from their respective classical traditions. The Uzbeks tended to perform the same four melodies, which, disappointingly for the organizers, included only one march, "Signal." The Russians performed pieces by composers like Tchaikovsky, Schubert, and Liszt—not even Beethoven the revolutionary.[107] One article even reported without comment that some Olympiad musicians had performed the Iroq *maqom*, precisely the one that Fitrat had denounced as conveying a mood too mournful for revolution.[108]

One of the few success stories at the Olympiad was "Signal," the only Soviet song to make the list of most-performed pieces. The composer, To'xtasin Jalilov, was a close collaborator of both Hamza and Qori-Yoqubov. Born in

Andijan to the family of a wagon-driver, Jalilov began his musical education as an apprentice to neighborhood musicians.[109] In Andijan in 1919, Jalilov joined Hamza in a series of popular performances consisting of a short satirical play and enlightening presentations from Hamza and his comrades. As part of these exhortations, Jalilov would perform selections from Hamza's "national songs."[110] Jalilov adopted a similar format when, beginning in 1919, he joined and eventually directed an "Agitational Wagon" that toured the countryside with popular performances and propaganda songs.

Ultimately, Jalilov became the progenitor of a cohort of musicians that composer Muxtor Ashrafiy somewhat patronizingly calls "melodists."[111] Neither professional musicologists nor formally trained composers, these singers produced their own versions of Soviet mass music. It was in this mode that he wrote his song "Signal," an instrumental recording of which appeared on the soundtrack to Dziga Vertov's 1934 film, *Three Songs of Lenin*.[112] In many ways, "Signal" is out of character for Uzbek folk music. Intended for choral performance, the song has been transcribed using a basic 4/4 time signature and a key of G major. The refrain comprises the crudest of agitational lyrics: "Cotton, cotton, cotton is the soul of factories / cotton is the pulsing blood of our time."[113] Formally, the song's rhythm reflects the "pulsing" heartbeat of the refrain: a driving melodic motif, repeated four times, is followed by a forcefully syncopated concluding line, bringing emphasis to key words in the song. The song's concluding line underscores the perceived link between musical meter and the rhythms of production: the factory machines "weave songs from their tempos, never stopping." Its lyrics weave continuity between the factory machines, the factory's workers, and the songs they sing together.

What could be more Soviet than a mass choral song about harvesting cotton? Yet the song's appeal likely derived in part from its proximity to pre-Soviet forms. In fact, the melody itself derived from "Mushkulot," a melody from the Shashmaqom—a derivation that goes unacknowledged in the description on the recording. Adopting a technique he had utilized elsewhere, Jalilov sped up the tempo of "Mushkulot" dramatically, rendering the melody all but unrecognizable to the uninitiated, but nevertheless familiar.[114] Furthermore, although a choral piece, the original arrangement is not harmonized: the 1935 recording comprises a mixed-gender choir performing entirely in unison.[115] Here was a song that both cultivated an insistent, regular rhythm and made space for "national" flavor. Jalilov and his fellow melodists' songs about cotton and collective farms pushed Hamza's argument—that a popular melody could carry any message—to its utmost extent.

The new repertoire circulated through popular live performances, as troupes appeared on stage in cities and traveled in brigades through the countryside, but it spread most widely in print notation and through recordings—both on records and on the radio. For these new mediums, it was essential that songs be standard and reproducible. While popular "folk" songs were based in fieldwork, they did not represent the unmediated voice of the "people." Before releasing folk songs back to the masses, cultural mediators arranged them for choral or orchestral performance rather than small ensembles and soloists. Songs that would once have been performed by a solo vocalist with a *doira* drum and a *tar* lute were now arranged for a choir and the piano; others were rewritten for newfound national "orchestras," comprising large numbers of musical instruments that would once have performed solo.

Making "Folk" Music Mass Music

To build the new, more lively repertoire, the culture and propaganda machine mobilized a sizable cohort of performers, folklorists, and composers to gather and arrange folk songs.[116] These works of folklore were just a few examples of the broader phenomenon of explicitly political folklore produced throughout the Soviet Union.[117] Such literary production has pejoratively been described as "fakelore" because, due to its Party content, standardized form and language, and sloganeering tone, it has been presumed to be inauthentic. Some works of "fakelore" have even been suspected of being fabrications by their purported "collectors."[118] More frequently, however, it appears that performers of folklore were encouraged to compose works on a given topic—say, the Five-Year Plan, or Lenin and Stalin. Then, with guidance from the "collector," these performers would compose a song expressing their (positive) dispositions toward the topic. The "collector" would transcribe the work and standardize its language before publication.

Given these circumstances, it is obviously pointless with respect to these texts to attempt to recover some kind of authentic "folk" voice speaking independently of state slogans and intelligentsia intervention.[119] Regardless of their authenticity, however, framing these texts as "folklore" means they can be interpreted as an official way to represent the "masses" and their experience of state policy. Rather than foregrounding ideological or theoretical terms, these works instead focused on everyday life as it was experienced in a Soviet context. The dispositions these works conveyed thus show what was becoming the expected norm for ordinary people's participation in the Soviet project.

To give one example of the process of "folklore" collection in Uzbekistan, in 1931 the Narkompros organized an expedition of four folklorists to gather songs from Ferghana: Uspenskii and musicologists Elena Romanovskaia, Xafiyaxon Muhamedova, and Ilyos Akbarov.[120] The collections of songs that emerged from the expedition were published under Romanovskaia's name, and Akbarov became a famous composer often through working with folkloric material. But Muhamedova, who would eventually marry Akbarov, has largely been erased in favor of her Russian research partner and her husband as a key contributor to the early development of Uzbek popular and "folk" music. Given her weak Uzbek language skills, Romanovskaia capitalized on Muhamedova's language ability and cultural affinity with her informants to gain access to woman musicians. Lacking a phonograph for this expedition, Romanovskaia transcribed all the songs by hand, often relying on Muhamedova to ask performers to repeat difficult lines over and over again. A later article by Muhamedova and Akbarov's son described the team's encounter with singer Lutfixonim Sarimsoqova in detail.[121] Residents of the Ferghana Valley town of Marg'ilon had recommended Lutfixonim to the team of musicologists. The team visited Lutfixonim in her house, and after Muhamedova introduced Romanovskaia as a Petersburg-educated lover of Uzbek culture who knew the Qur'an, they explained their mission to collect regional folklore. Muhamedova and Romanovskaia spoke of how difficult their work had been: even women recommended by their neighbors as talented singers would pretend they did not know how to sing, or defer to the "professionals." In the end, the team collected about two hundred songs from a range of informants, from professional singers to homemakers, factory workers and schoolgirls, and even a professional mourner.[122] Lutfixonim was not shy like many other women: a veteran of Hamza's performance troupe, at the time of Romanovskaia's expedition she was performing in a musical group based out of Marg'ilon. She immediately brought her *dutor* down from the wall as Romanovskaia and Muhamedova scrambled to take out their metronome and transcription paper. According to Akbarov, some of Uzbekistan's most famous "folk" songs emerged from this encounter between Romanovskaia, Muhamedova, and Lutfixonim.[123] As for Lutfixonim, she would soon become one of Uzbekistan's most beloved film actresses.

After the expedition returned, a brigade of musicologists from the Tashkent musical tekhnikum worked to harmonize the collected songs in a way that would make it possible for the pieces to "reach" listeners.[124] Marina Frolova-Walker has argued that harmonization was "nonnegotiable" in musical cultures throughout the Soviet Union, from Russian folk song to Azeri *mugam*.[125] Such may have been the official rhetoric, but in practice, a large proportion of the Uzbek popular songs of the 1930s were unharmonized or lightly harmonized. Romanovskaia describes how listeners resoundingly rejected the arrangements that the brigade presented for "public review" (*obshchestvennyi prosmotr*). "Ordinary European meters proved inappropriate; harmony overwhelms the listener, he loses the leading melodic line, and the large number of sounds shocks (*udivliaet*) him."[126] As a result, the musicologists' brigade had no choice but to come up with new, simplified arrangements. Romanovskaia stressed that among the song arrangements being produced at the time, audiences favored those produced by Uspenskii, who stressed the "rhythmic side" of the songs he arranged, as opposed to harmony. Although composers and arrangers never openly rejected the norm for harmonization, in practice, they minimized it. Ultimately, the 1931 expedition resulted in two new songbooks, both published in 1934.[127]

The 1934 songbooks were too little and too late for the Olympiad. In July 1934, drawing on their early lessons about the lack of repertoire and based on the results of the Olympiad, the Komsomol's Central Asian Bureau published a series of resolutions based on the results of the Olympiad. Along with improving musical education, the document called for new musical repertoires to be published.[128] The Writers' Union, in turn, laid out a plan for the second half of 1935, to publish a collection of folk (*narodnye*) songs in Uzbek, including both texts and melodies, under the direction of marginalized ex-Jadid Cho'lpon.[129]

More mass songs soon followed. Yunus Rajabiy (1897–1976), the son of a butcher from Tashkent and director of the Uzbek radio ensemble, was already becoming a leading figure in the effort to adapt Uzbek "folk" music for concert halls and choral circles. His 1930 song "Factory *Yalla*," transformed a traditional festive song genre from the Ferghana Valley, the *yalla*, for a decidedly Five-Year-Plan context, and "All of Us," an original composition, drew on his experience with oral performance tradition. Both songs were unharmonized, intended for amateur choirs unskilled with harmony; at the time, even Rajabiy himself was relatively inexperienced with the type of harmonization that top officials were beginning to demand.[130] Instead, Rajabiy boasted connections to renowned lineages of professional musicians from Transoxania, even appearing in Zafariy's diagram above, and unlike Qori-Yoqubov, he had received his training entirely in Central Asia. "All of Us" appeared on a record in 1935, performed by Rajabiy's radio ensemble. In the recording, a unison chorus alternates with solos from male and female vocalists. A driving percussion beat, a lively flute soloist, and an ensemble of stringed instruments accompany the singers. The song threads a needle between the official demands for choral singing and the clear popular precedent for solo or small ensemble vocals; while the choir is audible, the soloists, clearly quite skilled, lead the ensemble distinctly even during the chorus.

Tamara Khanum's most famous song of the 1930s, "My Scarf" (*Ro'molim*), exemplified the lightly edited "folk" songs that soon became essential to Soviet mass work in Uzbekistan.[131] Derived from a Khorezmian piece that emerged from a folklore expedition in the late 1920s, "My Scarf" followed a very simple structure; it comprised five quatrains, all with the rhyme scheme *aaab*; the last line of each stanza ends with the word *ro'mol*, "scarf." Compared to many mass songs of the era, the song is relatively lacking in ideological content. The lyrics of the song are simple: incrementally, the singer describes her scarf: where she got it, what it is made of, where she will wear it, how beautiful it is. Verses describe the "amulet" hanging from it; its silk fringes; its "half-moon decorations," and in the concluding stanza, the speaker regrets losing the scarf. Most lines are repeated twice. Only a single line about how the speaker's parents are poor offers the slightest hint of ideological content.

How, then, was the song grandfathered in to a Soviet repertoire, despite its lack of ideological content and its lightly Islamic imagery? A recording from 1935 gives a sense for how Tamara Khanum performed the piece.[132] Accompanied by a duo of accordion and *doira* (tambourine), Tamara Khanum performs the verses of the song with a distinctive panache: although the melody is repetitive, and each line is repeated twice, Tamara Khanum brings a lilt to key words; listening to the recording, one can imagine Tamara Khanum's coy dancing: how she might mime tying the scarf around her head or stroking its silk fringe. Some reports indicate that Tamara Khanum performed the song during the construction of the Ferghana Canal in 1939.[133] The Ferghana Canal was built nearly entirely with forced labor under punishing conditions. To perform a lively folk song like this one in such a context carried ideological weight, regardless of the lyrics.

Still, the Olympiad organizers specifically asked for songs with ideological content, and the new repertoire became increasingly overt. An instructive comparison to "My Scarf" is Muxtor Ashrafiy's arrangement of another song about a scarf, "On the Road to the Factory."[134] A choral song from the perspective of a female factory worker, the piece became, in Ashrafiy's own words, one of the most popular songs of the era.[135] Even today, many Uzbeks can hum the song on request, and in 2013, an opposition political group accused the authoritarian president's daughter, Gulnora Karimova, of rewriting the song as a propaganda piece of another kind.[136] The song is written from the perspective of a young woman who finds a red scarf while walking to work. "On the way to the factory I found a red scarf," begins the speaker, and a few verses later, corrects herself: "I didn't find it—I wove it with my own labor (*mehnat*)." The lyrics further drive home the by-then-cliché theme of the factory girl: "Uzbekistan's girls/ have come to the factories" (*fabrikaga joylandi*). As if to drive home the Sovietness of it all, the song is laden with borrowings from Russian: "Hydro water" (*hidro suv*) powers the factory's machines (*mashinalar*); the "first bell" (*pervoi gudok*) awakens the young woman for her factory shift.

And yet, although the vocabulary is so foreign and the agitational message so obvious, the song has exhibited remarkable staying power. Lyrically, this song represents a curious resonance between "folk" motifs and official ideology. Well before the Soviet period, women's folk songs told of young girls embroidering scarves and skullcaps, often in preparation for a lover. Here, performers adapt the motif for a Soviet moment: the speaker weaves in a factory rather than embroidering by hand, and the girl is preparing not for marriage, but for factory work. The song also taps into the broader "silk and velvet" discourse about Soviet women and luxury textiles. Comprising quatrains in *barmoq* meter, rhyming *abcb*, the song is punctuated by a largely meaningless refrain: "Gulyoraxon bo'ylaridin gulyor." While Ashrafiy would later add harmony to the arrangement, his very earliest transcription conveyed just the melody: a simple, lively tune in F major. Despite the heavy-handedness of the lyrics, the upbeat melody had genuine mass appeal. The song appeared in a song book in 1937 (Figure 4.5) and became a standard part of the official repertoire well into the post-Stalin years. Like the "silk and velvet" of collective farm speeches, this song of a factory girl's scarf set a tempo for Uzbek women and men's participation in the Soviet public.

"On the Road to the Factory," like most mass songs of the era, should be understood as the product of collaborative work by mediators on the ground in the Ferghana Valley. Well before Ashrafiy published his transcription, the song was being performed as part of Lutfixonim Sarimsoqova's repertoire in the Ferghana Valley, and she performed the song for Romanovskaia and Muhamedova when they undertook their expedition to the Ferghana Valley in 1931.[137] Neither a "folk" piece nor a work of "fakelore," it might better be understood as part of a grassroots repertoire developed in the 1920s by a cohort of performers with deep connections in the Ferghana Valley and its performance traditions. Even as they built careers within official Soviet institutions, their early bodies of work drew on their interactions with live audiences as they toured the countryside.

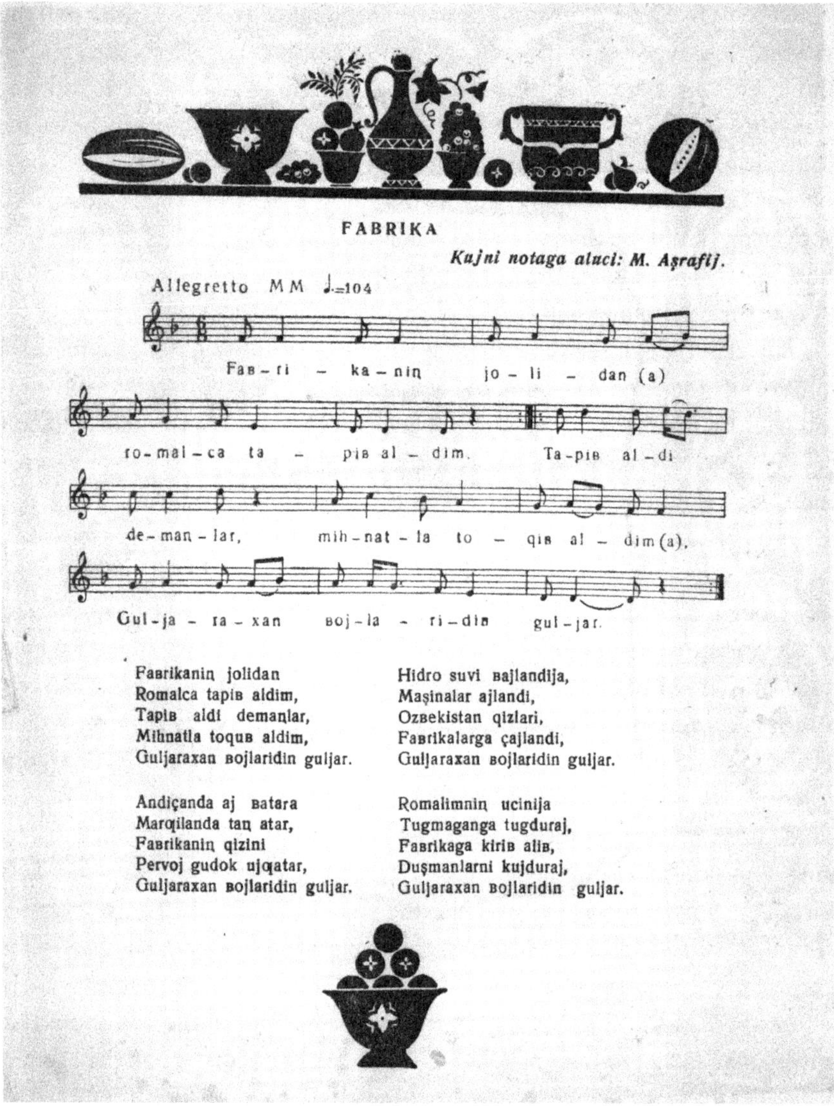
FABRIKA
Kujni notaga aluci: M. Aşrafij.
Allegretto MM ♩.=104
Faʙ-ri - ka-niꞑ jo - li - dan (a)
ro-mal-ca ta - piʙ al - dim. Ta-piʙ al-di
de-maꞑ-lar, mih-nat-la to - qiʙ al - dim(a).
Gul-ja - ra-xan ʙoj-la - ri-din gul-jar.
Faʙrikaniꞑ jolidan
Romalca tapiʙ aldim,
Tapiʙ aldi demaꞑlar,
Mihnatla toquʙ aldim,
Guljaraxan ʙojlaridin guljar.
Hidro suvi ʙajlandija,
Maşinalar ajlandi,
Ozʙekistan qizlari,
Faʙrikalarga çajlandi,
Guljaraxan ʙojlaridin guljar.
Andiçanda aj ʙatara
Marɋilanda taꞑ atar,
Faʙrikaniꞑ qizini
Pervoj gudok ujɋatar,
Guljaraxan ʙojlaridin guljar.
Romalimniꞑ ucinija
Tugmaganga tugduraj,
Faʙrikaga kiriʙ aliʙ,
Duşmanlarni kujduraj,
Guljaraxan ʙojlaridin guljar.

Figure 4.5 Muxtor Ashrafiy, "Fabrika" ("On the Road to the Factory") song music and lyrics, X. Rasulov and I. Akbarov, eds., *O'zbek Xalq Ashulalari* (Tashkent: O'zbekiston davlat nashriyoti, 1937).

The purpose of these popular songs was not to demonstrate Uzbekistan's modernity on a global or even an all-Soviet stage like the first national operas. Instead, these popular songs were intended more for internal performance within Uzbekistan than for exhibition on the illustrious dekada stages in Moscow or at festivals abroad.[138] Songs like "Signal" and "On the Way to the

Factory" were forged by performers who were trained in oral traditions often well before the Russian Revolution, some of whom cultivated their skills in mass enlightenment alongside Hamza. When those performers made common cause with the Bolsheviks, they brought their experiences to bear on building a repertoire that both appealed to regional audiences and set a Bolshevik tempo.

When the new "folk" songs set a Bolshevik tempo, they amplified some popular melodies, but drowned out other, older rhythms. The story of perhaps the most famous mass song of the interwar period, "Long Live the Soviets" ("Yasha, Sho'ro") interweaves the liturgical rhythms of Islamic collective prayer, the upbeat tempos of the Turkic nation, and the Soviet rhythms of production under Stalin. According to Soviet lore, Hamza composed "Long Live the Soviets" in 1918, an outpouring of his eager welcome for the coming of Bolshevik power.[139] The song supposedly appeared in *The Rose* (*Atir Gul*, 1919), one of the volumes of songs that Hamza published in the early years of Soviet rule, although that volume is no longer extant.[140]

Unlike "Signal" or "On the Road to the Factory," "Long Live the Soviets" lends itself to solo vocal virtuosity, and it became a kind of unofficial anthem for Soviet Uzbekistan already in the 1920s. Over the course of five verses, the song develops a stark contrast between the darkness of a pre-Soviet past and the revolutionary present. Successive verses amplify the contrast: the first two lines of the third stanza call on listeners first to meditate on their "slavery at the time of the tsar's rule" and then contrast it to their "joy that will never end."[141] The musical structure of each verse amplifies the message: in the first stanza, early, subdued lines about "blood shed" under past oppression give way to a soaring sixth to a high G on the word "enlightenment"—a whole step wider than the anthemic leap in the "Star-Spangled Banner." One can only imagine how stirring the melody might have been in Qori-Yoqubov's resonant baritone.

By all accounts, Qori-Yoqubov's performances made "Long Live the Soviets" famous, and conversely, those performances made Qori-Yoqubov's reputation as the "Uzbek Chaliapin."[142] One eyewitness of Qori-Yoqubov's early performances, Mannon Uyg'ur, described Qori-Yoqubov's "Long Live the Soviets" as the climax of his performances in Hamza's troupe: "the viewers stand and listen silently, with concentration, as if bowing."[143] For Qori-Yoqubov, the song came to mark his transition from the rhythms of Islamic worship to the socialist tempos of production. One of Qori-Yoqubov's collaborators, who hosted him during one of his visits to Moscow, describes how Qori-Yoqubov sang the song every morning when he awoke. When his host asked about the song, Qori-Yoqubov explained that as a boy training to be a Qur'an reciter, he had learned to perform the a'zan—the call to prayer—every morning. When he became a Soviet singer, he replaced the a'zan with "Long Live the Soviets," supplanting the routines of liturgical prayer with the rhythms of Soviet production. "I got used to pronouncing the words 'Long Live the Soviets' every morning instead of the *bismillah*."[144]

Such is the sacrilegious lore that accrued around Qori-Yoqubov and his signature song. And yet, all this lore obscures another, more complex story. As one of Hamza's earliest devotees, Qori-Yoqubov participated in his troupe not just as a supporter of the Bolsheviks, but also as an advocate for Hamza's project of national enlightenment—a project that predated and was superseded by the Soviet one. Indeed, one of Hamza's early collaborators claimed that Hamza wrote the song not as "Long Live the Soviets" ("Yasha Sho'ro"), but as "Long Live Turan" ("Yasha Turon"), referring not to the workers' councils but to the Turkic homeland.[145] At the time, Hamza was avidly churning out work in defense of a national project. For example, one song from the same year praises the Turkestan Autonomy, the short-lived independent government based in Kokand that the Bolsheviks soon overwhelmed. Condemning the tsar—a rapid about-face from his compositions earlier during the war—the song calls on all Muslims to unite in solidarity: "Unite Arabs, Turks—even India!"[146] If the song was indeed composed as early as 1918, the Turan variant is more plausible. Even the rhyme scheme works better with Turan: Soviet (*sho'ro*) rhymes poorly with "time" (*zamon*) and "world" (*jahon*) compared to Turan (*Turon*).

Is it possible that Hamza turned so quickly from Turan and the Kokand Autonomy to the Soviets and their government? Certainly, Hamza soon became an avid participant in early Soviet projects, but the posthumous martyrologies misrepresent the degree of his socialist orthodoxy. Hamza cooperated with the Bolsheviks because he saw them as the most likely ally for his project of national modernity—not necessarily because he began as a diehard supporter of the Soviets. By the time Qori-Yoqubov published the song in a collection from 1939, more than a decade after Hamza's death, the Soviet variant was long entrenched in performance practice, and the Hamza myth was already well established. Today, Uzbek musicologists agree that "Turon" was the original text of the song and suggest that Qori-Yoqubov was responsible for changing the official variant—even though Qori-Yoqubov may have personally preferred the Turan variant.[147]

The Soviet-era story of Qori-Yoqubov's trajectory as replacing religion with communist commitment is also likely oversimplified. In a later unpublished interview about their time in Paris, Tamara Khanum describes the two of them discovering a mosque when they heard the call to prayer during a walk around the city. Qori-Yoqubov entered and begin singing: he started with verses from the Qur'an, then sang, in turn, an Uzbek folk song and Hamza's "Oh, Workers!" He concluded this impromptu performance with "Long Live the Soviets."[148] Apocryphal as the story may be, it suggests that for Qori-Yoqubov and Tamara Khanum, at least in private and at least for a time, the transition from Qur'an reciter to Soviet Chaliapin was not substitutive but additive.

The story of "Long Live the Soviets / Long Live Turan," like the Paris mosque recitation, speaks to the alternative social imaginaries that Soviet publicity suppressed. By the end of the 1930s, Hamza and Fitrat were both dead, religion had been officially suppressed, and the Jadid vision for national music was all but gone. And yet, Soviet public culture suppressed these alternative visions not by completely eradicating them, but by swallowing them up—by mobilizing them on behalf of a refashioned way of social and cultural life.

Conclusion

When Zulfiya wrote her poem about the Bolshevik "tempo," she tapped into an all-Soviet propaganda language about tempos of production—a language that soon trickled down into all spheres of culture, from poetic meter to musical performance. Over the course of the 1920s and 1930s, Uzbekistan's cultural mediators worked to adapt these socialist tempos into the Uzbek "national forms" of music. In the stead of the "regressive" forms of the past, intermediaries developed a new repertoire of socialist songs for the Uzbek public: songs that carried ideological messages in their lyrics, to be sure, but that, more importantly, facilitated a socialist "mood." The folk song profoundly and permanently reshaped Uzbekistan's musical culture. While the opera dominated Tashkent's stages, I would argue that the popular song did more—it made a precedent for song as a political medium extending beyond the center, bringing regional face-to-face communities together around imagined publics. Music facilitated a kind of public participation focused not on rational-critical engagement but on affective engagement and mass mobilization. In this respect, ideology mattered little: what mattered, instead, was that the "masses" learn to step in time.

Socialism Mediated: The Making of Soviet Culture in Central Asia. Claire Roosien, Oxford University Press.
 DOI: 10.1093/9780198971153.003.0006

5

Silks and Velvets

Introduction

In late December 1935, the Soviet Writers' Union sponsored a "comradely meeting" between Soviet writers and shock-working cotton farmers from Uzbekistan. Speaking in front of luminaries of Soviet culture and politics, shock worker Tojixon To'rayeva emphasized her poverty prior to collectivization: "I could not even dream of having five meters of new fabric. I always wore the remnants and castoffs of my masters' clothes." "How is my life different now?" she asked rhetorically, and then answered immediately, "I dress in silk and velvet. Before I never had enough, but now I have plenty."[1] For Qahhor's antihero Saidiy, the luxury textiles in bourgeois interiors seduced into counterrevolution, but for To'rayeva, they attracted her to socialist construction. At another speech before assembled dignitaries during the same visit to Moscow, To'rayeva repeated her reference to clothing. After detailing the most tragic elements of her childhood, including the loss of her mother and several siblings to hunger, To'rayeva effused about how happy she was now to be a Komsomol member and a Stakhanovite. Now, in contrast to her dark past, she had a local power station, plenty of grain, and "many clothes" (*kiyim-kechagim ko'p*). All this, because the Party and Soviet power had freed her from "slavery" and given her a new life.[2]

To'rayeva earned her renown through feats of cotton production. Indeed, during the same visit to Moscow, she announced that she had managed to pick 150 kilograms of cotton per day in the previous season and stated her intention to raise that quota to 180 in the upcoming year. It may seem strange, then, that To'rayeva conveyed her attachment to the Party in terms of silk and velvet instead of cotton. According to the Party agenda for cotton autarky, cotton production was the main way for Central Asian women to perform their civic duty; the Party "emancipated" women so they could then be mobilized as *producers* on collective farms. But for To'rayeva, the Uzbek women in her audience, and the many other Uzbek women who effused about "silk and velvet" during the cruel 1930s, the rhetoric of luxury textiles complicated the discourse of hyper-production: it foregrounded sensuous consumption as a form of public participation for themselves and others like them.

In this chapter, I propose that we read the luxury textiles in To'rayeva's speech as a critical component in cultivating a sense of Soviet publicity in Central Asia. I argue that luxury textiles served to integrate some Uzbek women in the Soviet public because they elicited potent affective resonances, beyond the discursive, that often had very little to do with cottonization and collectivization.[3] The speech represents a clear image both of a relatable positive hero (To'rayeva) and of an intensely tactile "reality in its revolutionary development"—as smooth as silk, as soft as velvet. As such, luxury textiles comprised a key component in the discourse of Socialist Realism in Central Asia, offering a compelling vision of reality as it was ostensibly *coming to be* rather than reality *as it was*. By creating a tactile imaginary of "reality in its revolutionary development," textile reward revealed the unpredictable resonances of Soviet propaganda in Central Asia—resonances that the original architects of the textile reward may not have anticipated.

This chapter comprises four main parts. It begins by laying out a contrast between what I term a "Hujum aesthetic" and the aesthetic of Socialist Realism, making a case for a significant change in official culture between the 1920s and 1930s that tracks with all-Soviet developments while also exemplifying Central Asia's distinctiveness. Then, it parses the many cultural meanings attributed to textiles in Central Asia, concluding with an analysis of the Soviet unveiling campaign, or Hujum, as a complex social, discursive, and material phenomenon. Drawing on the 1930s press and the archives of the Central Asian Bureau, the ephemeral Machine-Tractor Station Political Divisions, and Uzbekistan's Narkompros, this section shows how clothing became freighted with new political resonances in the context of the Hujum and its aftermath. The third part examines how in the early 1930s, Party activists used textiles to mobilize women to participate in Soviet projects, from unveiling to collectivization. I demonstrate that the use of luxury textiles in official Soviet discourse was overdetermined by Orientalist and Ornamentalist tropes, Stakhanovite propaganda, the local gift economy around textiles and clothing, and the material conditions of women's lives in 1930s Uzbekistan.[4] Finally, I examine several examples of "textile-texts," a series of poems thematizing luxury textiles, all written by women, and published primarily in the women's press. A close reading of these textile-texts reveals how luxury textiles functioned as potent affective nodes for Uzbek women, both situating the state as a patriarchal provider and linking Central Asian women to an imagined socialist public of Soviet working women.[5]

This analysis reveals core tensions in the Soviet project of mass publicity and socialist transformation in Central Asia. Soviet policies asserted central Party control over Central Asia, rendering it a cotton monoculture against the protestations of local stakeholders; on the other, at the same time creating a space in which some Central Asian women represented themselves as equal participants in an all-Soviet public. These women comprised a new elite, embodying the privileges that a small segment of women enjoyed if they cooperated with collectivization and cottonization. In a moment when those policies demanded all hands on deck, silk and velvet conjured potent resonances that Moscow propagandists may not have anticipated. Consequently, although cottonization was the order of the day, not cotton, but silk and velvet became markers of Central Asian femininity. Attention to the discourse of silk and velvet, therefore, makes visible the latent potentialities in Soviet publicity, possibilities that remained unfulfilled in the context of Stalin-era authoritarianism.

Dress was a component in state publicity in many parts of the world, but it played a distinctive role in Soviet Central Asia. It has long been observed that the sartorial reforms that took place throughout the Middle East and Central Asia in the interwar period went far beyond unveiling. In Central Asia, as in Turkey and Iran, unveiling carried with it a raft of expectations about women's political participation. Removing the veil begged the question of how women would then dress, and the way that their "modern" dress would enable them to engage in modern society in new ways. In many Turkish regions, official decrees banned the wearing of the face- and body veil (*peçe* and *çarşaf*) that had become customary by the end of the nineteenth century, replacing them with a *manto*, or overcoat, and a headscarf (*eşarp*)—or with no scarf at all. In addition to eliminating the face veil—now coded as a sign of backwardness—Turkish nationalists also strove to suppress markers of "non-national" identity—anything perceived to be "ethnic, tribal, Islamic, or traditional."[6] In this context, identifiably Kurdish dress, for example, became intolerable, while "European" (*alafranga*) dress signified an unmarked national modernity.

The situation differed in Soviet Central Asia. While ambitious young activists sometimes turned to European-coded dress—tailored dresses, blazers, even men's *gimnasterkas*—the state did not promote such dress on a broad level. To the contrary: identifiably "national" dress, particularly for women, was critical to the pageantry of Soviet publicity, which both subsumed and superseded diversity. Luxury textiles in "national" designs encoded Central Asian women as modern participants in a Soviet public, but also marked their difference. Such garments thus straddled the uncomfortable tension between difference and universality in a way that other mediums struggled to do.

From the Hujum Aesthetic to the Aesthetic of Socialist Realism

The Hujum had profound effects not just on social life, but also on aesthetic culture in Central Asia. Based on a close analysis of the works published in *New Way* women's journal, in fact, we might argue that a "Hujum aesthetic" emerged, emphasizing women's emancipation as an ongoing struggle, and men as their abusers or valorous rescuers. Although the Hujum aesthetic holds out hope that Uzbek women will one day be free, it sits in a space of suspension, waiting on the Party to resolve ongoing injustice. As such, it is a fundamentally *negative* aesthetic, criticizing the vestiges of the past rather than imagining the future.

An agitational image that appeared in the October–November 1927 issue of *Yangi Yo'l* demonstrates several key features of the Hujum aesthetic (Figure 5.1). A woman with unveiled face stands triumphantly, holding aloft the Bolshevik banner. Under her feet she tramples a snakelike whip, the emblem of her oppression. From her wrists dangle the broken remains of the chains that once shackled her. Now emancipated by the power of the red banner of socialism, the woman stands as a solitary leader, showing the way to industrialization, as represented in the right portion of the image. In the background on the left, a mass of soon-to-be-unveiled women under a Bolshevik flag marches behind her. Although still veiled, these women too face toward their unveiled leader and will soon follow her lead.

While the image implies revolutionary change, it is strikingly preoccupied with the vestiges of the past. The women in the image reject the instruments of their oppression—the chains, the whip, the veil—and yet, those instruments of oppression occupy front and center in the image. Apart from the factories in the right background, the image fixates entirely on the process of unveiling, not what will come afterward. The image offers no concrete image of what unveiling is *for*; nor does it offer a compelling vision of what Central Asia's women are striving toward.

"Tuyg'un Oy," a story by Davron from the June 1927 issue of *Yangi Yo'l*, exhibits the Hujum aesthetic in narrative form.[7] The story begins with a childhood idyll: in an enclosed garden full of rustling trees and fragrant

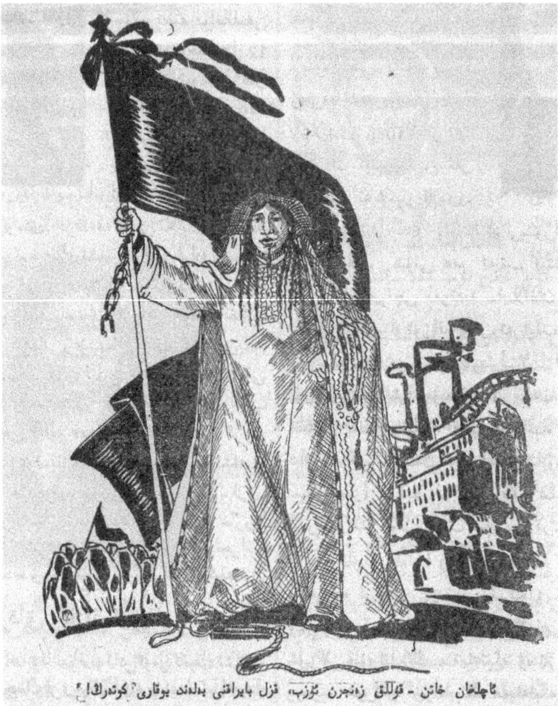
ئاچلغان خاتن - قزلق زەنجرن ئۈزب، قزل بایراقنی بەلەند یوقاری کوتدرك!

Figure 5.1 Editorial cartoon, "Unveiled women and girls, break your chains and raise the red banner high!" *Yangi Yo'l* no. 10–11 (1927), 27.

flowers, a group of young girls plays joyfully. The garden evokes the gardens of love characteristic of classical Persianate poetry, complete with "lovely-voiced nightingales." But a dark shadow follows fourteen-year-old Tuyg'un Oy when she enters the garden, dejected. The family of an old rich married man, Nurmat Boy, has come to ask for her hand in marriage. Tuyg'un Oy's friends attempt to cheer her up in vain, singing songs in their "lovely, thin voices," "playing, and jumping."

The opening scenes of the story emphasizes Tuyg'un Oy and her friends' infantile femininity. The girls sing songs in "lovely, thin" girlish voices, and they "play and jump" like children in the garden.[8] The song they sing underscores their girlish innocence:

> "One bloom among many flowers, I shall be bowed down," she said.
> "Innocence has left us, my beloved said he shall depart."
> Alas my friend, from her beloved sundered is she now!
> "Gone is my sweet way of life; I shall be sold," she said.[9]

Like many Hujum and later, Socialist Realist texts, this quatrain draws on an extended Persianate literary tradition in representing the woman as a flower.[10] The verse implies an anxiety about concealing the woman's face, which is "bowed down," turned away from the outsider's gaze—and from the gaze of the beloved. But the woman's hidden face is not the only discordant note here. The woman in this poem is betrothed to another against her will; she is to be "sold" to one she does not love. In these first months of Hujum, then, this poem reflects the ubiquitous association of veiling both with patriarchy and with capitalism. The veil is no mere piece of cloth; it is the oppressor's blinder and the girl-victim's shroud. In this respect, Tuyg'un Oy is one among a myriad of Hujum-era models for Shams's Nodira.

Despite her desperate pleas, Tuyg'un's parents agree to betrothe her to Nurmat. Tuyg'un racks her brain for a solution, but the only exit she can imagine is suicide. When the wedding day finally comes, Tuyg'un cannot answer the imam's thrice-repeated question: "Do you agree to marry Nurmat Boy, son of Toshmat Boy?" The imam asks again ("contrary to shari'ah," notes the narrator), and this time another woman from the audience answers "yes" in Tuyg'un's stead.[11] Unable even to speak for herself, the subaltern Tuyg'un is spoken for by others. Bursting into tears, Tuyg'un is ushered into a back room with her sister, Jo'raxon. Jo'raxon assists her in escaping the house, helping Tuyg'un to the banks of the stream where Tuyg'un has long contemplated drowning herself. But this time, there is another rescuer for Tuyg'un. A hitherto unmentioned young man, Hamdamjon, comes as a *deus ex machina* to release Tuyg'un from her oppressors, whisking her away to Tashkent on the horses he has standing ready. In Tashkent, the narrator tells us, the young couple studies for three years before returning to the village.

Almost everything in the story of Tuyg'un Oy is shrouded in darkness. Tuyg'un's entire village is situated in a "far, dark corner."[12] On the day of Tuyg'un's wedding, the darkness thickens. "As the day grew late and the world darkened, Tuyg'un's spirit darkened even more."[13] The bright garden that opens the story stands in stark contrast to this atmosphere of oppression. Indeed, when Tuyg'un escapes to her rescuer, she exits through the garden. The story thus indicates that Tuyg'un is capable of being rescued precisely because she remains so helpless and childlike. The garden of innocence is the young woman's entryway to Tashkent, the capital city and source of enlightenment.

Accompanying the representations of women in "Tuyg'un Oy" are their concomitant masculinities. The story implies that not all men are created equal. Tuyg'un Oy's father is hardly to blame for her forced marriage when he chose it out of economic necessity and at the behest of his wife. In contrast,

Nurmat Boy is utterly evil, not only making designs on a helpless young girl, but also ruining her parents when she runs away from him. The story of Tuyg'un Oy thus shows the Hujum's identification of gender with class. Tuyg'un Oy represents an economic underclass that is obliged, according to the song, to prostitute its daughters for survival. Tuyg'un's father is an underdeveloped, nameless character precisely because his situation is most fully expressed in the story of his daughter. The Hujum aesthetic thus feminizes poverty and masculinizes oppression. Tuyg'un Oy is the face of destitution; Nurmat Boy is the voice of capital.

The pseudo-chivalric character of Hamdamjon suggests, but does not enflesh an alternative masculinity. Despite Hamdamjon's importance to the plot, the majority of the story is still dominated by a negative aesthetic. Tuyg'un Oy and Hamdamjon return home only in the last paragraph; the rescue of Tuyg'un's family occurs in the single concluding sentence of the story. Readers get no detail about the young couple's time away from home other than that they were in Tashkent, studying. The story thus exhibits an uncertainty about what exactly Soviet socialism would look like. Instead, it recognizes that socialist power has a long way to go—it is, quite literally, distant from the story's setting—and the darkness of the past retains its hold over Uzbek women and men. "Tuyg'un Oy" draws on tropes about violent Uzbek masculinity and helpless Uzbek femininity, creating an opportunity for Soviet masculinity to assert itself as rescuer. But what is Uzbek socialism? Preoccupied with unveiling the past for what it is, the Hujum aesthetic is powerless to say. Into this gap steps Socialist Realism: the new aesthetic representing not the depredations of the past, but the hopes of the future.

An Oydin poem, "Tulips in Bloom," published in *New Way* just two years later, portrays a much different scene.[14] Now, instead of thematizing unveiling as an ongoing process, Oydin takes the women's unveiled faces as a given. Although the poem differs dramatically from Hujum poetry, unveiling—or, rather, the state of being unveiled—is still a major focus of Oydin's representation. In an almost untranslatable couplet, Oydin introduces the women as flowers: "The true faces of the tulips / Have broken into bloom today."[15] Drawing on the stock association of women's faces with flowers, in these lines Oydin moves fluidly between tulip as flower and tulip as woman's face. This association is furthered by a homonym: the Uzbek verb "ochilmoq," or "to be opened," applies both to the blooming of a flower and the unveiling of a woman. In this vein, the title of the poem might be translated, "Opened Tulips," or even "Tulips Unveiled." The verb tense, a past passive participle, emphasizes that the act of unveiling is complete. Instead of languishing in oppression while waiting for their rescuers, Oydin's women are active participants in socialist construction. Oydin emphasizes this in the slightly awkward phrase that I have translated as "true faces." The word Oydin uses here for "true," "amal," is likely a shortened form of the adjective "amaliy," meaning "real" or "true," but also "practical" or "applied," as in "applied science." Literally, then, this phrase could even be rendered as "active faces." The faces of Oydin's women are not merely decorative; they are faces at work. They use their newfound skills in "every office, every job" of socialist construction: "at factories, sovkhozes, and kolkhozes."[16] In March 1930, then, Oydin is already imagining the unveiling process as complete—even though significant numbers of Uzbek women still veiled at that time.

The contrast between Davron's story and Oydin's poem in the March 1930 issue of *Yangi Yo'l* are characteristic of a much broader transition that occurs in the magazine between the initiation of Hujum and the 1934 Writers' Congress declaration about Socialist Realism. Beginning in 1926, when the cultural and intellectual trends began to congeal that would lead to the Hujum declarations of March 1927, *New Way* changes in its representation of unveiling and unveiled Uzbek women. The emphasis shifts from the violent process of unveiling to the hard work of socialist construction, which is performed by unveiled women. Men change from violent oppressors and dashing rescuers to supportive older brothers and reliable sons. The distinction is not a strict binary, but rather a continuum, so the proportion of proto-Socialist Realist texts grows over time. However, the earliest significant change appears in about 1928, with the initiation of the first Five-Year Plan. Building over 1929 and culminating in 1930, Socialist Realist modes—production literature, stories focused on positive heroes—become ever-more common on the pages of *Yangi Yo'l*. Stories depicting patriarchal oppression still appear in the press, but they are often marked as describing an earlier time or set in foreign regions such as Iran or East Turkestan.[17]

This shift clearly corresponds to the expectations that would be associated with Socialist Realism: present a positive image of Uzbekistan "in its revolutionary development." Yet the practical implications of such an undertaking were in fact unclear, and produced at times puzzling results. A poem by Shukur Sa'dulla published in the Nov.–Dec. 1933 issue of *New Way* is one such self-contradictory expression of the emerging Socialist Realist mode. The title situates the (fictional) poem within a bigger prose genre of interviews with shock-workers and other heroes of production: "When I Am Asked, 'How Do You Pick 115–120 Kilograms of Cotton at the First Picking?' This Is How I Answer."[18] This two-page poem narrates a day in the life of an

Uzbek woman on a collective cotton farm. Waking with the dawn, the woman attends to the livestock and then her children in keeping with the principles of socialist everyday life. In four short lines, she wakes, washes, and dresses her children. She is fastidious about sanitation: she washes her face and hands before milking the cows, and makes sure her children are properly washed and their hair combed before delivering them to the collective farm's crèche. Then she heads off to the dew-covered cotton fields. The bulk of the poem portrays the woman's experience arriving at the cotton field and picking throughout the day. Finally, the day ends and the woman has her bundle of cotton weighed: "[It] / Comes out / To 115–120 kilograms!"[19]

The focus on hygiene, sanitation, and childcare is hardly unique to "When I Am Asked," but Sa'dulla uses cultured everyday life (*kul'tbyt*) as a mere backdrop for much stranger project to mobilize affect around the production process. Sa'dulla's poem traffics in sensory detail.[20] Walking to the cotton field, the woman sees moths taking off from the morning cotton. She describes the "dust and dirt"[21] that would settle on the cotton blossoms if not for protection from the morning dew, the cotton's "night watchman."[22] A white scarf bound around her waist serves as a vessel for collecting the cotton. The woman breathes deeply of the air at the cotton field, and wets her hands before picking the cotton bolls in order to keep them intact. If in Tuyg'un Oy's story socialism was both invisible and intangible in distant Tashkent, now the woman in Sa'dulla's poem experiences socialism and socialist labor with all her senses.

More strikingly still, the poem attaches an intense sense of embodiment to the process of production. When the woman picks cotton, she uses the same language to refer to her interaction with cotton plants as she had used with her children. Just as she combed her children's hair before taking them to the crèche, the woman "combs" the cotton plants' "hair"[23] to release the white bolls. Words using the root for "comb," *tara*, appear three times in the space of eleven lines, anthropomorphizing the cotton plant and underscoring the parallel with the woman's children. While the woman spent all of four lines describing how she cared for her children, she goes into great length about the cotton. "Coddling it / I make it laugh / And comb its hair!"[24] The woman cares for a cotton plant *as if for a child*, in fact, more lovingly than she cares for her own children.

The poem's coda amplifies the woman's maternal attachment to cotton. At the end of the day, she takes her pile of freshly picked cotton to be cleaned and weighed.

I press my cotton daughter
To my breast.
I lick her
Clean.
I wash my newborn
daughter, then
I dress
and swaddle her.
And in the evening
I have her weighed!
How much does
my daughter weigh?
I am a mother,
She knows me well.
Her weight
Comes out
To 115-120 kilos.[25]

With tongue, with breast, with embrace, the woman displaces the affective energies of birth and childcare onto the process of cotton production. Yet the poem produces an uncanny sense of excess: from the outrageous length of the title, to the monstrous size of the "baby," to the absurdity of a mother tenderly caressing a bundle of raw cotton, the poem straddles a tenuous line between socialist feeling and grotesque self-parody. The poem is markedly less convincing as an example of gendered ventriloquism: how convincing is it, really, for a Tashkent-based male poet to suggest that cotton-picking might mobilize the affect of mother-love? If Socialist Realism was supposed to bring the sensory to socialism, this poem runs the risk of doing precisely the reverse. Textile rewards and the textile-text offered something of a solution to this affective conundrum.

Unveiling as Getting Dressed

Soviet activists' use of textiles in 1930s Uzbekistan was rooted in the longer history of women's dress in Central Asia. Well before the Bolshevik revolution, women's dress in the region was subject both to economic pressures and changing social dynamics. Generally, at least in the Tashkent area, women's clothing consisted of a long tunic (*ko'ylak/ko'ynak*) over loose pantaloons (*ishton*), sometimes covered with a robe or jacket.[26] Women usually wore scarves on their heads. Color had social significance: bright colors such as red were reserved for young women, while older women wore more subdued colors such as gray and light blue.[27] The type of textiles women wore also reflected social status. Wealthier women could afford fine textiles, such as silk, semi-silk, velvet, and brocade. Women of lesser means were restricted to cheaper cotton garments, but those who could manage it tried to keep a silk dress for special occasions; the most popular silks came from Central Asia.[28] During the Russian imperial period, the most widespread textiles were cotton fabrics woven by local artisans, but in the late nineteenth century, factory-made chintz from Russia began to be sold at low prices in Turkestan. Under Soviet manufacturing practices, Russian-made textiles only became more dominant.[29]

Atop these items of clothing, many women wore veils or otherwise covered their faces and hair in public. By the early twentieth century, the most common form of veil, at least in cities, consisted of a face-veil made of horsehair (*chachvon*) worn underneath a head-veil (*paranji*).[30] Rural and lower-class women who could not afford a *paranji* and *chachvon* simply pulled their robes over their faces when in the presence of non-kin men.[31]

In prerevolutionary Central Asia, textiles and clothing were part of gift exchange practices in a variety of contexts. For example, ritualized exchanges of clothing or fabric were a key component of marriage engagements. Once an engagement was agreed upon, the family of the groom was expected to visit the bride's home with gifts, including food items and "various presents (depending on their wealth), such as galoshes, looking glasses, cotton or silk fabrics, etc."; the bride's family then returned gifts of similar value, such as "scarves, sashes, [and] robes." *Qalin*, the payment(s) made from the groom's family to that of the bride after the engagement, was often accompanied by gifts of clothing and textiles for the entire family, while the bride's family was expected to reciprocate in kind.[32] The wealthier the families, the finer the textiles. The most expensive and prestigious fabrics were, of course, silk and velvet.[33]

Robes made from luxury fabrics like silk brocade also comprised a long-standing feature of political ceremonial throughout the Persianate world, from Qajar and Safavid Iran to Mughal India. Central Asia was no exception.[34] Robes (*khil'at*) served as an expression of legitimization, deputization, or patronage. Accepting a robe from a political leader, Sufi *pir*, merchant, or *'alem* signified a willingness to serve them; granting a robe to a subordinate conferred the gift-giver's prestige, and bestowed legitimacy on the recipient as an authorized representative. Although there are some indications that robing rituals were receding in prominence elsewhere in the Islamic world by the end of the nineteenth century, they nonetheless remained salient as political imagery. In prerevolutionary Central Asia, then, gifts of luxury fabrics or clothing made from them could serve as markers of political legitimation and subordination, patronage, kinship, or economic attachment. The Soviet-era discourse of silk and velvet in Central Asia re-activated all of these resonances.[35]

For Central Asian women, clothing and textiles attained new significance in the context of the Hujum. In early Soviet Central Asia, veiling was more than a sartorial choice: it was a complex social, religious, and political phenomenon. Not all Central Asians practiced veiling, and not all those who practiced it did so in the same way. Generally, however, veiling represented a social order in which the sexes were strictly segregated, and "respectable" women covered their faces in the presence of non-kin men. Veiling thus enabled women to venture out in public when they would have otherwise been confined to their homes, but it also reinforced a social order in which women's behavior was tightly regulated by their male kin.[36] This system of women's seclusion had cultural associations with religiosity, although there was in fact a range of views about whether Islamic piety required veiling.[37] As the Bolsheviks undertook increasingly intensive campaigns against both Islam and veiling in the late 1920s, the two became more tightly linked: opposition to unveiling became imbricated with opposition to Russian/Soviet colonization, and that opposition was often expressed in Islamic terms. This came to a head in 1927, when the Party announced an outright "attack" (*Hujum*) on women's veiling and seclusion. Women who participated in this moment of social transformation tore off their veils and burned them in public. In this context, men who saw themselves as protectors of Islam, of local cultural identity, and of their female kin considered it their responsibility to oppose women's unveiling and their participation in the public sphere.[38] The chauvinism of some European activists, who saw veiling as evidence of the primordial backwardness of Central Asians, served only to exacerbate this dynamic.[39]

Yet in addition to these sociopolitical resonances, unveiling had real material consequences for Central Asian women and the men who were expected to provide for them. When women unveiled, the clothes that were normally concealed by a veil suddenly became visible. Now, women needed more clothes that would be presentable on the street on an everyday basis. This put unprecedented economic pressure on women and their families. Even if men were able to overcome their anxieties about unveiling as a threat to their religiosity, political views, or their masculine role as protectors, some still resisted unveiling because they feared they would not be able to afford the new clothing their unveiled female relatives would need.[40] For example, one secret police report noted the widespread complaint that unveiled women needed dresses, a coat, stockings, shoes, and underwear—a wardrobe that cost far more than many families could spare.[41] Veils were themselves expensive, so discarding or destroying one was hard to justify. Unveiling put pressure on Uzbek men in their patriarchal role not just as defenders of women's honor or protectors of the faith, but also as economic providers. Paradoxically, it made some women more dependent on their male kin to provide and maintain this newly expanded wardrobe.

Clothing and Politics in Central Asia

Textiles had long carried strong affective resonances in Central Asia. But in post-Hujum Uzbekistan, textiles—in particular the fabrics of which women's clothes were made—took on new significance for national identity, class ascription, and political allegiance. Throughout the 1920s and 1930s, rallying around Stalin's slogan "national in form, socialist in content," denizens of the new nations were expected to forge national cultural forms, including "national" costume. Some types of textiles—especially *atlas* silk—thus became attached to newfound categories of "Uzbekness," "Kyrgyzness," "Tajikness," and so forth. All-Soviet pageantry, such as the Moscow reception where To'rayeva delivered her speech, tapped into longstanding Orientalist associations between Asian women and opulent material culture, a web of associations that scholar Anne Anlin Cheng has theorized as "Ornamentalism."[42] In these contexts, Central Asian women frequently appeared in their national garb—the brightly colored silks and decorative patterns that were now markers of their nationality (Plate 8). As these Ornamentalist representations percolated down through the Soviet media and interacted with local cultural realities, they were appropriated by Central Asian women as a way to perform their nationality in public.[43] Although the texts I discuss in this chapter do not explicitly thematize nationality, they appear in publications in the new literary "Uzbek," and describe women's attachments through textiles to other women in cities throughout the newfound republic. They are thus among the first documents in which luxury textiles such as *atlas* silk become attached to the Uzbek nation, with women as its representative.

Textiles lent themselves to "national form," but in the context of Uzbekistan, they were particularly well-suited to "socialist content" in the form of cotton. Most Central Asian cotton left the region after minimal processing and was manufactured elsewhere, but the production of consumer textiles from cotton remained prominent in Uzbekistan's press. To Uzbek-speaking audiences, cotton was explicitly linked with textile production, and those textiles were represented as the birthright of all who participated in fulfilling the Five-Year Plans. In a speech he delivered alongside To'rayeva, whose speech opened this chapter, Akmal Ikromov, then First Secretary of the Central Committee of the Communist Party of Uzbekistan, insisted that Uzbekistan produce enough cotton for Uzbek women to own eight dresses each, and men to have half that number of shirts.[44] For Uzbekistan's workers, to a far greater degree than, say, for a Russian collective farmer, textiles were supposed to symbolize not only the prosperity that was supposedly now available, but also the congealment of their own labor power.[45] Cotton production, Ikromov and others insisted, would ultimately manifest in opportunities for Central Asians to engage in opulent consumption.

The use of silk textiles in Central Asian political discourse was particularly significant for women. In the prerevolutionary period, women had often participated in silk production, especially the cultivation of silkworms.[46] Beginning in the 1920s, however, the state began creating separate women-only silkmaking cooperatives and silk factories (Figure 5.2). Work in textile production was consequently less of a threat to women's social respectability than other forms of work. As a result, at a moment when Soviet activists were still struggling to get women out to work in the collective farm fields alongside men, women constituted a majority in textile and clothing production. A newspaper article from 1932, for example, reported that women comprised 64% of workers in silk production, 45.3% in weaving, and 77.7% in sewing factories.[47] This disproportionality was not seen as a problem: in fact, in 1935 the chair of the Uzbekistan Council of Trade Unions wrote to the Party Central Executive Committee of Uzbekistan recommending that the proportion of women in silk production be increased to 90%.[48] Agitation for increased participation in textile production was a priority in Party work among women throughout the early 1930s.[49] Accordingly, the press frequently reported on the successes of women's factories and workshops. Female textile workers were uniquely visible in the women's press, where articles, photo essays, short stories, and poems about them appeared throughout the decade.[50]

Women played an important role with respect to textiles not only as producers, but also as consumers. Given that the vast majority of Uzbek cotton

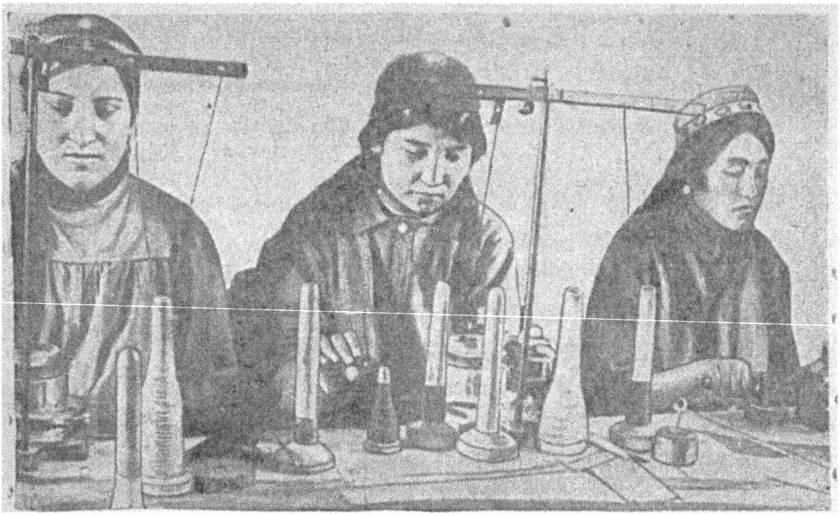

Figure 5.2 Uzbek silk workers, *Yangi Yo'l* no. 3–4 (1933), 27.

would never return to Central Asia for consumption, Ikramov's emphasis on consumer cotton was quite disingenuous. In contrast to cotton, however, luxury fabrics like silk were both produced and consumed closer to home. By the late nineteenth century, and continuing into the Soviet period, most ready-made cotton fabric came from mills in Russia.[51] According to Thomas Skallerup, Uzbekistan's silk production increased significantly during the 1920s, and most of that increase was oriented toward meeting local demand for "unique colorings." If the late 1920s are any indication, a much larger proportion of silk than cotton stayed in the local market: in 1926–27, silk fabric comprised 3.3% of Uzbekistan's total gross product in the crafts industry, and that silk was intended "exclusively for local consumption."[52] Sukhareva also indicates that the most common silk fabrics were produced locally: by the 1930s, the silks most widely used for shirts and dresses came in striped patterns from Ferghana.[53] This was particularly significant because, unlike in Russia, dressmaking was officially permitted in Uzbekistan.[54] As opposed to cotton, silk and velvet represented a fully Central Asian cycle of production and consumption.

Given unveiled women's material need, the outsize role of Central Asian women in textile production, and the symbolic value of textiles as a marker of nationality and gender, textiles proved an ideal tool for advancing the Soviet agenda in Central Asia. As Botakoz Kassymbekova notes with respect to Tajikistan, which was an autonomous republic within Uzbekistan until 1928, gifts of textiles were a recurring incentive for Central Asians in joining the

Bolshevik cause.[55] When the Hujum began, women were sometimes given clothing and footwear at unveiling demonstrations.[56] This trend continued with the First Five Year Plan, when the hyper-ambitious quotas for agricultural and industrial production gave rise to a system of incentives for top production. Soon, with the start of the shock worker movement in the late 1920s, and the subsequent Stakhanovite movement, the Party-state began promoting hyper-production in Uzbekistan through material rewards, including shoes, clothing, and bolts of raw fabric.[57] Propaganda situating the Party as material provider was, of course, ubiquitous throughout the Soviet Union. Tatiana Kondrat'eva has argued, for example, that Stalin-era political discourse and administrative practices tapped into longstanding expectations that political authority was rooted in the ability to feed one's subordinates.[58] E. A. Osokina identifies hierarchical systems for the allocation of resources as a key feature of the Stalin-era economy throughout the Soviet Union after 1928; these systems, she argues, privileged the top workers and other elite categories of the population, creating a highly unequal system of distribution.[59] The textile reward is thus one example in a broader system of resource allocation, but one that took on distinctive features in the cultural context of Central Asia.

In the early 1930s, the Uzbek press began to report frequently on prizes that women received for exemplary work.[60] In 1931, for example, an article in *Yangi Yo'l* reported that shock worker women from Mirzacho'l had been rewarded with galoshes, fabric, and scarves.[61] But the textile prize as a genre reached its apex in the mid-1930s, as the shock work and subsequent Stakhanovite movements came into their own. A January 1934 report in *Truth of the East* (*Pravda Vostoka*), for example, announced that exemplary collective farm brigades in Central Asia would be rewarded with prizes including wool suits (*kostiumy*), women's scarves, bolts of factory-made fabric (*manufaktura*), robes (*khalat*), and sewing machines.[62] In this case, both men and women were rewarded, but women received textiles and clothing most of all. For example, during the festivities around International Women's Day on March 8, 1934, collective farms throughout Central Asia awarded female shock workers with various textiles, clothing, and footwear, including satin and other fabrics, scarves, and galoshes.[63] A report from one Machine-Tractor Station described awarding shock worker women with "[sewing] machines, samovars, calico [*chit*], velvet [*baxmal*], scarves, and coats."[64] At the Hamza Theater during the 1930s, women could exchange their veils for silk scarves provided by the Women's Division of the Communist Party; the theater would then use the cast-off veils as costumes.[65] Regional authorities were often required to report the yardage of fabric and the numbers of articles of footwear and clothing that had been distributed. Because these awards were made in mass assemblies and then reported on in the press, they reached Uzbekistan's women twice: first, in the assemblies; and, second, in the mass media where they were pictured and discussed.

The architects of the textile reward in Central Asia and elsewhere in the Soviet Union may not have anticipated the local cultural resonances of the bolts of silk they distributed to top Stakhanovites. But as the textile rewards were distributed in Central Asia and represented in the mass media, they took on new, locally specific meanings. There is no unmediated source that would elucidate the extent to which "ordinary" Central Asian women sincerely believed the rhetoric about newfound prosperity. It is clear that most women did not own multiple dresses made of luxury fabrics; these were reserved for shock workers, Stakhanovites, and Party elites. We also know that many Uzbek women suffered from food shortages and even famine during the years of collectivization.[66] Nevertheless, even when individual experiences contradicted the media narrative about "silk and velvet" prosperity, the ubiquitous presence of that narrative shaped the way some women represented the imagined communities to which they belonged. Even though everyday life did not always correspond to the media narrative, women foregrounded the ways that their lives did correspond to that narrative in an effort to articulate a place for themselves in the Soviet public.

A 1934 collection of twelve (self-)nominations for a prize "for the best work in the spring sowing campaign and in the cultivation of cotton" of Central Asian MTS political division women's organizers serves to illustrate this point.[67] The nominations apparently reflect a prompt from the MTS political divisions requesting information on the woman's class background, the time and conditions under which she joined the collective farm, and the nature of her work on the collective farm.[68] The biographies are clearly highly mediated sources, conveying the self-representation of activist cadres, some of whom were even literate in Russian. They cannot be assumed to represent any private or disinterested beliefs. In the context of collectivization and the media blitz surrounding it, female Central Asian activists understood how they should describe their relationship to a broader community of collective farm women, and how textiles figured in the representation of that relationship.

Most of the biographies follow a predictable narrative arc, describing the poverty and privation the woman experienced prior to joining the collective farm, the hard work she has undertaken on behalf of cotton, and the ways her life has improved since collectivization.[69] A large proportion of the writers adduce evidence of a difficult background: several of the nominees lack parents or a father; others merely report that they harken from a "worker" or "poor" family.[70] One woman elaborates her background at length, telling a story straight from the Hujum playbook.[71] Her father was a wage worker, and her family lived "very poorly"; there was nothing to eat, and because she was an extra mouth to feed, her parents married her off at age sixteen to an older man who beat her and forced her to wear her *paranji* constantly, permitting her to unveil only when she lay down to sleep. After five years of marriage, the woman fled to her parents' home in 1927, the Hujum year. Until collectivization, the woman earned meager pay embroidering skullcaps. In 1930, she joined the local collective farm, becoming a Party member in 1931, and taking on responsibility as the director of the collective farm nursery.

Of the twelve nominations, half mention textiles explicitly. In each case, the biographies adduce the woman activist's clothing as evidence both of her dedicated work on behalf of the Party and of her newfound prosperity. The woman who once made a living embroidering skullcaps, for example, enumerates that she now owns three silk dresses, two silk scarves, three velvet robes, one silk robe, and not just one, but *two* sewing machines.[72] This woman goes into unusual detail, but she is not the only writer to specify that she owns several outfits of silk or velvet.[73] Another nominee is described as now owning "several festive outfits of clothing for her entire family," with the primary Central Asian festive textile being, of course, silk.[74] Writers favorably compare these new wardrobes to their previous poverty and report that they received some of the items as rewards for their dedicated labor. These phantasmagorias of consumption thus paradoxically reflect the women's feats of hyper-production in service of cotton autarky.

Given the widespread coverage of textile rewards in the mass media, obviously these women did not autonomously decide to speak of their "silk and velvet." Instead, drawing on what they had heard of and seen in the mass media and at mass institutions, they described their personal prosperity as part of a broader trend across their entire republic. After enumerating all the fine clothing she now owned, the former skullcap-embroiderer put it directly: "Our woman collective farmer (*nasha kolkhoznitsa*) of Uzbekistan has stepped onto a bright path and is building a new collective farm life."[75] This last flourish indicates how textiles functioned in a broader project to induce Uzbek women to understand themselves as belonging to an imagined community of women like themselves. By describing her own life trajectory, and then extrapolating it to "*our* woman collective farmer of Uzbekistan," the writer envisions herself one of a growing public of prosperous, cotton-growing, Soviet and Central Asian women.

The Stakhanovite's Silk Dress

As I have shown, luxury textiles appeared frequently in the women's press throughout the 1930s—often foregrounding women as textile-producers. In the late 1930s, however, a number of poems appeared that foregrounded women as consumers of luxury textiles. These poems comprise a rare source for the affective resonances of textile rewards among Central Asian women. For example, a poem published in the official Uzbek literary journal in June 1935, "My Silk Dress" by Nortoji Abdullayeva, expresses the combination of sensual enjoyment and labor congealment that made textiles a productive medium for women's participation in the 1930s Soviet public. In the opening three lines, the speaker conveys her subjective visual experience of the silk fabric.

> Its warp is blue, its woof is pink;
> It shimmers in the sunlight's rays.
> It shimmers out, beauty upon beauty.[76]

When the poem begins, one imagines the speaker walking alone outdoors, noticing how the sun shimmers on the fabric. The opening lines of the poem thus establish the speaker as a seeing *subject*. Before she is seen by others, she sees herself. The speaker's own subjectivity, her own sensuality, makes up the core of the poem.

Only after establishing her own subjectivity does the speaker turn to herself as an object, as one who is seen. She concludes in the first stanza's final line: "Whoever sees it [the dress] stops to look." In the Uzbek, the object of seeing is ambiguous—the line could more accurately be translated, "Whoever sees stops to look." The dress and the woman are one: when passersby see the woman, they see the dress, and vice versa. Later in the poem, the speaker re-emphasizes this feeling of being seen: even the birds flying above her "sing in praise." For the speaker, being seen adds to her pleasure in wearing the dress. This has a particular significance in the context of post-Hujum Uzbekistan. Every reader of the poem would be aware that, for many Uzbek women, stepping out unveiled in public was an exercise in being seen. The great anxiety for newly unveiled women was that they would be looked at invasively, indecently. As one woman who unveiled early in the Hujum put it, speaking in the 1990s with oral historian Marianne Kamp:

> In the mahalla [NB: neighborhood], I was the only one [who unveiled then]... I used to do this with a newspaper [she demonstrates walking with a newspaper in front of her face]. I didn't tell you about that. Everyone was staring at me. At the little bazaar I would get on the tram. There was a tea-seller there... They [the men at the teahouse] watched. There was one who stared really badly. He'd look at everyone and say, "Look at that!" They'd say, right in front of me, "Must be some Russian's wife, unveiled like that." So then, poor me, I walked with a newspaper.[77]

In drawing attention to the *dress* the unveiled woman wears, rather than the woman's face or body, Abdullayeva proposes one way a woman can be seen in public, even admired, while remaining respectable. For newly unveiled women, it was embarrassing, even violating to be stared at in the face. In contrast, being noticed for a beautiful dress was flattering, particularly since part of a dress would have been visible even under a *paranji* and *chachvon*. The dress's shimmering conveys this dual sense of being seen without being violated. The shimmering renders her at once visible and unseen. In reflecting sunlight, the dress also deflects the penetrating gaze—of men and other outsiders.[78]

The dress is a tactile pleasure as well as visual. When the woman walks, her dress swirls around her "softly." The tactile experience of wearing the silk dress sharply contrasts to the experience of wearing the veil, which propaganda represented as coarse, uncomfortable, and restrictive. If the oppressive past felt coarse and unpleasant, the new era was smooth and free. "When I wear my silk dress," the speaker continues, "My soul (*ko'ngil*) opens like a flower." In most Persianate poems the "flower" is the face of the beloved, gazed upon by their lover. Abdullayeva thus expands the trope, becoming a lover as well as a beloved, opening her heart as well as her face. In the poem's concluding couplet, Abdullayeva signs off as a sensuous subject: "My loving heart is bound to you / I honor you with great regard, oh my silk dress."

Abdullayeva's affective attachment to the dress is clearly rooted in her embodied and sensual experience of wearing it. And yet, that subjective experience does not disaggregate her as an individual, but inducts her into a collective. After all, the dress represents the skilled labor of her fellow women workers. In the second stanza, Abdullayeva notes specifically that the dress was made at a factory in Ferghana. Describing for a second time the colorful, shimmering fabric, Abdullayeva notes that the factory "has no blame in the art (*hunar*) of weaving." In speaking of "art" rather than labor (*mehnat*), Abdullayeva conveys the women's skill—for her, they represent no mere brute labor power, but self-fulfilled, creative, and productive subjects much like herself. Later, Abdullayeva says she "loves" the dress that has come from "her women friends' labors." When Abdullayeva concludes with a statement of her "love" for the beautiful silk dress, then, that love is caught up in her attachment to fellow female workers. Soviet reality, Abdullayeva suggests, is not only productive and just: it is pleasurable. In contrast to Party propaganda that represented Uzbek women as so many cotton-picking machines, and foregrounded the Five-Year Plan as a gift from Comrade Stalin, Abdullayeva offers a vision of socialism rooted in solidarity among workers and generative of embodied pleasure.[79]

One of the places where textiles appeared most prominently is in the "folklore" gathered by Writers' Union members and published in the periodical press. One representative work of folk/fakelore is the song "Tursunoy," published in the Uzbek women's magazine, then called *Bright Life*, in 1936.[80] It appeared alongside several short biographies of exemplary collective farm workers, including, on the previous page, a female collective farm director pictured wearing white. An explanatory caption identifies the text as "the song of a collective farm girl"; the author/composer is otherwise anonymous. It praises an Uzbek female Party activist named Tursunoy, and is comprised of seven quatrains with varying rhyme scheme and a memorable syllabic (*barmoq*) meter. This meter lends credence to the claim of the song's oral composition and oral performance. Indeed, a significant proportion of the audience for "Tursunoy" was likely illiterate women who had the song read or sung aloud to them. Most of the stanzas include enigmatic folkloric motifs, often making sense primarily because they generate a singsongy rhyme: the moon, a pipe, water, the earth, a stone. These motifs are then combined with descriptions of Tursunoy's admirable qualities, which the singer claims she has seen for herself. For example, several stanzas point out Tursunoy's leadership role in the singer's own community: "She is young, but that matters not:/ She is boss (*bosh*) to all of us." Tursunoy, we learn in the course of the song, is both educated and an avid Party activist.

It is no surprise, given Tursunoy's admirable qualities, that the singer describes her as being "like Tojixon," presumably referring to celebrity Stakhanovite Tojixon Shodieva.[81] But unlike Tojixon, whom we can assume to be accessible to the singer only through the mass media, Tursunoy is personally known to the singer. In one stanza, the singer reports that Tursunoy personally invites her to official functions: "Come, let's go to the meeting!" The penultimate stanza remarks that Tursunoy can hold her own even in front of men, including "Mahkamboy my brother" (*akam*).[82] Later, in pointing out Tursunoy's literacy and political awareness, the singer emphasizes Tursunoy's personal accessibility: "If you ask Tursunoy / She reads newspapers every day." Later, the singer underscores this again: "If you ask Tursunoy, / She is a Party member." Although the song is suffused with admiration for Tursunoy's boldness among men, her literacy, and her Party activism, Tursunoy remains accessible to the singer on a personal level.

The poem underscores Tursunoy's link to working girls like the singer using references to textiles: in the final stanza, the singer reports that "Tursunoy's dress / Is made of fine white silk (*oq shoyining tozasi*)." As in Abdullayeva's poem, the silk dress is beautiful. It adds to the description in the first stanza, which concludes that beauty like Tursunoy's can be found only "on the moon, not on earth." On a subtler level, the silk dress and the physical description of Tursunoy advance political attachments, not just personal dispositions. In Persianate poetry, the moon was a frequent poetic trope to describe a woman's face; the epithet "oychehra," or moon-faced, was and is used in Uzbek to describe a woman with a beautiful face.[83] Because of her Party activism and work among men and women, we can assume Tursunoy to be unveiled. The physical description thus reminds the reader that unveiling was a precondition for Tursunoy's other admirable traits. Similarly, Tursunoy's silk dress can be assumed to be a reward or payment for her dedicated socialist labor. The poem underscores Tursunoy's connection to other working women with a direct reference to women's participation in textile production: "Girls at the factory / Weave scarves every day." In wearing a silk dress, Tursunoy exhibits not just her beauty, but also her political rectitude and the affluence that comes along with it.

This point is important, because Tursunoy's other admirable features were not easy for the average collective farm girl to emulate. When the poem was published in 1936, literacy initiatives were just beginning to reach rural populations, particularly rural women. A collective farm girl might be able to look at pictures in the newspaper, to hear it read aloud, and perhaps to read the headlines occasionally—but to read it daily for herself was another matter altogether. Being a leader in public, particularly in a co-ed group, was daunting for some women who had unveiled only recently, and who had been taught to behave with modesty in mixed company. Tursunoy's silk dress thus serves as an attractive, intensely tactile gateway into imitation of Tursunoy's other qualities, and into Party loyalty more broadly.

Space does not permit a full examination of all references to textiles in the Uzbek press of the 1930s, but two more examples will help to confirm the point. Another "fakelore" poem, "Tojixon," also published in 1936 in *Bright Life*, begins with a quatrain in the same folkloric meter as "Tursunoy":

> Long live those who wove
> My dress of white silk.
> Long live Tojixon,
> Shock worker of women and girls.[84]

For the speaker in this song, as for Tursonoy and Abdullayeva, the silk dress again serves as an affective link to a collective of working girls and women, including both silk-makers and cotton workers like Tojixon. In still another poem, by the prominent woman poet Oydin whom I discussed in Chapter 2, a young activist woman named Adolatxon is described as wearing "a black elastic vest," a "satin dress," a "red wool scarf," and leather boots.[85] Adolatxon is the dedicated leader of a work brigade—so dedicated that she walks around from door to door at dawn each morning, awakening the women in her brigade. The fine fabric of Adolatxon's dress suggests that her hard work on behalf of socialism has paid off, while the modern vest and leather boots remind the reader that Adolatxon is no ordinary, rank-and-file worker: she is a modern, capable administrator.

The discourse about textiles as a marker of prosperity was thus more than a mere attempt to "buy out" needy or greedy women. Instead, the tactile and visual pleasures they produced generated political affect in two main ways. On the one hand, they placed the Party-state in the position that patriarchal family would once have held, situating the Party as benevolent provider and wise tutor.[86] Such representations of the Party as provider were particularly prominent in the all-Soviet press and on the front pages of flagship newspapers such as *Red Uzbekistan* and *Truth of the East*. This hierarchal, authoritarian political disposition stood in tension with another, lateral attachment: textiles communicated women's contribution to socialist construction, and linked them to other working women throughout Uzbekistan and in the Soviet Union more broadly. In other words, textile-texts both conveyed a spirit of lateral solidarity among Central Asian women and promoted their collective participation in top-down Party initiatives for the production of textiles and raw cotton.

Conclusion

Cotton was king in 1930s Uzbekistan. It filled the front pages of newspapers and turned former wheat fields white. Cotton blossoms appeared on teapots and tapestries, at parades and in poems. The entire collective farm calendar centered around an annual litany of sowing, irrigation, cultivation and harvest. In volume and value, cotton far exceeded the other products of Soviet Uzbekistan. Nevertheless, not cotton, but silk and velvet became the textiles of choice when Stakhanovites spoke of the rewards for their work (picking cotton) or when collective farmers composed poems about their new, "joyous" lives in the (cotton) fields.

In the 1930s, as the Hujum aesthetic gave way to an aesthetic of Socialist Realism, luxury textiles became part of a major multimedia effort, appearing in posters and poems, newspapers and journals. Through the material culture and mass-mediated representations of luxury textiles, all-Soviet discourses about productivity and the material prosperity of Stakhanovites resonated with longstanding political practices in Transoxania. For some activist Central Asian women, the rhetoric of silk and velvet represented a notional political and economic order that would benefit themselves and others like them—despite the reality that most Central Asian women did not have access to the luxury textiles or material provisions of their Stakhanovite comrades, nor did they have the political power to shape the conditions of production in Central Asia or the Soviet order more broadly. At the same time as they evoked rituals of political legitimation and situated the Party-state as a patriarchal provider, textile rewards conjured an imagined public of other Soviet Central Asian women. For some Central Asian women, textiles—and textile-texts—thus became a medium to make some elements of official discourse palatable, if not attractive. The discourse of "silk and velvet" created a space in which some women represented themselves as powerful during a moment of their collective disempowerment.

Socialism Mediated: The Making of Soviet Culture in Central Asia. Claire Roosien, Oxford University Press.
 DOI: 10.1093/9780198971153.003.0007

6
Celebrity

Tojixon: Person and Persona

Over the course of five chapters, we have traversed much ground. We first visited the Red Teahouse, where Central Asia's mediators staged a confrontation between "Red" and "Black" teahouse patrons and their practices of public life. From the teahouse we turned to the Writers' Union, where Uzbekistan's writers built their personas as representatives of the masses even as they formed a new elite. We have explored the diverse mediums that served to build, or at least to imagine a Soviet public in Central Asia: the Socialist Realist novel, the luxury textile, the lyric poem, the popular song. Each medium imagined and addressed an emergent Soviet public while at the same time revealing its inner tensions: between universality and difference, between participation and control, between vanguardism and mass mobilization. By engaging in the newfound system of Soviet publicity, Central Asia's mediators both made a space for themselves in the new revolutionary order and highlighted the inherent contradictions in that order.

Perhaps no one better exemplifies these tensions than the woman who introduced us to it all: Tojixon Shodieva. Tojixon brought all these mediums together. She worked in the press; she organized woman activists; she hobnobbed with writers and poets. She was a mediator, sometimes, but more frequently a *medium* in her own right. Her image bedecked Red Teahouses, and stories, poems, and popular songs told and retold her story. By returning to Tojixon, we can understand the real stakes of seeing socialist construction in Central Asia as a process of mediation.

Socialist exemplars like Tojixon are often understood as convenient vehicles for state propaganda messages: socialist labor, collectivization, women's "emancipation." I argue here that Socialist Realist celebrities like Tojixon might better be understood as sites of mediation. Tojixon Shodieva's persona evokes anxieties about the limits of state control and the extent of Soviet decolonization, emerging not as a vehicle for propaganda messaging but as an archive of the social contradictions that produced her. In this respect, she bears much greater similarity to the celebrities of other parts of the non-socialist world than has hitherto been acknowledged.

The shared dynamics of western celebrity and Soviet heroism can be attributed to a number of common features. First, the technologies of the modern mass media—the mass circulation newspaper, the radio and cinema, and the mass-distributed poster, to name a few—were common to systems of mass publicity worldwide, regardless of ideological context.[1] Scholars of celebrity in Europe and the USA have long linked celebrity to the rise of the mass media. Just as the rise of mass print culture and the cinema contributed to the advent of the celebrity in the liberal west, so it also facilitated the development of a kind of celebrity culture in the Soviet Union.[2] If these Soviet celebrities at first seem unrelated to the celebrities of the capitalist west, it is because they have usually been described in terms that distance them from it—as Stakhanovites, shock workers, propaganda figures, and so forth. Despite the widely recognized ideological differences between these mass media systems, they produced parallel celebrity cults with a shared genealogical relationship and some shared dynamics.

Perhaps the most definitive shared dynamic has to do with modern ideologies of political legitimation. Soviet and western celebrity cultures share a common intellectual genealogy in the Enlightenment ideas of popular sovereignty, which were common to both western liberalism and Soviet socialism. Fred Inglis argues that the earliest modern celebrities arose in Europe during the latter half of the eighteenth century, corresponding to a shift from old-order monarchies to the "rise of urban democracy."[3] As the locus of sovereignty shifted from *ancien regime* nobility to the ordinary citizen, Inglis suggests, celebrities appropriated some of the charisma that once surrounded pre-modern aristocracies. The celebrity, in other words, represented the common man who now legitimized the modern state. As Chris Rojek puts it, "Paradoxically, the move to eliminate privilege unintentionally laid the foundations for the emergence of new forms of distinction. Celebrity culture [is the direct descendant] of the revolt against tyranny."[4] Celebrity culture, in other words, arose from a new notion of sovereignty rooted in the *mass public* rather than the nobility.

Likewise, the Soviet cults of the shock worker, the Stakhanovite, the war hero, and so forth owe their existence to Soviet revolutionary ideology, rooted in the notion of popular sovereignty, and dependent on ideological claims about the bourgeoisie as usurpers of the working masses' legitimate right to self-rule. A Soviet hero thus represented the legitimate and legitimizing public—first and foremost the sovereign proletariat, but also, in Central Asia, the national public and the community of women. As an Uzbek Soviet woman, Tojixon thus triply articulated the ideology of popular sovereignty along lines of nation, gender, and class. In a moment when anti-colonial revolt was a recent memory in Central Asia, Tojixon had great significance as a legitimizing figure.[5]

To be sure, many features of Soviet celebrity culture should be distinguished from modes of celebrity in the liberal west. Most significantly, the Soviet culture industry functioned according to the dictates of the Party-state, not the market. The primary object of Shodieva's persona was to promote mass mobilization among Central Asian women on behalf of the Party-state.[6] In this respect, Shodieva's celebrity might also be effectively compared to mass-media representations of exemplary women in other nonliberal and nonwestern contexts. Interwar Turkey, for example, saw a rise in the mass circulation press and an increase in representations of women in the press. The mass circulation newspaper *Cumhuriyet* sponsored beauty contests that promoted women as a new kind of public figures. The beauty queens' public personas at once reflected the state-led efforts to modernize Turkish womanhood and also promoted a place for women as autonomous subjects in the public sphere.[7] In interwar Iran, likewise, feminist activists published biographies of exemplary women throughout history, marshaling them as evidence that women were entitled to education and endowed with political rights. Beginning in the late 1920s, under the authoritarian Pahlavi regime, representations of exemplary women were mobilized to demonstrate the largesse of Pahlavi monarch Reza Shah while also staking a claim for women's participation in the public sphere.[8] In Egypt, biographies of exemplary women began to circulate in the late nineteenth century and reached a fever pitch by the interwar period, contributing both to the formation of new national movements and to the remaking of gender roles.[9] In interwar Egypt, women celebrities contributed to an oppositional counterpublic; such is the case of Safiyya Zaghlul, who carefully curated a media persona as "Mother of the Egyptians" during the struggle against British colonial rule, even as her husband and leader of the nationalist movement Sa'd Zaghlul faced repression and imprisonment.[10] In each case, representations of exemplary women in the mass media—a new culture of mass-mediated "celebrities"—served to mobilize women as participants in the public sphere, while also integrating them in efforts for nation-building and state-led modernization. The Soviet project for celebrity-making in Central Asia exemplified a parallel tension between authoritarian modernization and women's self-determination.

To compare is not to identify: I am not arguing that Soviet celebrity culture was identical to Hollywood celebrity culture or those of Turkey, Egypt, or Iran. Still, the technologies and practices of mass mediation and the shared ideologies of popular sovereignty created a number of common dynamics in celebrity cultures worldwide. Among these is one of the central paradoxes of modern celebrity: the dialectic between immediacy and distance.[11] Like celebrities elsewhere, Socialist Realist heroes represented the possibilities now available to the "common man," but also exemplified a new form of distinction—distinction that was really only possible for a select few. The celebrity, after all, is famous because she is somehow exceptional: talented, beautiful, rich, notorious, or, in the case of Tojixon, powerful and productive. At the same time, she can only truly be popular if she in some way represents the people—if she can be understood to be "one of us." Hence the prominence of the "girl next door" celebrity: the sense of immediacy amplifies her celebrity status, rather than mitigating it. The visual technologies of mass mediation further the sense of immediacy: close-up shots in magazines and on screen, or detailed coverage emphasizing the celebrity's everyday life and affinity with "ordinary" people.

The Soviet context only amplified these dynamics. As a model for mobilization, Tojixon needed to represent her public: cultural directives were quite clear that Central Asian women needed to be able to see themselves in her and follow her example in the cotton fields. Yet the very qualities that made her exemplary also rendered her inaccessible. The mediated representations of Tojixon reveal anxieties about whether that mobilizational project was in fact feasible, or whether Tojixon would always remain an unattainable vision to her Central Asian public. Furthermore, examining Shodieva's celebrity offers insights into the racial dynamics of representation in the early Soviet context. In the works of Central Asian mediators, Shodieva's racialized physiognomy made her a *model* for her Central Asian public, but for the broader European and all-Soviet audience, the dynamics of racialization made her the object of oversight rather than an object for imitation.

As mediated as it was, Shodieva's life story must be understood as myth as much as biography. Still, the basic contours of Shodieva's biography are generally reliable.[12] Born in Ferghana to a large, poor family in 1905, Shodieva was married to a much older man as a girl, possibly as young as twelve. Her husband was an early Communist Party member, and she moved with him to Tashkent, where she unveiled and attended a Party-sponsored school; at some point during these years, she divorced her husband, who physically abused her[13]. The earliest published biography of Shodieva indicates that, like Oydin, she was educated at home as a girl.[14] Shodieva became a Communist Party member in 1925, at a time when female Party members in Uzbekistan numbered in the mere hundreds, and she soon became a member of its Central Committee. In the late 1920s, Tojixon Shodieva worked for the

Women's Division in Kokand and Xorezm, joining the committee that organized the Hujum in 1927, and serving as an editor for *New Way*, the Uzbek women's journal.[15] She quickly became well known as a powerful orator. In 1928, for example, she delivered an impassioned speech at the 3rd Komsomol Convention of Uzbekistan, in which she argued that the Komsomol had neglected its duty to eliminate bride-price (*kalym*) and polygamy, and that women and girls remained marginalized in the educational system. Shodieva specifically pointed out that the vast majority of Uzbek students who had been sent to Moscow were men, a proportion she would help to shift when she traveled to study at the Communist University for the Toilers of the East in Moscow in the early 1930s.[16]

Shodieva was a vocal advocate for women's inclusion, but also chafed against a system that forced her into gendered roles when she envisioned herself as an activist on a broader stage. Some sources indicate she specifically asked to be removed from her duties in "women's work," which had dominated her career during the 1920s.[17] From the early 1930s until her death, Shodieva appears to have avoided the women-focused occupations that had dominated her early years. In 1933, Shodieva became the Director of the Ferghana Machine-Tractor Station Political Division, which was responsible for agitation and propaganda at collective farms in the region.[18] She became a ferocious defender of collectivization; one magazine article proudly indicated that she was personally responsible for the purging of 563 kulaks from Ferghana Valley Collective Farms.[19] But soon, like so many Soviet activists, she turned quickly from a perpetrator of state-sponsored violence into its victim. Shodieva's close political ally, Akmal Ikromov, the First Secretary of the Communist Party of Uzbekistan, was purged in 1937, and Shodieva fell with him.[20] Unlike most of her male counterparts, who were sentenced to death, Shodieva was sent for hard labor in the camp at Magadan and remained there until her rehabilitation and release in 1956. She then became the chair of a state farm in the Ferghana Valley, where in 1981 she died. The state farm she ran was posthumously named after her, and Shodieva died as the bearer of many other honors, including the Order of Lenin, the Order of the October Revolution, and the Order of the Red Banner.

Tojixon the Star

Shodieva's life story circulated widely through a variety of media in Uzbek, Russian, and many other languages. But few representations of Shodieva's life express the visual dynamics of her persona as evocatively as an Uzbek-language poem by one B. Aziziy, published in 1935 in illustrated journal *Guliston* (The *Flower Garden*). By the time Aziziy's poem was published, Shodieva's name was so widely recognized that she required no introduction: the poem was titled, simply, "Tojixon."[21] The text reports the key components of Shodieva's mythos, drawing on well-established components of her biography: her childhood in poverty, her labor as a domestic and then a factory worker, her marriage-cum-"enslavement" to a much older man, and her "deliverance" through the revolution.[22] The poem exhibits Tojixon's life story not only as a tale of her emancipation, but also of her visual exposure. It thus sets the stage for understanding Shodieva's persona as the focal point for an emergent mass public in Uzbekistan. It also offers an example of the persistent tropes that surrounded Tojixon's persona, and the representation of Central Asian women in the discourse of Socialist Realism more broadly.

Aziziy structures the entire poem around an astronomical metaphor, relying on images of moonless night and the "sun" of revolution. In the opening lines of the poem, the image is literal, communicating the physical darkness of the mines where Shodieva's father worked: "Beneath the earth, a narrow street / Terrifying and pitch-dark" (ll. 1–2). But this physical darkness also serves as a metaphorical image for workers' lives in prerevolutionary Central Asia.

> For years and years, the sun and moon
> Illuminated earth's face.
> But they could not illuminate
> The workers' everyday (*turmush* [Rus. *byt*]).

Hidden away in the mine and shrouded by the darkness of oppression, Tojixon's father and his fellow workers are rendered invisible. Not only are they invisible, they are also unable to see: "Not a glint of light from sun or moon/ Can be seen here" (ll. 13–14).[23] The contrast between a dark past and a bright future is typical of the Hujum aesthetic. In Tojixon's case, however the blindness/invisibility trope conveys not only the evolutionist assumptions of Soviet enlightenment, but also the dynamics of public-formation around her newfound Socialist Realist celebrity persona. Tojixon becomes visible in order to be seen; she is cured of her metaphorical blindness in order to participate in the public.

If the blindness/invisibility trope appears first in the story of Tojixon's father, Aziziy's representation of Tojixon herself amplifies it greatly. Even before her veiling, Tojixon is invisible, living in near-complete isolation. She begins working as a young girl in the home of a wealthy man who keeps her hungry, giving her scraps of bread "in a corner." Soon, she finds work at a silk factory, where she is so bereft of friends that she makes herself a doll and calls it her "girlfriend," until her factory boss cruelly destroys it. Her isolation is made complete when a mullah tells her father to marry her off, forcing Tojixon to be "imprisoned in seclusion" (lit. "inside" [*ichkari*]). Because of their invisibility/ blindness, Tojixon and her father's only relationships are hierarchical: prerevolutionary darkness obstructs friendship, comradeship, and lateral family relations. Even Tojixon's mother and siblings barely figure in the story.

This blindness has real bodily consequences. Aziziy points out with reference to the mine, "Those who work ceaselessly here/ have sallow faces." In 1930s Uzbekistan, it would be impossible to miss the parallel between the faces of miners, turned sallow because of their invisibility as oppressed workers; and the faces of women, turned sallow through their invisibility as the subordinate sex. Hujum-era propaganda about the veil emphasized the supposedly detrimental health effects of veiling: the *paranji* and *chachvan* were supposed to inhibit physical activity and obstruct fresh air and sunshine, causing disease, premature aging, infertility, dangerous births, and weak offspring.[24] Unhealthy sallow (lit. "yellow," *sariq*) faces were a common trope in Hujum-era portrayals of veiled women. The parallelism is underscored through the image of the whip (*qamchin*), which the miners' boss uses to beat them, but also appeared as a common motif in representations of the violent husbands of veiled wives. The darkness that makes Tojixon and her father blind also physically disables them.

Into this dark isolation breaks the "sun of revolution," illuminating agricultural fields, mineshafts, and veiled women's domestic prisons alike.

> Not only did the workers' mineshaft
> Become light;
> The farmer's field
> Also became light.
> Every woman in four walls
> Was illuminated
> Uzbekistan's women and girls
> Moved toward the light.

Aziziy's reference to the "light" of revolution owes much to the linear narratives of progress and discourse of enlightenment that were ubiquitous in the Soviet 1930s.[25] "Enlightenment" entailed a whole host of "modern" behaviors in everyday life (*turmush*), from hygiene and sanitation, to education, to labor discipline. But for Aziziy, illumination also marks the installation of "Uzbekistan's women and girls" as a collective historical subject, moving as one, rather than as a group of isolated and individual victims.

The light of revolution also helps Tojixon to *see* the suffering of other Uzbek women:

> Tojixon once tasted
> the bitterness of captivity [*asiralik tuzini*];
> when she saw [others in] captivity,
> how could she close her eyes?

In Aziziy's representation, Tojixon was once both blind and invisible, capable only of tasting the bitterness of captivity. Now, able to see her oppressed sisters, Tojixon is initiated as the vanguard of a lateral public, a community of equals. Seeing the suffering of her fellow Uzbek women motivates Tojixon to a host of accomplishments in their behalf, and indeed, the remainder of the poem reads like a flowery resume: Tojixon joins the Komsomol and the Party; she gives a speech before the Central Committee; she is elected as a representative (*vakil*) to multiple official institutions; she heads up the Political Division; she wins a Lenin Prize.[26] Tojixon's restored vision empowers her to the feats of production and activism that made her famous, making her the first among "Uzbekistan's women and girls" in their march toward the light of revolution.

In restoring Tojixon's sight, then, the light of Revolution also confers *visibility* on Tojixon. Once "rescued" by the Revolution, Tojixon is no longer shrouded in darkness and isolation; she is permanently in the public eye. Indeed, Aziziy's poem appeared alongside a photographic close-up of the unveiled Tojixon, showing her in her usual costume of *gimnasterka* and cap, hair cropped short and gaze intense, with the Lenin prize affixed to her breast (Figure 6.1). The poem's concluding lines serve as a kind of ekphrasis on the photograph: "A Lenin prize / was fixed on her breast."

Tojixon's portrait suggests a certain tension between her individuation and her status as representative. The visual language of the close-up was loaded with ideological significance in early Soviet photography and cinema. Film theorist Béla Balázs, whose works were widely influential in the Soviet Union already in the 1920s, and who resided in Moscow from 1933, argued in 1930 that close-ups not only represent an individual; they also represent, as synecdoche, the collective to which their subject belongs. Two main categories

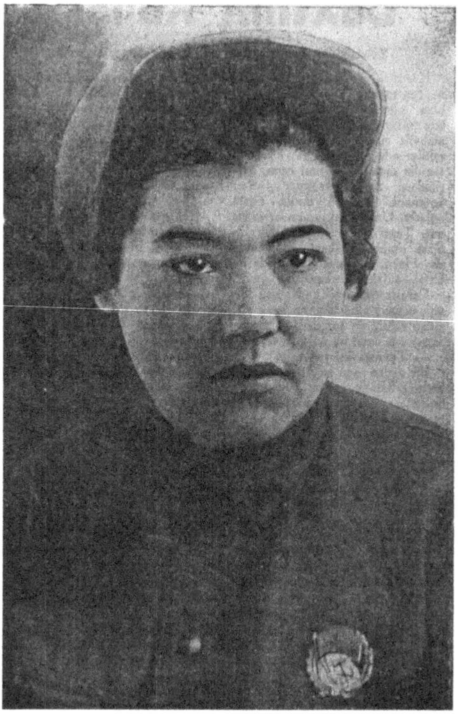

Figure 6.1 Portrait of Tojixon Shodieva published with Aziziy poem, *Guliston*, no. 3 (1935), 9, uncredited.

were of particular significance for Balázs. First, class: a close-up photograph, according to Balázs, could convey the "supra-individual face of different classes."[27] Montages of close-up shots, such as those in Eisenstein's *October* or Dovzhenko's *Arsenal*, offered a "physiognomical cross-section of social stratification." "The worker, the soldier, the ordinary craftsman, the small trader, the factory owner and the rich merchant... nothing but close-ups of all these faces, and yet we know precisely what they are." Physiognomy expressed social realities beyond language. And yet, for Balázs, class is not the primary physiognomic category. If the physiognomy of class came late, as "the great achievement of film," Balázs contended, "the supra-individual face of different races has always been known." Tojixon's physiognomy was burdened with representation: not only of her class, but also her race, and, insofar as race was gendered and gender racialized in the Central Asian context, her gender. Tojixon was Uzbek, she was proletarian, she was woman, and only then was she Tojixon Shodieva.

Despite the heavy burden of racial/national and gender representation, Tojixon appears to have asserted some degree of control over her self-presentation. Unlike most other Uzbek women Stakhanovites and shock-workers, Tojixon appeared in public not in luxury textiles or feminine dresses, but in the *gimnasterka* more characteristic of Politburo members than of Uzbek women's activists.[28] Originally a component of military dress, the *gimnasterka* became the uniform of Soviet power under Stalin. Written descriptions of Shodieva often remarked upon her cap and *gimnasterka* as unique features of her dress: features that projected (masculine) power and (European) distinction at the expense of her racialized and gendered representational role. Tojixon's face—not her costume, not her behavior—bore the full burden of her role as representative.

Shodieva's representational role was to stand in for an Uzbek proletarian public that included women as well as men. But in practice, just like her unusual sartorial choices, Shodieva's story calls into question just how much Shodieva resembles her public.[29] The first half of the poem's insistent linkage between Tojixon's plight and the broader plight of women and workers emphasizes her similarity to other Uzbek women. But as Tojixon becomes more exceptional—as she emerges into visibility—it becomes increasingly difficult to articulate how she resembles her public. Indeed, Aziziy suggests that the public itself demands a kind of substitution: "The public / expected great service of her" (*ko'p xizmat/kutar edi jamoat*). The public expects Tojixon to do in their stead what they are incapable of doing, to *serve* them.

Ultimately, of course, the propaganda utility of a Stakhanovite like Shodieva was to mobilize her public, if not to equivalent feats of production, then at least to some degree of socialist productivity. Indeed, Aziziy suggests that "many women and girls / bound their hearts to her." At the same time, the promise of mass mobilization around Tojixon has yet to materialize. This tension is articulated most clearly in the concluding stanza:

> Full of courage [*botir*], master of all she does,
> Tojixon is a shining star.
> The CC [Party Central Committee] has brought us
> Many hundreds [*necha yuz*] just like her.

On the one hand, the stanza's first two lines emphasize Tojixon as an exceptional hero. The word I have translated "full of courage," *botir*, evokes larger-than-life folkloric heroes—it can be translated "strongmen," with all the gendered and embodied implications of the term.[30] Tojixon is "a shining star," suggesting that she shines more brightly in the firmament than the other heavenly bodies around her.

Yet in the concluding line, Aziziy reverses this emphasis on Tojixon's exceptional status, suggesting that in fact, Shodieva merely represents "many hundreds just like her." The assertion that Tojixon stood in for a nascent new cadre of exemplary Central Asian women became something of a trope in the Uzbek-language press. For example, in a speech he delivered to the 1936 Komsomol Convention of Young Women (*qiz-juvonlar qurultoyi*), First Secretary of the Uzbek Communist Party Akmal Ikromov praised Shodieva for achieving her successes through great struggle (*kurash*). He insisted that if his audience showed the same energy and initiative as Shodieva, they would soon become "hundreds, thousands of Tojixons."[31] When the speech was published in the Komsomol newspaper *Young Leninist*, it appeared below a collage of photographs of young Uzbek activist women with the headline "Tojixon Shodievas Are Growing Up," as if the transformation was imminent. Like Aziziy, Ikromov suggested an inherent tension in Shodieva's public persona. Clearly Shodieva is a vanguard, a substitution for a still-inchoate public; on the other hand, she supposedly resembles her public, the "many hundreds" like herself who had yet to reach their purported potential.

Tojixon the Representative

A poem about Shodieva by Oydin vividly bears out the anxiety about whether it would ever be possible for Shodieva to resemble her public, and more importantly, for the public to resemble her. The poem, "My Congratulations to You!" appeared in June 1934 as part of a cluster of pieces on Shodieva in the official literary journal of the Soviet Writers Union of Uzbekistan.[32] If any cultural mediator were qualified to portray Tojixon in the Uzbek press, it was Oydin. As former co-editors of *New Way* along with several other women, Oydin and Shodieva belonged to a small circle of Uzbek activist women who joined the Soviet cause even before the Hujum. As a woman who had succeeded in a man's world at great personal cost, Oydin was particularly sensitive to the risks of being a woman and a public figure in early Soviet Uzbekistan. Oydin's "My Congratulations to You!" can thus be read as a personal address as well as a public document.

Yet in "My Congratulations," Oydin foregrounds not her own personal encounters with Shodieva, but the imagined public that would encounter Tojixon through the mass media. Indeed, the public is as much the subject of this poem as Tojixon herself: although the poem is dedicated "To Tojixon Shodieva," of its four parts, only two concern Tojixon directly. The other two sections comprise a frame narrative in first-person voice, written from the perspective of a young factory-working woman. As a whole, this frame narrative takes up a full third of the poem. Along with other "emancipated" women, the woman encounters the story of Tojixon's successes in a newspaper. By learning of Tojixon through the newspaper and seeing her portrait on its pages, Oydin suggests, the young speaker and the other women in Tojixon's public will be inspired to emulate her feats of socialist labor:

> If you work like she worked,
> You will receive a Lenin prize.
> You'll receive a hero's great name,
> Bring glory to the people.

On the surface level, then, the poem posits a strictly mimetic relationship between Tojixon and her public, much like Aziziy and Ikromov suggested. Uzbek women see Tojixon's iconic photograph; they are reminded of her deeds in the periodical press; they imitate her and achieve the same. But a closer reading of the poem reveals a greater disjuncture between Tojixon and her public than a literal reading would admit: the opening "if" bears a great deal of weight. In fact, Oydin's poem is suffused with anxiety that "ordinary" working women may never achieve the same heights of socialist productivity as Tojixon.

The poem opens with a lyrical springtime scene that threatens to distract the young speaker from her socialist duties. In the opening stanza, Oydin evokes the freshness and beauty of nature as the woman encounters it on her way to work:

> Spring has come! Tender (*mayin*) breezes
> Make the fresh new tendrils (*maysalar*) tremble
> Among the willow branches, a pair of mynas (*maynalar*)
> Have been twittering since dawn.

In the two playful and highly alliterative stanzas that follow, the babbling canal responds in kind to the birds' chatter, and the woman dreams of wandering through the springtime meadows, dotted with flowers. The lyrical prologue was well established in Persianate literary tradition from which Oydin came, but this is no traditional Persianate lyric. Nor is it a romantic lyric extolling the beauties of nature over and against industrial development. Ultimately, nature is a distraction: the beauties of springtime tempt the woman to delay, to stop and roam the lovely spring meadows, even at the expense of missing work. But in the end, the consciousness of her inner disciplined worker prevails. "No, I must go, my beauties," she responds to the birds and the canal and the meadows, "I must go quickly to my work." The obstacles to socialist participation come not only from within, but also from without: the woman usually takes a tram to work, but the tram fails to arrive. Forced to rush on foot the long distance to work, the woman says anxiously to herself, "I'm late."

The prologue thus sets up an implicit problem. Oydin's speaker is committed to socialist labor, she is unveiled and working outside her home, and yet a host of obstacles stand in the way of her participation in socialist construction. She lacks the proper sense of time-discipline; she constantly rushes to keep up with the tempo of socialist labor; and even when she tries, the infrastructure around her, still under construction, thwarts her efforts to keep time.[33]

It is at this moment of anxiety about catching up to socialist progress that the speaker encounters a new issue of the newspaper:

> Someone is looking at the newspaper
> Over there in rapt attention.
> Nodding her head, gnawing her lip,
> Saying, "Well done!" about one page.

That page, we learn, contains an announcement that Tojixon Shodieva has just been awarded a Lenin Prize. A few stanzas later, Oydin remarks that Tojixon earned her recognition by leading Ferghana to fulfill the plan just one year after it had produced cotton at a shamefully slow pace, a "city riding on a tortoise." Tojixon's exemplary achievements thus confront the speaker as a contrast: the speaker may be running late, but Tojixon is on time for socialism.

The poem devotes eight stanzas to this scene of encounter with the newspaper. On Oydin's part, the framing of Tojixon's story articulates a certain anxiety about how Uzbek women less educated and well-connected than herself might be integrated into the Soviet public. The speaker points out, for example, that some of Tojixon's admirers are likely to be illiterate: "One will take it [the newspaper], another will not / Another may not know how to read." Oydin consequently describes the encounter in terms that emphasizes their experience of the newspaper as not only a literary, but a multisensory and highly affective experience. When the narrator first encounters the newspaper, for example, she describes it as "shouting right beside" her (*yonginamda qichqirib*). Mixing metaphors, she then describes the newspaper in visual terms, as "strutting" (*javlon urar*) beside her. Finally, the women jostle for an opportunity to hold the newspaper themselves, suggesting a tactile experience: "Some of them shout, excited / Pass the newspaper!"[34]

Of these three senses, however, vision again dominates this scene. Oydin reports that Tojixon "blooms forth" from the newspaper page, indicating that the women are not only *reading* of Tojixon, but seeing a photograph of her. When the speaker asks another woman for the newspaper, her eager visual language emphasizes this point: "Let me *see* the one who's been awarded / Who's become a sincere Leninist!"[35] Again, Tojixon's portrait serves as an iconographic shorthand for her story, with which the speaker is already familiar:

> The boss [*nachalnik*] bloomed forth
> In the row of heroes.
> Your history came to my mind.
> Let's begin our tale right here.

Readers of the literary journal where "My Congratulations to You!" appeared had a clear point of reference for that story and that "blooming" image: the article immediately preceding Oydin's poem was a biographical essay about Shodieva, written by Valeriia Gerasimova. Accompanying that article, on the page immediately preceding Oydin's poem, appears a photographic close-up of Tojixon that closely matches the word-portrait Oydin offers shortly after: "Brow furrowed, eyes wide, / Her worker's cap is tilted up." The poem thus offers another ekphrastic moment, much like Aziziy's. Tojixon's photographic portrait—her icon—is both a potent reminder of her achievements and an exhortation to imitate her.

In his early writing on close-ups, Balázs stressed the affective power of the photographic close-up:

> Close ups are a kind of naturalism. They amount to the sharp observation of detail. However, such observation contains an element of tenderness, and I should like to call it the naturalism of love... In films with many good close-ups you often gain the impression that these shots are the product not so much of a good eye as of a good heart.[36]

For Oydin and her lyric persona, Tojixon's photographic portrait carries a similar affective weight. The illiterate viewers of Tojixon's close-up encounter her not as a propaganda slogan but as an affective invitation to socialist construction.

Tojixon, like her public, is unveiled. If Tojixon's "furrowed brows" are exposed, the text emphasizes that all the women who see Tojixon in the newspaper encounter her with unveiled faces: they are "pomegranate-faced girls."[37] For unveiled women, participation in the Soviet public was not without its risks. The newspaper now "shouts" of Tojixon's Stakhanovite honor, but when Tojixon first began her work, Oydin's poem says it was surrounded by hostile whisperings—a conspiratorial counterpublic. "Quietly, the enemy / whispers in the ear" that Ferghana is now "gone to pieces." Although their hostility may seem threatening, Oydin minimizes the threat by undermining the authority of the whisperers: "They said some things, some kind of thing / Let them say them, what they say." In Uzbek, the text is onomatopoeic, repeating "m's" and "n's" to create a murmuring effect, and repeating "de," the verb stem for "say" ("Dedi kimlar, kim nimalar / Desa, desun har nima"). In this stanza, the repetition is completely devoid of content; the lines do not indicate what precisely the enemy is saying, nor does it seem to matter. Tojixon did not care what the whisperers said, Oydin suggests, so neither should her admirers. In a context when women were subject to beatings, murder, and rape merely for unveiling, let alone participating publicly as activists, for many women it was not so simple to ignore gossip, whispered though it may be. Oydin instead suggests that what the men said was completely lacking in substance: she minimizes the possibility that they might have any legitimate criticism of cottonization and collectivization. Just as workers' correspondent reports excised "black" teahouse users from the legitimate, "Red" public, so Oydin implies that these murmurers have no place in the state public.

For the most part, the whisperers' complaints are vague and undefined. But in one respect, Oydin articulates them specifically: "These are very strange [*ajab qiziq*] days / A woman is the boss [*nachalnik*]." In using a borrowed term from Russian, *nachalnik*, the gossipers point up the strangeness of Tojixon's work. The position she works in is "strange" in the obvious sense that it is foreign and it promotes a foreign agenda. But Tojixon's work was strange not only because it was foreign. In Russian, the word *nachal'nik* is gendered masculine, reflecting the gender dynamics of Party administrative positions in Central Asia and in the Soviet Union more broadly. Tojixon's role as a boss, particularly at the level on which she operated, was completely unprecedented for a woman in Uzbekistan, and rare even for the Soviet

Union writ large. In the *Pravda* report that announced her award, for example, Tojixon's was the only female face in a row of male Political Division directors that had won the Lenin Prize. In this sense, the word *qiziq* might be translated not only as "strange" or "interesting," but as "queer," with a distinct connotation of gender-bending. This impression of Tojixon's queerness is underscored by Oydin's use of the adverb "bravely" or "manly" (*mardonadek*), which is derived from the strongly gendered Persian word for man, *mard*. In the last stanza, in fact, Oydin concludes that Tojixon has done her work "like a man" (*bir er kabi*). Tojixon's success makes her appear both less Central Asian and less feminine.

Despite Tojixon's perceived unfemininity, Oydin stresses that Tojixon has managed to remain respectable despite her role as a public figure. Pressing her subordinates to work harder, Tojixon uses the language of honor that was also widely used to describe feminine honor: "If we don't fulfill the Plan today / It will be bad for our honor [*nomus*]."[38] Later, she calls on workers to avoid "a hundred shamings" (*uyot*) by fulfilling the Plan, and describes collective farm work as "respectable work, honorable work [*sharaf ishi, shon ishi*]."[39] When applied to women, this language had strong connotations of sexual respectability. But in Oydin's representation, Tojixon has completely reframed the gendered language of respectability and honor. No longer does honor reflect a woman's sexual propriety; for Tojixon, respectability—for both men and women—comes through socialist labor, and through labor alone. The only dishonor worth fearing is the dishonor of failing to fulfill the Plan.

Just as Oydin's Tojixon reframes the language of feminine respectability in the terms of socialist labor, by the end of the poem, Oydin also reinterprets the lyrical language of spring. No longer will spring be a seductive distraction from the work at hand. Now, spring represents the joyous life that comes through Tojixon's dedicated labor:

> Summer is gone; the fall has passed;
> The spring is overtaking winter
> Building strength on strength,
> Ferghana is now again in bloom.

Under Tojixon's direction, no more does spring delay the march of socialist progress, as it threatened to do in the prologue. To the contrary: the spring "overtakes" winter, outpacing the frozen relics of the past. Blooming flowers no longer distract women from their work; instead, they serve as a metaphor for the joyous advance of socialism in Ferghana.

In order to succeed on Soviet terms and remain honorable in a man's world, Oydin suggests, Tojixon has redefined the terms that once framed her existence. She has relinquished her femininity, or at least the constructions of femininity that shaped her childhood. She has identified with a state that is associated, at least for her enemies, with foreign domination. She has even reimagined spring—not as a season of natural beauty, but as an image for the arrival of socialism. Perhaps this approach made sense for Tojixon, but for readers that more resembled the women in the frame narrative, however, it is highly implausible. Tojixon achieved her renown by adopting a masculine-coded self-presentation, but what of the women with their feminine "pomegranate faces" and their "sweet" voices? What of those for whom gossip was more than a harmless whispering? And what of those more prone to seduction by the beauties of Transoxania in the spring, not just the springtime of socialism?

Ultimately, Oydin never addresses the problems raised in the frame narrative at the beginning of the poem. Instead, the poem ends abruptly, as the speaker congratulates Tojixon: "Congratulations to you, my friend / You have achieved a hero's name." The reader never learns whether the speaker made it to her work, and in the context of all the obstacles presented at the beginning of the poem, one questions the veracity of the promise made near the beginning: "If you work as she worked… / You'll achieve a hero's great name." At best, the poem offers an invitation to readers, an open existential question: will you indeed work as she worked? The poem thus posits, not an unreliable narrator, but an unreliable public.

Tojixon the Overseer

A 1930s film about Shodieva's life, Liudmila Shezhinskaia's *Tadzhikhan Shadieva*, similarly emphasizes Shodieva's unveiling not just as a social phenomenon, but as an event of public-formation. Unlike the other representations of Tojixon I have discussed so far, however, this film was addressed not only to an Uzbek-speaking Central Asian public, but to a broader, all-Soviet audience. Like the other representations I have discussed so far, the film at once imagines a mobilizing Central Asian public, and calls the tractability of that public into question. For the all-Soviet European public, in contrast, the film puts forward visions of an exotic and backward locale, functioning primarily as an "engaging" (*zanimatel'naia*) rather than a mobilizational work. In this respect, it destabilizes the notion of a lateral, multinational public in which Central Asians participate as equals. Tojixon holds a liminal position, alternately appearing as a representative of a nascent Central Asian Soviet public, and as a disciplining overseer of that public.

Tadzhikhan Shadieva was one of five films produced in Central Asia by the agitational Film Train organized by cinema luminary Aleksandr Medvedkin.[40] Beginning in 1931, the Film Train traveled throughout the Soviet Union to a variety of workplaces, such as collective farms and factories. In Medvedkin's vision, the Film Train was to create a cinema that would break down the boundaries between art and life, not just making art but also aiding in the fulfillment of the Five-Year Plan. The train's filmmakers would produce a film about the workplace they visited and then screen it immediately to workers at the production site as a way of motivating them. To that end, the Film Train employed non-professional actors from each site it visited. Filmmaking and screenings were just a component of a larger program of "mass work": the film train produced a print newspaper, wall newspapers, posters, and "satire windows"; hosted agitational seminars and cultural events for workers' correspondents and shock workers; and organized meetings on hygiene and sanitation.[41] Medvedkin was the son of a railway worker, and he used the Film Train to advocate for efficient railway operation. In Kokand, for example, the film train was instrumental in ensuring that trains full of raw cotton be shipped in a timely and organized manner.

The earliest Film Train films tended to take a critical stance, exposing lapses in socialist production. In Medvedkin's plan, when the worker-performers saw the films in which they appeared, they would be ashamed of their failures and spurred to rectify their behavior. Emma Widdis suggests it was this uncomfortable negativity that prevented the films from receiving wider distribution outside of the locales in which they were made.[42] The goal of these early films was agitation, and Medvedkin believed shame to be a powerful motivator.

Despite his dedication to critique and agitation, Medvedkin believed in the importance of engagingness (*zanimatel'nost'*) as a mobilizational tool. In his writings on the film train, he foregrounded *zanimatel'nost'* as crucial for attracting "mass audiences."[43] The agitational message, he suggested, could come across only to spectators whose attention had already been captured. In addition to documentary films (*ocherk*, or sketch, was a common genre and the genre to which *Tadzhikhan Shadieva* belonged), Medvedkin also experimented with agitational fiction films. Medvedkin had left the film train by the time it arrived in Central Asia in late 1934. Under the rising star of Socialist Realism, which had been officially promulgated just months before at the

First Congress of the all-Soviet Writers' Union, the films came to emphasize *zanimatel'nost'* more than ever before. Under the direction of Liudmila Snezhinskaia, *Tadzhikhan Shadieva* put forward not a negative example, but a positive hero in the spirit of Socialist Realism.The film clearly draws on Gerasimova in telling Tojixon's story, beginning with Tojixon's exemplary achievements in the Ferghana collectivization effort, and flashing back to her child marriage and her "emancipation" by the Party.[44] The film thus brings together the Film Train's early emphasis on documentary with the new narrative expectations of Socialist Realism.

Like the other works on Shodieva, the film reflects an acute concern with Shodieva as a public figure, rather than an individual subject. Clearly, the film was produced with multiple viewerships in mind. The film's bilingual intertitles in Russian and Uzbek, as well as a soundtrack including Uzbek music and lines delivered in Uzbek, suggest that the film was produced to be screened for a multinational, multilingual audience.[45] Local participation was a major component of the film's production: Shodieva performed as herself, including, apparently, delivering her own sound lines in Uzbek. Most of the other actors and extras seem to be non-professionals, and portions of the film appear to have been shot on site, at a cotton-growing collective farm. It is unclear when, where, or whether the film was screened, or even whether Shodieva ever saw the completed film.[46] Whether it was screened at the time of its production or not, the film rewards close analysis. When brought into conversation with the many other mass-media representations of Shodieva, the film's disparate treatment of Central Asian publics and European observers conveys a broader pattern in the Soviet system of mass publicity: the tension between the Central Asian public as an object of mobilization and a tool for legitimation, and the invisible oversight of outsiders, many of whom were Russian-speaking Europeans. In the film, Shodieva addressed multiple imagined publics—among them a public of Muslim women, an Uzbek national public, an all-Soviet Russophone public, and an international socialist public—and for none of those publics was it an uncomplicated delivery.

For the local public in the Ferghana Valley, *Tadzhikhan Shadieva* was intended as an agitational film. For Uzbek collective farmers, Shodieva represented a vanguard-representative, whose life was to serve as an inspirational model for their own lives. Given Shodieva's fervent dedication to the causes of collectivization and women's emancipation, she likely considered her performance in the film an agitational effort. Shodieva's scenes portray her doing what she was most passionate about: running a collective farm, supervising Central Asian workers, delivering rousing speeches.

On the other hand, for non-Central Asian viewers, the film offered an ethnographic snapshot of life in distant, exotic locales. In a pamphlet surveying the film train published from Kokand in 1934, shortly after *Tadzhikhan Shadieva* was shot, Iakov Bliokh put it:

> The spectator is interested in knowing how people in the Fergana Valley live, what the Khorezm Oasis looks like, what Nagornyi Karabakh is [...], how people hunt for tigers, how people live on the Murmansk coast. As we move around 'on wheels' we spend time in all these places, see all of this, and we have a duty to show it all to the spectator, who has long hoped for that genre which we call the 'local interest' (*kraevedcheskii*) film.[47]

Bliokh puts forward an imagined geography of Soviet empire, spanning from the Caucasus to the Far East, from the Arctic to Central Asia. Here, agitation is far from Bliokh's purview: instead, he articulates an imperial gaze, reflecting a metropolitan demand for images of "local color," tigers and all. Indeed, the cover of the pamphlet represented the film train's travels as a network of routes radiating outward from Moscow, with each stop on the film train's route represented as a node on the network. The Central Asian stops lie along the Tashkent line, which was completed in 1906. Like the Russian Empire's rail infrastructure, the Film Train's route reflected the fact that all (rail)roads led back to Moscow. While *Tadzhikhan Shadieva* was conceived as a sketch (*ocherk*), rather than a "local interest" film, it also included strong components of the exoticizing gaze Bliokh articulates here. As a Russian outsider participating in a Film Train that was founded to promote socialist construction but evolved to satisfy the metropolitan demand for exotic perspectives, Snezhinskaia toggles between an Orientalizing gaze and an agitational mode. The film thus reflects an uncomfortable tension in the project of mass publicity in Central Asia: the legitimizing Central Asian public is the primary object of representation, while the European consumer-cum-supervisor is all but invisible.

From the first frames of the film, the filmmakers draw attention to Shodieva's unveiled face as a focus of media attention. After the opening credits, the camera cuts to a lingering close-up of another photographic close-up of Shodieva wearing her *gimnasterka* and worker's cap, smiling as she gazes into the distance. The shot emphasizes the photograph as a material object, framing it in a diagonal position that emphasizes its square shape against the background, and including the white border surrounding Shodieva's portrait (Figure 6.2). Then, the film cuts to intertitles quoting the Party Central

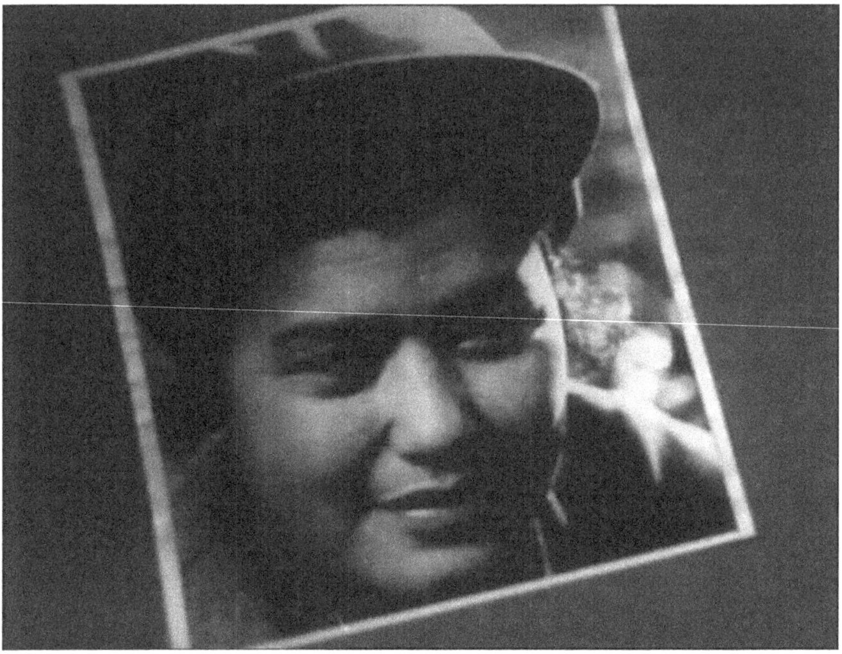

Figure 6.2 Still from *Tadzhikhan Shadieva*, dir. Liudmila Snezhinskaia (1934).

Committee resolution to award Shodieva the Lenin Prize for "the fearless fighter for women's liberation," and commending her "heroic, selfless execution of the Party and government directives about the socialist reorganization of the countryside." Between intertitles, the film cuts to close-ups of the medals Shodieva received, and concludes the sequence with another lingering shot of the photograph of Shodieva.[48] The film thus opens with a series of mediated quotations, both visual and verbal: not with Shodieva the living woman, but with her close-up portrait; not with Shodieva's famed oratory, but with the Party resolution that was reproduced and distributed in newspapers throughout the Soviet Union; not with an image of Shodieva wearing her medal, but of the prize by itself, unattached, with its equally decontextualized portrait of Lenin.

Snezhinskaia's film traffics in intensely affective close-up shots of both Tojixon and the members of her public. But the opening sequence—not a close-up, but a close-up of a close-up—fundamentally reverses the close-up effect Balázs described. Rather than creating intimacy, the shots of Tojixon's photograph alienate and decontextualize. Throughout the short film, the dialectic between Tojixon's immediacy and her distance persists.

Like Oydin's poem, in the film, Tojixon's story is embedded in a frame narrative. Directly following the opening credits, an intertitle conveys that the year is 1934, the same year the film was produced. Tojixon is supervising the work of her subordinates at a collective cotton farm in the idyllic Ferghana Valley. She berates them for cutting corners in their cotton picking, but no matter: they surround and greet her with smiling, upturned faces. The camera lingers on each close-up, each individual's line of sight oriented somewhere off-screen, at Tojixon. If for Balázs, close-ups represented a variety of urban social types, so they do here for the Uzbek countryside: an old *dehqon*, a young woman, an adolescent boy—all cotton workers. These are the first among many gazes that will be turned toward Tojixon in this 19-minute-long film: Tojixon's public is as much the subject of Snezhinskaia's film as Tojixon herself.

Shortly, the film camera follows the public's gaze and lingers on another shot of Shodieva. The shot rhymes visually with the photographic portrait from the opening credits, but this time it is a live tableau. Such long, still close-ups of Shodieva the celebrity appear repeatedly in the film, even studded within flashback scenes, as if to remind viewers that the past has been fully superseded. Just as for Oydin's narrator, the image of Tojixon triggers a narrative about her past. Surrounded by the upturned faces of her collective farm subordinates, Shodieva begins sharing the inspirational story of her past.

If Shodieva of 1934 is a media celebrity, the film situates prerevolutionary Tojixon as a helpless girl-victim, subjected to the patriarchal gaze rather than public view. Opening the flashback sequence about Shodieva's violent childhood, an intertitle announces, "Tojixon's past is the past of thousands of Uzbek women." The intertitles announce the date as 1916. The next scene shows Shodieva as a young, prepubescent girl frolicking among friends. But the fun quickly comes to an end when two veiled women enter the courtyard. "Don't cry," they tell Tojixon, "It's a good bride-price: two hundred *so'm* and a sewing machine." They then proceed to lower a thick horsehair face-veil, followed by a head-veil, over her body. Financial necessity is forcing Tojixon to marry a much older man, a local folk healer (*tabib*).

This scene exemplifies the cinematic quality of (un)veiling: the camera captures how the veil slowly descends over Tojixon's childish frame, obscuring first her face, and then her entire body. Tojixon's playmates watch in sad sobriety as she walks away. In the film, then, Tojixon's grandmother regains her sight at the cost of Tojixon's freedom. Because the veil obscures Tojixon's sight, it might even be argued that the grandmother's sight is exchanged for

Tojixon's. And yet, the grandmother is a hapless victim herself: her blindness is curable, and yet she is too impoverished to pay for the sought-after cure. Visually, as represented by the veil, patriarchal and class-based violence renders Tojixon and all other Uzbek women both blind and invisible to all but the patriarchal gaze.

In the scene of Shodieva's veiling, the veil completely obscures Shodieva's body: it functions as a barrier, both from non-kin men who might threaten her feminine honor, and from the camera. But with the arrival of revolution, the veil soon becomes not a barrier, but a screen. The tabib, introduced now as the Soviet police chief of Kokand, is hosting several local officials inside his guest room. Central Asia is in a liminal state between backwardness and revolution: the tabib has still not been unmasked as an enemy of the people. Today, the intertitles explain, that tabib/police chief has taken his ninth wife.[49] When Tojixon enters to serve the men, she recognizes one of them as the local Party chief (*rais*). Tojixon runs up from behind and desperately grasps his arm, asking him urgently, "*Rais*! Is there a government that can protect women?" As the chief nods tentatively in assent, Shodieva responds, "If there is such a government, I will become its servant (*cho'ri*). On its behalf, I will turn the stones on the road into gravel."[50] When her husband sees her whispering to the *rais*, he advances menacingly toward her, and Tojixon hunches over, covering her veiled head with her arms—a gesture that will be repeated later in the film. Most likely, Gerasimova invented these words, since it is in Gerasimova that they are first attested. Certainly they are characteristic of Gerasimova's flair for the floridly dramatic. No matter their provenance, their function in the film is clear: in addition to conveying Shodieva's intense commitment to the Soviet cause, the line suggests that Shodieva's "emancipation" has turned her over from one form of submission to another, from patriarchal oppression to service to the Party-state.[51]

This moment of Tojixon's transfer from patriarchal control to Party control coincides with the moment of her becoming visible. When Shodieva first enters the room, and in the shot of her grabbing the *rais*'s arm, her veil is opaque as ever. But when she begins to speak, the veil no longer functions as a barrier, but as a screen: Shodieva's face is visible through its fabric. An ordinary horsehair veil would not permit such visibility, so evidently, it has been replaced by the filmmakers with another, more translucent fabric. Strategic lighting exaggerates the effect of transparency. In this scene, showing Tojixon's face through a veil serves to emphasize her liminal position, between the infantile, oppressed victim she once was, and the Stakhanovite hero we know she will become. The veil-as-screen, in other words, becomes the segué for

Shodieva's exposure on the silver screen. The transparency of the veil mirrors the liminality of Tojixon's position between the patriarchy and the Party. The veil marks her as a servant of the patriarchy; her bare face conveys her service to the Party.

The cinematic quality of Shodieva's veiling is matched only by the drama of her unveiling scene, which follows soon after the scene with the *rais*. The unveiling displays not only Tojixon's personal transformation, but also the organization of a public around her. In the scene, Shodieva ascends the podium at a rally, wearing a face veil. As she begins speaking, the crowds of men and mostly veiled women watching her rise eagerly to their feet. With the veil still covering her face, she delivers an impassioned speech calling on her brothers and sisters (*akalar* and *singillar*) to struggle against the enemies of the "worker-peasant" government. Her speech concludes with uproarious applause, and as the audience continues to clap, its members begin shouting for her to remove her veil. She lifts the face-veil, and frowns with downcast eyes as the crowd continues cheering. Overwhelmed, she covers her face with her hands and runs down from the podium. Dropping her veil, Cinderella-like, on the stairs from the podium, Shodieva jumps onto a waiting donkey-cart, which she rides home, hunched over her knees in order to hide her face. Shodieva wears a long dress with pantaloons and a scarf over her hair: of Shodieva's body, viewers can see only the hands covering her face.

Although Snezhinskaia is clearly invested in representing a mobilizational public around Tojixon, the film suggests a more complex dynamic. At the moment of her exposure, Tojixon experiences the gaze of the Central Asian Soviet public much like she experienced the prerevolutionary patriarchal gaze: as an invasion. Indeed, the footage of the crowd, particularly the footage of the larger crowd, leaves an impression of more than just enthusiasm. Some men and women staidly clap their hands, but others—men in particular—shout, wave, and pump their fists, demanding that Shodieva unveil. The context indicates they are shouting in support of Shodieva, but based on their body language alone, they may as well be hecklers. Likewise, Shodieva's body language after unveiling—her hunched-over frame, arms shielding her face and head—recalls her defensive body language when anticipating a blow from her husband the *tabib*. The intensity of exposure overwhelms her. The scene suggests a latent anxiety that the public is perhaps not as organized, not as controllable, as Snezhinskaia would like to represent it. There is an uncanny slippage between the unruly crowd and the aspirational public, organized and mobilizing behind the Party.

In addition to the anxiety about organization, the unveiling scene foregrounds a clear discrepancy between the Central Asian public and their European Soviet observers. The crowd at Shodieva's unveiling is comprised completely of Central Asians, with nary a European to be seen. Likewise, Shodieva's speech, the only sound speech in the film, is also entirely in Uzbek, and plays completely without interpretation into Russian. Here, Russians are exclusively behind the camera, subjecting Central Asians to an outside gaze, but unable to understand Shodieva's own words without learning her language. In this film, the Central Asian public is the main object of representation. The non-Central Asian outsiders are more outside overseers than members of the public. They watch while remaining invisible, rather than participating alongside the Central Asian public.

Shodieva's speech drives home this distinction. The speech is simple: Shodieva proclaims that the "government of workers and peasants" has granted women the opportunity for a "bright life" (*turmush* / Rus. *byt*). She exhorts her "brothers" to fight against an unspecified enemy, and her "sisters" to overcome "oppression" (*zulm*). Shodieva does not mention the Party, Soviet power, or the Bolsheviks, which figure prominently elsewhere in the intertitles. Nor does she use the language for class categories that had been widely adopted by the mid-1930s, comprising largely borrowed terms or calques from Russian. Instead, she uses language that emphasizes her project as an indigenous one, belonging to nonspecific workers (Uzb. *ishchi*, not the borrowed and more heavily ideological *proletar*) and the generic term for farmers (*dehqon*).[52]

In contrast with Tojixon's Uzbek-language speech with their strong commitment to an indigenous revolutionary project, the intertitles suggest that Tojixon is submitting to Party tutelage and control. We have already seen Tojixon's insistence, likely originating in Gerasimova, that she would become the "slave" of any government that could protect women. The intertitles that follow the scene of unveiling convey a similar sentiment of submission to the Party, which is identified not with the Uzbek public but with Moscow authority. "The first step was very hard," says Shodieva in the intertitles; "But our great friend and protector, the Party had my back. They sent me to study in Moscow." Unlike Tojixon's Uzbek-language speech, the bilingual intertitles emphasize Tojixon's indebtedness to Moscow-based Party tutelage. The tension between Moscow control and locally rooted public participation comes out most clearly in the following intertitle, which includes a glaring discrepancy between the Russian and the Uzbek. In the Russian, Tojixon proclaims, "Party cultivation made me a human being and a Bolshevik." The Uzbek, on the other hand, omits one key word: "Party cultivation made me a Bolshevik." The single word, "human being," suggests that Tojixon owes not only her activist career, but her very humanity to the Party. The two discrepancies—the untranslated speech and the missing Uzbek word in the intertitles—lend themselves to disparate interpretations for the film's different audiences. For Russian-speaking viewers, the film conveys a deep sense of Central Asia's indebtedness to European Party tutelage; for Uzbek-speakers, the film suggests that the Central Asian public is at the helm. In both cases, the film insistently represents a Central Asian public while eliding the invisible European presence.

In this sense, when analyzing this work it is difficult to discuss a European "public." In Snezhinskaia's film, Europeans comprise an audience, consuming exotic images of Central Asian women and men, but not a mobilizing public. They also function as overseers, offering tutelage and administering control while remaining invisible to the Central Asian public. The Central Asian public is subordinated to a Party-state that, at the central Moscow level, is controlled not by Central Asian women like Shodieva but mostly by European men. Europeans, in this case, function not as a lateral public but as representatives of a hierarchical state.

Indeed, this problem is suffused through the representations of Shodieva. If we return to Halle's account of Shodieva's unveiling, for example, the distinction between the European observer and the Central Asian public is quite distinct. For Shodieva's Central Asian comrades, gazing expectantly at Shodieva on the stage, she represented *one of them*. In looking at Shodieva, they were supposed to see her as a model for mobilization and an emblem of their bright future. For Shodieva's European observers, on the other hand—the factory workers and Ukrainian collective farmers, Krupskaya and Halle—Shodieva was a relic of the past, shrouded in an artifact of medieval superstition and patriarchy, and requiring their assistance to enter modernity. If the Central Asian audience is a mobilizing public, the European audience is a surveilling, disciplining, or at best, tutoring observer.

At the same time, the film reflects a more complex dynamic than a binary opposition between European overseers and the Central Asian public. This is perhaps most evident in the scenes when Shodieva looks back at her public, rather than merely being seen by it. I have already discussed one such scene: the scene of Shodieva's unveiling, in which she is terrorized by the public's gaze. But by 1934, when Shodieva is a supervisor at a collective farm, that perspective has changed. "Director, friend, comrade" (Rus. *rukovoditel', drug, tovarishch* /Uzb. *rahbar, do'st, o'rtoq*) reads the intertitle introducing the Tojixon of 1934. The intertitle suggests an inherent tension in Tojixon's relationship with her public: on the one hand, she interacts with it as an equal—a friend and a comrade. But her position as director of the collective farm unsettles these lateral relations.

A scene near the end of the film visually emphasizes Shodieva as invisible overseer rather than public figure, friend, or comrade. As Shodieva makes her rounds of the cotton fields, she walks up on an unsuspecting young couple flirting during work time. A strapping young farmer offers a cotton blossom to a young cotton-picking woman, who bashfully accepts the gift. The couple surreptitiously embrace as Tojixon comes upon them from behind. When the couple part from their embrace, they are embarrassed to notice that Tojixon has been watching them. Tojixon wags her finger at them in mock reproach, and the young couple smilingly return to their work. Again, Tojixon walks a fine line between director and comrade. On the one hand, she surveils and disciplines, at one point urging a subordinate to fine delinquent workers two work days' worth of pay. On the other, she plays the role of a benevolent comrade, affably reminding her fellow workers to stay on task.[53]

In a film that has so strongly thematized Shodieva being made visible, this scene shows the reverse: Shodieva again becomes invisible. But instead of being rendered both blind and invisible by a veil, Shodieva now willingly hides herself to surveil others. In so doing, she embodies a new kind of power relation, one that entails an identification with the panoptical state: only a select few are entitled to see without being seen.

Shodieva's position as invisible supervisor creates an uneasy tension with her status as a Soviet celebrity. The major premise of the Hujum was that unveiling would empower Central Asian women. Visibility inducted Uzbek women into the public, and visibility was a kind of power. But Tojixon's story suggests something more complex—that unveiling itself did not grant Tojixon power, and that her power came later, when she identified herself with the surveilling Party-state. What empowered Shodieva was not her visibility, but her access to the state's monopoly on violence: her ability to fine "delinquent" workers, to dispossess those she deemed *kulaks* and to send wreckers to labor camps. Shodieva's case exemplifies the limitations of Soviet publicity: as much as the mass media represented a participatory public, in the end power remained rooted in the panoptical surveillance state.

The Invisible Tojixon

To conclude, I return to Halle, whose cinematic scene of Tojixon's unveiling opened this book. When Halle visited Central Asia, she made a point of visiting Ferghana in hopes of meeting Tojixon Shodieva in person. But when she arrived in Ferghana in the fall, Shodieva was nowhere to be found. The cotton harvest was in full swing, and a directive had just come out to bring in the entire crop in time for the anniversary of the October Revolution. Halle waited for days in Ferghana, but Shodieva was busy traversing the district "to direct and supervise the 'campaign.'" Occupied with her supervisory duties, Halle reports, Shodieva "remained invisible for days." Finally, Shodieva arrived in the city at three o'clock in the morning, but by that time Halle was both ill and obliged to depart with the ticket she had already purchased. Shodieva, for whom the photographers had once "placed their apparatus," was now impossible to see: she was far too busy with her supervisory duties.

There is some indication that Shodieva preferred things this way. She was passionately devoted to her work and a powerful speaker, but often gave the impression that she was frustrated by the obligation of performing as a representative of Central Asian femininity when there was so much important work to be done and so many people to be managed. In the context of the Soviet media system, however, Shodieva became a celebrity, attaining larger-than-life proportions in the barrage of representations of her that appeared in Soviet newspapers, journals, books, posters, and film. I have argued that these representations were as much concerned with representing and mobilizing a Central Asian public around Tojixon as with portraying Tojixon herself. Like the novels, songs, textiles, and workers' correspondence notes in earlier chapters, these representations imagine a participatory mass public of Central Asians, even as they articulate anxieties about that public's level of organization. Into this disjuncture peers the disciplining, surveilling, and often foreign gaze of the state: a gaze that Tojixon both adopted and was subjected to.

Socialism Mediated: The Making of Soviet Culture in Central Asia. Claire Roosien, Oxford University Press.
 DOI: 10.1093/9780198971153.003.0008

Conclusion

When presenting my research, I have often been asked if this book is about the "Sovietization" of Central Asia. The question seems straightforward, but in fact it presumes a great deal. It presupposes, first and foremost, that at some point there existed an established Soviet "outside" that could then be imposed on an authentic Central Asian "inside." "Sovietness," implicitly, was made in Moscow and exported to the peripheries, where it then encountered, conflicted with, repressed, or otherwise interacted with an essential "Central Asianness." The expected outcome of a study of the "Sovietization of Central Asia" is some kind of emphasis on hybridity, or, conversely, on cultural erasure. Here, we might say, are the elements of "Central Asianness" and there are the elements of "Sovietness." There, they intertwine neatly and there they seem to be at odds. That encounter between "Sovietness" and "Central Asianness" has been described, on the one hand, as a mostly harmonious process of hybridization, as Ali İğmen argues in his book about early Soviet culture in Kyrgyzstan, *Speaking Soviet with an Accent: Culture and Power in Kyrgyzstan*.[1] On the other hand, it could be a confrontation characterized by violence and cultural erasure, as generations of Cold War scholars emphasized, and a new generation now turns to in fresh ways.[2] In both cases, the "Central Asian," the "Uzbek," the "Islamic," or whatever else you might call it can be juxtaposed, *in toto*, with a Soviet alterity. William Mazzarella has called this problem the "*hybridity paradox*, namely, the way that talking about how two entities are always already in hybrid relation with each other ends up re-reifying them as, precisely, two entities."[3] The problem with the "Sovietization in Central Asia" approach is that it reifies both the "Soviet" and the "Central Asian."

In today's climate, both these approaches have become highly politicized. Either emphasize the fundamental hybridity of Soviet cultural practices, potentially implying that they were somehow less violent than they actually were; or stress the dynamics of cultural erasure and violence, thereby foregrounding the colonial hierarchies of repression but at the risk of essentialism. In the crisis that has shaken the study of Russia, Eastern Europe, Eurasia, and the Soviet Union after Russia's full-fledged invasion of Ukraine in 2022, "decolonization" is sometimes taken to mean the latter approach, while advocates of the former have argued against "decolonization" as excessively reductive, lending itself to a fruitless search for "national or civilizational authenticity."[4]

By foregrounding the processes of mediation, this book has taken a different approach. It has analyzed the efforts of cultural mediators in organizing and imagining what I have termed a "state public," a shared space of officially sponsored discourse. I took early inspiration in this project from a broad body of scholarship on missions and empire, especially Vicente Rafael's *Contracting Colonialism*, which emphasized Spanish mission in the Philippines as a process of translation. Much as I resist the language of "Sovietization," Rafael resisted the language of "Christianization." For Rafael, translation was not a transparent process of transferring stable ideas from one containing language to another. Instead, Rafael argued, "translation tended to cast intentions adrift, now laying, now subverting the ideological grounds of colonial hegemony."[5] Writing as he did at the peak of the linguistic turn, Rafael emphasized linguistic mediation, but as I have demonstrated here with reference to Soviet Uzbekistan, material culture or music could prove just as potent a medium as spoken or written language.

Because of its temporal displacement from many other colonial civilizing missions, and because of the Soviet state's ideologically anti-colonial self-representation, the culture and propaganda effort in Soviet Central Asia differed in important ways from colonial enlightenment projects. Most significant, perhaps, is the newly central place of the mass media. The Soviet Union perfected the techniques of mass communication, distributing mediums like newspapers, radio, film through mass institutions that were designed to reach the maximum audiences possible. The Soviet system of culture and propaganda can thus be seen as a cultural enlightenment effort, continuous with those of earlier empires, but recalibrated for the age of mass publicity.

Combined with the top-down nature of Soviet archives, the vast reach and unprecedented uniformity of Soviet media technologies mean that Soviet culture and propaganda often appear, to the untrained eye, to be homogeneous messages emanating from Moscow and received in the periphery by new "converts." Like Catholic missionaries, who first used the term "propaganda," Soviet Party leaders perfected messaging that they hoped their targets in Central Asia would receive with enthusiasm. What both Catholic missionaries and Soviet ideologues tended to miss is that the very process of conversion was, by definition, a process of mediation. Soviet culture and propaganda created a public, and therefore, a space of participation, interpretation, and creativity that the Party could not and did not fully control. When it came to the material agendas that culture and propaganda were supposed to support—the campaigns for cottonization and collectivization, first and foremost—mediators sometimes succeeded in producing works that resonated with the public, and other times did not.

By emphasizing the role of mediators in the work of imagining and organizing a Soviet public, I stake a renewed claim for the significance of culture in early Soviet Central Asia. Culture functioned not as a repository for authentic "Uzbekness," "Tajikness," or "Kyrgyzness," but as an ideological tool for underscoring the Soviet Party-state's ostensible commitment to national self-determination. And yet, by constructing a vast apparatus for state publicity, the Soviet system of culture and propaganda created space for (mis)interpretation and appropriation. Occasionally, mediators expressed resistance, but in many cases, it is fruitless to look for resistance in a public sphere designed to render resistance invisible.[6] Instead of merely looking for marks of resistance or accommodation, I have highlighted the unpredictable moments of resonance and reaction that go beyond such categories.[7] The purpose here is not to minimize hierarchy and state violence, but to understand the myriad ways cultural producers from Central Asia invested "Sovietness" with new meaning.

By framing my argument in terms of publicity rather than subjectivity, I bracket the questions of sincerity and authenticity, belief and dissidence that continue to haunt the study of Soviet culture, particularly since the heyday of the subjectivity school in the 1990s. When Stephen Kotkin introduced "speaking Bolshevik" in 1995, he could hardly have predicted the myriad adaptations to which it would lend itself. Subsequent scholarship has amplified some of the assumptions that underpinned Kotkin and the subjectivity scholars' work, and certainly the assumptions of many of their readers: namely, that "Bolshevik" was a language one could learn from the authorities, with its established grammar and vocabulary that Soviet people could master, and a body of fixed phrases that one could assent to in public or question in private. Such assumptions underpin Ali İğmen's argument that Kyrgyz cultural producers spoke "Bolshevik with an accent." In reaction to İğmen and the broader revisionist historiography to which Kotkin belonged, meanwhile, Botakoz Kassymbekova has argued that most Party collaborators in Tajikistan did not really understand the ideological terms they were given: "Soviet words were used as recently seized *foreign* words, not quite understood and not quite mastered, any time speakers wanted to appear communist regardless of the awkward nonsense they produced."[8] Despite their differences of interpretation, both İğmen and Kassymbekova share an assumption that "Bolshevik" was a foreign language that Central Asians tried to master, or at least pretended to master. Despite their differences, all these approaches nevertheless assume an established grammar and vocabulary, which can be spoken poorly or fluently, and with varying degrees of comprehension and levels of commitment. Turning to mediation, rather than "Sovietization," serves to redirect analytical attention both from the liberal subject and from the implicit assumptions that have accrued around "speaking Soviet." Instead, it recognizes Central Asians as mediators, rather than true believers, secret dissidents, victims, or collaborators. "Soviet publicity," in my analysis, does for the Soviet collective what Soviet subjectivity has done for the individual: it both acknowledges the heavy hand of the state and shows the limits of its reach.

Mediators both imagined and organized the Soviet public in Central Asia. The mediums they brought to bear in that project did not always smoothly align with the mobilization agendas of the Party-state—the Red Teahouse proved less tractable an institution than some mediators had hoped—but they sometimes produced unexpected resonances for a few, as in the case of silk textile rewards for shock-working women. The efforts of mediators legitimized the Soviet state as answerable to the will of the "masses," but in fact, as I have argued, mediators constituted a new social and cultural elite, both beholden to and benefiting from state support. In the Writers' Union, emerging national writers strove to represent the "masses" even as they laid the groundwork for a new cultural hierarchy centered in Tashkent. As they participated in the effort to co-construct both Soviet and national cultures, mediators at once reproduced imperial discourses and—perhaps unwittingly—pointed up their contradictions. The very mediums that were supposed to transparently convey socialist content instead refracted it in unpredictable ways: Uzbekistan's first Socialist Realist novels highlight the contradictions inherent in adapting a European literary form, the novel, in the context of a cultural project that would be "national in form, socialist in content." Soviet popular song, like silk and velvet, appropriated pre-Soviet modes of publicity, from courtly musical traditions to national modernization projects; and at the same time mobilized popular affect among broad segments of the population around the Party in a then-semiliterate society. At the same time, "culturedness" became the accoutrement of a new Stakhanovite elite. Tojixon Shodieva, whose story brackets this book, was the member of just such an elite. The many mediated representations of Shodieva, circulated in a variety of languages and before a variety of publics, help to illuminate the contradictory valences of Soviet publicity—and the fraught significance of Shodieva as model of socialist construction, exemplum of women's emancipation, and eventually, as we will see below, as enemy of the people.

The men and women who made Soviet culture in Uzbekistan could not have predicted the long-term legacies of their work. Certainly, many of the biggest names of the 1930s faded into oblivion. Oydin died in relative obscurity just a couple months after Stalin, despite the efforts of her most famous student, the woman poet Zulfiya, to memorialize her legacy.[9] Shams, similarly, died an obscure death under unknown circumstances in 1943, and despite the efforts of some Uzbekistani scholars to revive his reputation during the 1970s, he remains largely unknown.[10] Others became canonical representatives of their national communities—Abdulla Qahhor, who built a literary empire lasting until his death in 1968, is required reading for middle-school students in Uzbekistan. Ayni has become the founding father of Tajik national literature, and his statue adorns a central square in Dushanbe, Tajikistan. The presence of his underresourced home-museum in the historic center of Samarkand remains a reminder of that city's longstanding status as a capital of a multilingual Persianate culture, in the context of a post-Soviet Uzbekistan that has stressed Uzbek as its constitutionally designated state language. Muhiddin Qori-Yoqubov built a brilliant career, surviving through the Terror, only to be indicted for "counter-revolutionary" activity in July 1952, just before Stalin's death, and condemned to a long imprisonment. Although he was exonerated in 1955, his career never fully recovered and he died after a fall in February 1957.[11] Today, nevertheless, Qori-Yoqubov is remembered as a founding father of modern Uzbek music. His ex-wife, Tamara Khanum, fared better, becoming the face of Soviet Central Asia at many an international festival well into the Cold War and until her death in 1991.[12] Her home museum remains a popular site of pilgrimage in Tashkent to this day.[13] Perhaps more enduring than any one of their reputations is the system of state publicity they helped to build: one that enforced the hegemony of a Soviet state governed from Moscow even as it carried the seed of its own contradictions. The patterns of participation and control, the tensions between state-manufactured eliteness and mass address, and the unpredictable resonances of cultural address remain defining features of post-Soviet publicity in Central Asia.

Perhaps no individual better exemplifies the contradictions of Soviet publicity than the woman whose story opened this book, Tojixon Shodieva. We left Shodieva in her position as Stakhanovite heroine and Stalinist overseer. But ultimately, after serving for a time as its representative, Tojixon fell victim to the depredations of the Soviet state. Her career abruptly halted in 1937, when at the height of the Great Terror, Shodieva was condemned with 164 others from Uzbekistan. Of these 165, only three were women.[14] 155 of the total were sentenced to death. In this respect, Shodieva was lucky: she was sentenced to the Gulag in Siberia, where she served an eighteen-year sentence. Still, Shodieva remained enthusiastic. In her memoir of the Gulag, Evgeniia Ginzburg recalls encountering Shodieva on a prisoners' train in Siberia. "Her face seems familiar to many from films and the covers of *Ogonek* and *Prozhektor*." To Ginzburg's astonishment, Shodieva spent the ride telling her fellow inmates about "long-ago plenums" and how she embarrassed a certain Biktagirov for his errors about the cotton harvest.[15]

Shodieva vanished from public view for eighteen years. When she returned, she was a woman changed. According to Saodat Shamsieva, a woman who had worked with Shodieva in her early years of activism but escaped the Great Terror herself:

> After amnesty, [Shodieva] returned, freed from almost twenty years of imprisonment. "I'll go to my own village, Saodat," she began to say, breathing with difficulty. "For me, the streets of this city, and the offices of administration have no value anymore. They remind me of the suffering that my companions and I underwent..."
>
> Tojixon's troubled and heavy expression at that moment even now will not pass from my eyes...I could say it still burns, here, in me...[she indicates her heart]. What must those eyes have seen.[16]

To Shamsieva, Shodieva's face communicated her bitter experience of betrayal and secret suffering. Tojixon's persona, on the other hand, remained largely unaltered. Gerasimova published another *Pravda* article on Tojixon's achievements in honor of International Women's Day, 1963; its representation of Tojixon's life was nearly identical to the ones Gerasimova had published thirty years earlier.[17] In 1966, one S. Normatov published a book-length biography of Shodieva.[18] His biography followed the arc of the earlier biographies, from childhood victimhood to adult achievement. The only addition is a glancing reference to the enemy saboteurs who supposedly sent her to the Gulag, and the chapters delineating her career after rehabilitation. For Normatov, unlike for Shamsieva, Tojixon picks up after rehabilitation essentially where she left off. When she returns to Uzbekistan, she seeks out the least productive collective farm in the Ferghana Valley and turns it around, much as she had done decades before. On the cover, a stylized portrait of a much-aged Tojixon looks intensely outward, somewhere beyond the reader. She casts her gaze sternly downward, as if she has been captured in the midst of her supervisory duties, and cannot be bothered to sit for a formal portrait; as if a delinquent cotton-picker has just caught her eye. Tojixon may look like a supervisor, but in his concluding sentences, Normatov insists, like all Tojixon's other biographers, that she is not just a supervisor, but a model for an aspirational public. "Here is the mandate for all of us: to learn from Tojixon, to try to become like her. Always and in everything!" The book is entitled, simply, *Tojixon*—she needs no further introduction.

Socialism Mediated: The Making of Soviet Culture in Central Asia. Claire Roosien, Oxford University Press.
 DOI: 10.1093/9780198971153.003.0009

Endnotes

Preface

1. This spectacular scene of Shodieva's unveiling may in fact be staged or apocryphal: other accounts place Shodieva's unveiling in Central Asia, or on a train between Central Asia and Moscow. Valeriia Gerasimova reports that Shodieva unveiled in 1926; see Valeriia Gerasimova, "Raskreposhchennyi Genii," *Pravda* (Moscow), March 8, 1937, 2. For a full summary of the different stories about Shodieva's unveiling, see Marianne Kamp, *The New Woman in Uzbekistan: Islam, Modernity, and Unveiling under Communism* (Seattle: University of Washington Press, 2006), 106. A photograph of Shodieva unveiled appeared in *Yangi Yo'l* in 1927: "Shodievaning qisqacha tarjima-i holi," *Yangi Yo'l*, no. 10–11 (1927), 28.
2. Fannina W. Halle, *Women in the Soviet East* (E.P. Dutton & Co., Inc., 1938), 310. In the later biography by S. Normatov, Shodieva unveils at the request of M. I. Kalinin; see S. Normatov, *Tadzhikhon* (Tashkent: Izd-vo "Uzbekistan") 1966, 51.
3. Halle's account of the unveiling scene appears unattributed, in quotation marks; but it immediately precedes a reference to Shodieva's "biographer," Gerasimova. I have yet to identify Gerasimova's source for this scene.
4. On labor heroes and Soviet exemplars, see Mary Buckley, *Mobilizing Soviet Peasants: Heroines and Heroes of Stalin's Fields* (Lanham, Md.: Rowman & Littlefield, 2006); Lewis H. Siegelbaum, *Stakhanovism and the Politics of Productivity in the USSR, 1935–1941* (Cambridge: Cambridge University Press, 1988).
5. On Tojixon Shodieva as one among a social cohort of Central Asian women's activists, see Kamp, *The New Woman*, 106. On Soviet heroines in Central Asia more broadly, see Ali F. İğmen, *Speaking Soviet with an Accent: Culture and Power in Kyrgyzstan* (Pittsburgh: University of Pittsburgh Press, 2012), 120–39.

Introduction

1. On the intensified campaign against Islam in 1927–29, see Shoshana Keller, *To Moscow, Not Mecca: The Soviet Campaign against Islam in Central Asia, 1917–1941* (Westport, CT: Praeger, 2001), 141–74.
2. "Vmesto mecheti - klub." *Pravda Vostoka*, April 15, 1929, 5.
3. RGASPI f. 62, op. 2, d. 1957, l. 18. The Shumiatskii mentioned here is almost certainly Boris Zakharovich Shumiatskii, who in 1929 was rector of the Communist University for Toilers of the East (KUTV) and a member of the Central Asian Bureau; in 1930, he was to become the influential director of Soiuzkino, the official state institution for film production.
4. On rural activists for collectivization, see Marianne Kamp, *Collectivization Generation: Oral Histories of a Social Revolution in Uzbekistan* (Ithaca, NY: Cornell University Press, 2024), 83–103.
5. The term "masses" was a constructed ideological category and a central figure of Soviet discourse. I have used scare quotes here to stress this point, but henceforth in my usage, it should be assumed that the term reflects the usage of my actors and not my own analytical category. On collectivization in Uzbekistan, see Kamp, *Collectivization Generation*.
6. V. I. Lenin and I. V. Stalin, "Ko vsem trudiashchimsia musul'man Rossii i Vostoka," *Izvestiia*, November 22, 1917, 1–2.
7. On the Soviet Union's self-representation as a benevolent alternative to other empires, see Botakoz Kassymbekova, *Despite Cultures: Early Soviet Rule in Tajikistan* (Pittsburgh, PA: University of Pittsburgh Press, 2016), 71–80.
8. Here I concur with Kassymbekova's claim that official Soviet language did not "produce meanings, standards, and categories that could be understood and internalized by all." Unlike Kassymbekova, however, I argue that Central Asia's mediators attempted to make sense of this often incomprehensible language; indeed, to create a language (and a material culture, a musical idiom, and so forth) that would make sense of socialist discourse. In this respect they did not completely *disregard* official discourse; instead, they remade it. See Kassymbekova, *Despite Cultures*, 7.

9. Bruno Latour, *Reassembling the Social: An Introduction to Actor-Network-Theory* (Oxford: Oxford University Press, 2005), 39. Latour's use of "intermediary" should be distinguished from the historiographical term, the "colonial intermediary."
10. On the script change, see Adeeb Khalid, *Making Uzbekistan* (Ithaca: Cornell University Press, 2016), 262–66.
11. Latinization had been discussed in the wider Turkic world since the 1850s and appealed to reform-minded intellectuals across the South Caucasus, Central Asia, and Middle East. In the Soviet period, reforms to make the Arabic script easier to learn preceded the shift to Latin; see Michael J. Erdman, "Vehicularizing the Vernacular: Using the Periodical Press to Popularize Vernacular Languages in Soviet Turkic Communities," *Central Asian Survey* 42, no. 3 (2023): 1–19.
12. In fact, due to similar concerns about "modernity," mass literacy, and state propaganda, the Turkish Republic also shifted to a modern Latin script in 1928. On the Turkish script reform, see Hale Yılmaz, *Becoming Turkish: Nationalist Reforms and Cultural Negotiations in Early Republican Turkey, 1923–1945* (Syracuse, NY: Syracuse University Press, 2013), 139–78.
13. For one example of the ongoing influence of Islamic manuscript traditions in the Soviet Union, see Alfrid K. Bustanov, "Muslim Literature in the Atheist State: Zainap Maksudova between Soviet Modernity and Tradition," *Journal of Islamic Manuscripts*, 9, no. 1 (2018): 1–31.
14. A major purge of so-called "bourgeois nationalists" took place across the Soviet national republics in 1929; on the purge in Uzbekistan, see Khalid, *Making Uzbekistan*, 370–78.
15. For one powerful example of such a critique, see M. A. Tchokaieff (Chokaev/Shoqay), "Fifteen Years of Bolshevik Rule in Turkistan," *Journal of the Royal Central Asian Society*, vol. 20 (1933), 351–59.
16. 1930 statistics are in RGASPI f. 62, op. 2, d. 2479, ll. 19–23; 1932 statistics are in RGASPI f. 62, op. 2, d. 2970.
17. The following statistics come from Kh. Pulatov, *Kul'turno-vospitatel'naia deiatel'nost' sovetskogo gosudarstva v Uzbekistane* (Tashkent: Gosudarstvennoe izdatel'stvo uzbekskoi SSR, 1959), 54–55.
18. Ibid.
19. RGASPI f. 62, op. 2, d. 2007, l. 58 ob.
20. Kh. Pulatov, *Kul'turno-vospitatel'naia deiatel'nost*, 55. The definitive work on early Soviet film in Uzbekistan is Cloé Drieu, *Cinema, Nation, and Empire in Uzbekistan, 1919–1937* (Bloomington: Indiana University Press, 2019). In its attention to the process of film production, as well as aesthetic analysis and reception history, Drieu's approach complements mine. However, because film had a much smaller reach than the print media and music, and because film production was dominated by Russians until the late 1930s, I have opted largely not to include it in my analysis here.
21. On archival sources for the study of Soviet Central Asian culture and the importance of published sources, see Claire Roosien, "Not by Archives Alone: The 'Revolution' in Soviet Central Asian Literary Studies," *Iranian Studies*, 55, no. 3 (2022): 777–85.
22. Contra the anarchists of his time, Lenin argued that the state was necessary during the process of destroying the vestiges of bourgeois statehood. Only the proletarian state, once fully stabilized, would create the conditions for its own "withering." See Frederic Engels, *Anti-Dühring*, in *Marx and Engels Collected Works* (London: Lawrence & Wishart, 1987), 254–71; V. I. Lenin, "Gosudarstvo i revoliutsiia," in *Sobranie sochinenii*, vol. 14, no. 2, *Burzhuaznaia revoliutsiia 1917 g.* (Moscow: Gosudarstvennoe izdatel'stvo, 1923), 308–13.
23. Still, a stark binary between capitalist consumption and socialist production would be out of place here. Leo Löwenthal distinguishes between celebrity culture in the interwar and postwar periods, arguing that early popular culture focused on heroes of business, the professions, and "serious" culture, while the postwar moment turned starkly to consumption. See Löwenthal, "The Triumph of Mass Idols," in *Literature and Mass Culture* (New Brunswick, NJ: Transaction Books, 1984), 203–36.
24. Central Asia can be called a "wardrobe" in precisely the same sense as Ukraine was called a bread basket—not because it produced or consumed ready-made clothes locally, any more than all Ukraine's grain was baked into bread or consumed in Ukraine. Rather, in using this expression, I intend to convey how Central Asia was incorporated in an all-Soviet economic system that relied on it for the raw material to produce those consumer goods.
25. On cottonization in Central Asia, see Julia Obertreis, *Imperial Desert Dreams: Cotton Growing and Irrigation in Central Asia 1860–1991* (Göttingen: V&R, 2017).
26. Until 1936, the territories of modern-day Kazakhstan and Kyrgyzstan were Autonomous Soviet Socialist Republics within the Russian federation. Although both regions had many cultural and historical connections with the rest of Central Asia, their administrative structure differed significantly from those of the other republics. Tajikistan attained the status of a full Union Republic in

1929. See Terry Martin, *The Affirmative Action Empire: Nations and Nationalism in the Soviet Union, 1923–1939* (Ithaca, NY: Cornell University Press, 2001), 31. On the status of Tajikistan, see Adeeb Khalid, "Tajik as a Residual Category," in Khalid, *Making Uzbekistan: Nation, Empire, and Revolution in the Early USSR* (Ithaca, NY: Cornell University Press, 2015), 291–315. For a summary of the process of national delimitation in Central Asia, see Adrienne Lynne Edgar, *Tribal Nation: The Making of Soviet Turkmenistan*. Princeton: Princeton University Press, 2004), pp. 43–59; Arne Haugen, *The Establishment of National Republics in Soviet Central Asia* (Basingstoke: Palgrave Macmillan, 2003).

27. On this process, and the role of Central Asians in defining and territorializing these national categories, see Khalid, *Making Uzbekistan* (2016). On the role of imperial ethnographers, see Francine Hirsch, *Empire of Nations: Ethnographic Knowledge and the Making of the Soviet Union*, Culture and Society after Socialism (Ithaca, NY: Cornell University Press, 2005).
28. On the history of Khoqand up to and including its conquest, see Scott Cameron Levi, *The Rise and Fall of Khoqand, 1709–1876: Central Asia in the Global Age* (Pittsburgh, PA: University of Pittsburgh Press, 2017). On the conquest of Central Asia, see Alexander Morrison, *The Russian Conquest of Central Asia: A Study in Imperial Expansion, 1814–1914* (Cambridge, UK: Cambridge University Press, 2021); A. M. Malikov, "The Russian Conquest of the Bukharan Emirate: Military and Diplomatic Aspects," *Central Asian Survey*, 33, no. 2 (2014): 180–98; Sergei Abashin, "The 'Fierce Fight' at Oshoba: A Microhistory of the Conquest of the Khoqand Khanate," *Central Asian Survey*, 33, no. 2 (2014): 215–31. On the conquest and administration of Russian Turkestan, see Alexander Morrison, *Russian Rule in Samarkand, 1868–1910* (Oxford: Oxford University Press, 2008); Beatrice Penati, "Notes on the Birth of Russian Turkestan's Fiscal System: A View from the Fergana Oblast,'" *Journal of the Economic & Social History of the Orient*, 53, no. 5 (December 2010): 739–69.
29. On the complex interactions between Russian colonial courts and shari'a law during the Russian colonial period, see Paolo Sartori, *Visions of Justice: Shari'a and Cultural Change in Russian Central Asia*, vol. 24, *Handbook of Oriental Studies* (Leiden: Brill, 2016).
30. On the motivation for the Russian conquest of Central Asia, see Morrison, *The Russian Conquest of Central Asia*, 1–28. Morrison argues, convincingly, that the motivations for the imperial conquest of Turkestan must be sought locally, rather than attributed to economic incentives (i.e., the "cotton canard") or to the Great Game.
31. On Russian imperial and early Soviet Tashkent, see Jeff Sahadeo, *Russian Colonial Society in Tashkent, 1865–1923* (Bloomington, IN: Indiana University Press, 2007).
32. On the problem of Central Asia's early modern "decline," and for an argument against the notion, see Levi, *Khoqand*.
33. Confusingly, the ancestors of those known as "Kazakhs" today were commonly designated as "Kirgiz" in nineteenth-century Russian-languages sources. Today, the term "Sart" is sometimes used as a slur for Uzbeks.
34. On the debates that produced Bolshevik nationalities policy, see the concise summary in Martin, *The Affirmative Action Empire*, 2–9.
35. V. I. Lenin, "K voprosu o natsional'noi politike," *Polnoe sobrani sochinenii* (5th ed., Moscow: Izdatel'stvo politicheskoi literatury, 1969), vol. 25, 66.
36. See Khalid, *Making Uzbekistan*, 1–2.
37. Until 1938, Central Asia's "local Jews" (*mestnye evrei*) enjoyed a periodical press in Judeo-Tajik and dedicated cultural institutions; after 1938, they lost the status of a separate nationality, including the privileges that came along with it. On the troubled status of the Jews of Central Asia in the early Soviet period, see Zeev Levin, *Collectivization and Social Engineering: Soviet Administration and the Jews of Uzbekistan, 1917–1939* (Leiden: Brill, 2015). On non-titular nations in the Caucasus region, see Krista A. Goff, *Nested Nationalism: Making and Unmaking Nations in the Soviet Caucasus* (Ithaca, NY: Cornell University Press, 2021).
38. Paul Bergne, *The Birth of Tajikistan: National Identity and the Origins of the Republic* (London: I. B. Tauris, 2007), 108–9.
39. The fourth characteristic, "ruled by a sovereign claiming absolute sovereignty," is less immediately applicable to the Soviet Union, although the cult of personality under Stalin can arguably fit under the rubric. Valerie A. Kivelson and Ronald Grigor Suny, *Russia's Empires* (New York: Oxford University Press, 2016), 4.
40. Leah Feldman, *On the Threshold of Eurasia: Revolutionary Poetics in the Caucasus* (Ithaca, NY: Cornell University Press, 2018), 2–3. The purpose of the nation was to *integrate* Soviet nationalities into a broader (neo)-imperial project. In this respect, Soviet nationalities policy differed significantly from other nationalizing projects such as the Turkish, which stressed autarky and independence from foreign domination. In practice, the Soviet Uzbek nation underpinned a

neo-imperial project that preserved many hierarchies of the Russian imperial order; in theory, it worked in service of world revolution.

41. In taking categories of masculinity and femininity as the outcome of historical negotiation rather than as a given, I rely on Joan Scott's foundational argument: Joan W. Scott, "Gender: A Useful Category of Historical Analysis," *The American Historical Review*, 91, no. 5 (1986): 1053–75.
42. Kamp, *The New Woman*.
43. On the similarities between the Soviet Hujum and other imperial projects for women's "emancipation," see Douglas Northrop, *Veiled Empire: Gender and Power in Stalinist Central Asia* (Ithaca, NY: Cornell University Press, 2004). On the parallel campaigns in other modernizing states, see Adrienne Edgar, "Bolshevism, Patriarchy, and the Nation: The Soviet 'Emancipation' of Muslim Women in Pan-Islamic Perspective," *Slavic Review*, 65, no. 2 (July 2006): 252–72; Hale Yılmaz, *Becoming Turkish: Nationalist Reforms and Cultural Negotiations in Early Republican Turkey, 1923–1945* (Syracuse, NY: Syracuse University Press, 2013), 78–138; Camron Michael Amin, *The Making of the Modern Iranian Woman: Gender, State Policy, and Popular Culture, 1865–1946* (Gainesville: University Press of Florida, 2002), 80–113.
44. On collectivization in Russia, see Lynne Viola, *Peasant Rebels under Stalin Collectivization and the Culture of Peasant Resistance* (New York: Oxford University Press, 1996); Moshe Lewin, *Russian Peasants and Soviet Power: A Study of Collectivization* (Evanston, IL: Northwestern University Press, 1968).
45. On this topic in broader Soviet perspective, see Sheila Fitzpatrick, "Ascribing Class: The Construction of Social Identity in Soviet Russia," *The Journal of Modern History*, 65, no. 4 (1993): 745–70. On early Soviet Khujand, which became part of Tajikistan but whose process of class ascription bore key similarities to that of Uzbekistan, see Flora J. Roberts, "Old Elites under Communism: Soviet Rule in Leninobod" (Ph.D. Diss., Chicago, University of Chicago, 2016), 109–74.
46. On this process, see Kamp, *Collectivization Generation*, 104–31.
47. Jürgen Habermas, *The Structural Transformation of the Public Sphere: An Inquiry into a Category of Bourgeois Society* (Cambridge: The MIT Press, 1991).
48. For a critique of the ideal civil society as completely separate from the state, see Nancy Fraser, "Rethinking the Public Sphere: A Contribution to the Critique of Actually Existing Democracy," *Social Text*, no. 25/26 (1990). On race, see The Black Public Sphere Collective, *The Black Public Sphere: A Public Culture Book*, ed. The Black Public Sphere Collective (Chicago: University of Chicago Press, 1995); on class, Alexander Kluge and Oskar Negt, *Public Sphere and Experience: Analysis of the Bourgeois and Proletarian Public Sphere* (New York: Verso Books, 2016; initially published in German in 1972); on gender, Joan B. Landes, *Women and the Public Sphere in the Age of the French Revolution* (Ithaca, NY: Cornell University Press, 1988). See also Robert Fine, "Civil Society Theory, Enlightenment and Critique," *Democratization*, 4, no. 1 (March 1, 1997): 7–28.
49. Anthony J. La Vopa, "Conceiving a Public: Ideas and Society in Eighteenth-Century Europe," in *Enlightenment Past and Present: Essays in a Social History of Ideas* (Liverpool: Liverpool University Press, 2022), 84.
50. This scholarship is far too extensive to discuss in full here. Key contributions include Vadim Volkov, "Obshchestvennost': Russia's Lost Concept of Civil Society," in *Civil Society in the Baltic Sea Region*, eds. Norbert Götz and Jörg Hackmann (Aldershot, Hants: Ashgate, 2003), 63–75; Laura Engelstein, "The Dream of a Civil Society in Tsarist Russia: Law, State, and Religion," in Nancy Bermeo and Philip Nord, eds., *Civil Society Before Democracy: Lessons from Nineteenth-Century Europe* (New York: Rowman and Littlefield, 2000), 23–41; Joseph Bradley, "Subjects into Citizens: Societies, Civil Society, and Autocracy in Tsarist Russia," *The American Historical Review*, no. 4 (2002): 1094–1123; Vera Kaplan, *Historians and Historical Societies in the Public Life of Imperial Russia* (Bloomington, IN: Indiana University Press, 2017), 12. See also the useful definitions in Catriona Kelly and Vadim Volkov, "Obshchestvennost', sobornost': Collective Identities," in *Constructing Russian Culture in the Age of Revolution, 1881–1940*, eds. Catriona Kelly and David Shepherd (Oxford: Oxford University Press, 1998), 26–27.
51. Matthew Lenoe, for example, translates the term as "official society"; see Matthew E. Lenoe, *Closer to the Masses: Stalinist Culture, Social Revolution, and Soviet Newspapers* (Cambridge: Harvard University Press, 2004), 52, 56. For a clear summary of the history of the concept across the revolutionary divide, see Yasuhiro Matsui, ed., *Obshchestvennost´ and Civic Agency in Late Imperial and Soviet Russia: Interface between State and Society* (Houndmills: Palgrave Macmillan, 2015), 82–108. Nikolai Bukharin was a leading theorist of *obshchestvennost'* as a mediating sphere between the Party and the masses. See Zenji Asaoka, "Nikolai Bukharin and the Rabsel'kor

movement," in *Obshchestvennost' and Civic Agency*, ed. Yasuhiro Matsui (Houndmills: Palgrave Macmillan, 2015), 82–108. After the agitprop conference of 1928, the usage of the term shifted significantly, as Party organizers shifted the emphasis from "convincing" the masses of Party doctrines through dialogue to "organizing" them around a predetermined Party line. By the 1930s, the term came to be much more closely identified with the Party and its sympathizers rather than the broad masses, although until his arrest in 1937, Bukharin continued to defend the autonomy of the workers' correspondence movement and of *obshchestvennost'*. See also Lenoe, *Closer to the Masses*, 247–48. Furthermore, while in practice *obshchestvennost'* often coincided with Party activists and officials, the underlying expectation was that *obshchestvennost'* was an omnivorous category: as the masses reached the appropriate level of consciousness, the now-enlightened, organized masses would ultimately all become subsumed within *obshchestvennost'*. For the reverse translation (from "public sphere" to *obshchestvennost'*), see, for example, Olga Rozenblium, "'Diskussii ne bylo...' otkrytye pis'ma 1960-x godov kak pole obshchestvennoi refleksii," in *Nesovershennaia publichnaia sfera: istoriia rezhimov publichnosti v Rossii*, eds. Timur Atnashev, Mikhail Velizhev, and Tatiana Vaizer (Moscow: Novoe literaturnoe obozrenie, 2021), 418.

52. A 2014 *begriffsgeschichte* offered both *publichnost'* and *obshchestvennost'* in a list of synonyms, including Habermas's German "öffentlichkeit" as a parenthetical. See Lucian Hölscher, "Publichnost'/ Glasnost'/ Publichnaia Sfera/ Obshchestvennost' (Öffentlichkeit)," in *Slovar' osnovnykh istoricheskikh poniatii: izbrannye stat'i*, ed. D. Sdvizhkov and I. Shirle, vol. 1 (Moscow: Novoe literaturnoe obozrenie, 2014). More recently, an edited volume on the topic consistently uses "publichnost'," in the ideal-normative sense of a deliberative democratic space. Atnashev et al., eds., *Nesovershennaia publichnaia sfera*.
53. For the critique of Habermas's public sphere as "unmistakably nostalgic and eminently mandarin," see Anthony J. La Vopa, "Conceiving a Public," 85.
54. For two popular examples of such an approach, see Masha Gessen, *Surviving Autocracy* (New York: Riverhead Books, 2020), 5–6; Timothy Snyder, *On Tyranny* (New York: Crown, 2017).
55. Bradley, "Subjects into Citizens"; Kaplan, *Historians and Historical Societies*; Stuart Finkel, *On the Ideological Front: The Russian Intelligentsia and the Making of the Soviet Public Sphere* (New Haven: Yale University Press, 2007), 1–12.
56. For a similar argument with respect to early Soviet newspapers, see Konstantin Bugrov, "Industrializatsiia, gazety, i rozhdenie sotsialisticheskoi publichnoi sfery v sovetskom gorode," in *Nesovershennaia Publichnaia Sfera* , ed. Atnashev et al., 312–40.
57. The term *jamoatchilik* also tapped into long-standing associations with Jadid and broader Islamic culture. *Jamoatchilik* derives from the Arabic *djamāʿa*. Historically, *djamāʿa* designated both the worldwide community of Muslims (similar to its correlate, the *umma*), and the face-to-face congregation of believers assembled in prayer. In this respect religious imaginaries might be understood as a premodern precursor of the modern public sphere, with the key difference that they lack mass mediation and the sense of simultaneity that comes with the latter. When Uzbek Bolsheviks translated the language of *obshchestvennost'* into their own language, then, they used the language of *jamoa* and *jamoatchilik*; while today, the Uzbek-language term for "public opinion," *jamoat fikri*, uses the same root. H. Fleisch, "D̲jamʿ, D̲jamāʿa," in P. Bearman (ed.), *Encyclopaedia of Islam New Edition Online (EI-2 English)*, (Leiden: Brill, 2012), Consulted online on June 26, 2023.
58. In this respect, Michael Warner argues, religious imaginaries unite believers as "people-whom-one-does-not-yet-know," as opposed to modern publicity, which is premised on permanent relations of "strangerhood"; see Michael Warner, "Publics and Counterpublics," *Public Culture*, 14, no. 1 (2002): 57.
59. Khalid, *The Politics of Muslim Cultural Reform: Jadidism in Central Asia* (Berkeley: University of California Press, 1999), 114–15. Before 1917, Jadids often used the root in the older senses. In the years before 1917, leading Jadid Abdurrauf Fitrat frequently uses the term *jamoa* to describe the "community of Muslims" (*musulmonlar jamoasi*) or a specific Muslim congregation (Abdurrauf Fitrat, *Tanlangan asarlar*, 54, 75, 94); but elsewhere to refer to society in general (46, 99), or to "enlightened society" (*donishmand jamoa*, 116), while Jadids begin forming associations (*jama'a*) for charitable and educational causes. Within the first five years after 1917, another leading Jadid, Behbudiy's usage is beginning to align more consistently with the meaning of *obshchestvennost'*, that is, the progressively minded intelligentsia; see the references to *jamoat* in Mahmudxo'ja Behbudiy, *Tanlangan Asarlar* (Tashkent: Ma'naviyat, 1999), 207, 254.
60. Jadids' understanding of "Turkic" included Turkic language speakers from Central Asia, East Turkestan, Iran, the Caucasus, and Anatolia; the later delineation of the Turkish nation was much narrower.

61. On Sufi networks, see Waleed Ziad, *Hidden Caliphate: Sufi Saints beyond the Oxus and Indus* (Cambridge, MA: Harvard University Press, 2021); on *madrasas*, James Pickett, *Polymaths of Islam: Power and Networks of Knowledge in Central Asia* (Ithaca, NY: Cornell University Press, 2020).
62. Alexei Yurchak, *Everything Was Forever Until It Was No More: The Last Soviet Generation* (Princeton: Princeton University Press, 2013); Kyrill Kunakhovich, *Communism's Public Sphere: Culture as Politics in Cold War Poland and East Germany* (Ithaca, NY: Cornell University Press, 2023).
63. Michael Warner defines a public as a relation among strangers, "self-organized through discourse," particularly through the mediated circulation of texts. It is a structural feature of public discourse that, when addressed as the member of a public, one understands oneself to be part of an indefinite community of strangers one may never meet face-to-face. Michael Warner, "Publics and Counterpublics," in Michael Warner, *Publics and Counterpublics* (New York: Zone Books, 2002), 74–76. This type of imaginative self-identification with a collective is the marker of a public, as opposed to a bureaucratic or legal designation imposed from above—say, citizenship or passport nationality. Warner's theory of public and counterpublics resonates with Benedict Anderson's theory of the nation as an "imagined community," taking shape through "print capitalism"; but it expands the frame of collective identification beyond the nation to any number of potential categories. It should be noted that Warner highlights two dimensions of publics that do not entirely correspond to what I describe here: their universality and their autonomy from the state. First, Warner distinguishes publics from "nations, religions, races, guilds," which have membership criteria and are thus not as universal as a "public." I would argue, instead, that a nation (or the "proletariat") is a kind of public, insofar as it constitutes a relation among strangers that is self-organized through discourse, even though it may be exclusionary.
64. For a major recent exception, see the recent *Slavic Review* research cluster, Evgeny Dobrenko and Klavdiia Smola, eds., "(Multi)national Faces of Socialist Realism," special issue, *Slavic Review*, 81, no. 4 (Winter 2022).
65. The field is too vast and the debates far too complex to summarize in a single footnote, but a foundational text in North American media studies is Marshall McLuhan, *Understanding Media: The Extensions of Man* (London: Routledge, 2001). Frankfurt School thinkers might be seen as a continental expression of a similar concern with form and mediation; see, for example, the foundational essay by Walter Benjamin, "The Work of Art in the Age of Mechanical Reproduction," in Walter Benjamin, *Illuminations*, ed. Hannah Arendt, trans. Harry Zhon (New York: Schocken Books, 2007), 217–52.
66. By emphasizing the future-orientedness of Socialist Realism, it is important to stress that the producers of Socialist Realism in Central Asia believed it to be a tool for advancing material transformation in the world, not just a "replacement" for reality, as Evgeny Dobrenko has argued in E. A. Dobrenko, *Political Economy of Socialist Realism* (New Haven: Yale University Press, 2007). On the discourse of Socialist Realism, see Sheila Fitzpatrick, "Becoming Cultured: Socialist Realism and the Representation of Privilege and Taste," in Fitzpatrick, *The Cultural Front: Power and Culture in Revolutionary Russia*, Studies in Soviet History and Society (Ithaca, NY: Cornell University Press, 1992), chapter 9. On "laterality" as a feature of early Socialist Realism, see Christina Kiaer, "Fairy-tales of the Proletariat, or, Is Socialist Realism Kitsch?," in *Socialist Realisms: Soviet Painting 1920–1970* (Milan: Skira, 2012), pp. 183–89.
67. On early Soviet theater, see Saodat T. Nazarova, "XX Asr 20-30 Yillaridagi Ijtimoiy-Siyosiy Muhitning o'zbek Sahna San'atiga Ta'siri" (PhD diss., Tashkent, Uzbekistan Academy of Sciences History Institute, 2024).

Chapter 1

1. Rossiiskii gosudarstvennyi arkhiv sotsial'no-politicheskoi istorii (RGASPI) f. M-1 (Central Committee of the All-Union Leninist Young Communist League [VLKSM, 1918–1991]), op. 23, d. 835a, l. 109.
2. More precisely, we might refer to a tea- and coffeehouse belt: in the lands of South, East, and Central Asia, tea was the order of the day; in the Ottoman Empire, with its imperial holdings in the Arabian peninsula, coffee was the drink of choice, while in Iran, most coffeehouses converted to teahouses at some point in the nineteenth century. See L. P. Elwell-Sutton, "Čāy-Ḵh̲āna," in in P. Bearman (ed.), *Encyclopaedia of Islam New Edition Online (EI-2 English)*, (Leiden: Brill, 2012), accessed January 19, 2018.
3. In nomadic regions, the Red Teahouse's counterpart was the Red Yurt; see Rebekah Ramsay, "Nomadic Hearths of Soviet Culture: 'Women's Red Yurt' Campaigns in Kazakhstan, 1925–1935,"

Europe-Asia Studies, 73, no. 10 (2021): 1937–61. On Soviet mass institutions, see also Ali F. İğmen, *Speaking Soviet with an Accent*, 37–82; Bruce Grant, *In the Soviet House of Culture: A Century of Perestroikas* (Princeton: Princeton University Press, 1995), 90–119.

4. Vorukh is now a Tajik exclave in Kyrgyzstan, disputed by the governments of Tajikistan and Kyrgyzstan. This event is described in detail in RGASPI f. 62, op. 2, d. 1815, ll. 29–30 ob.
5. RGASPI f. 62, op. 2, d. 1815, ll. 41, 41 ob. The episode is also mentioned in Khalid, *Making Uzbekistan*, 350–51.
6. O'zMDA f. 94, op. 1, d. 202, l. 196.
7. Red Teahouses were promoted in many Central Asian republics, especially Tajikistan and Uzbekistan, but also in sedentary regions of Turkmenistan and Kyrgyzstan. Although my analysis relies primarily on Uzbek sources, the dynamics seem to be similar in other republics as well. On Red Teahouses in Tajikistan, see Alisher Latypov, "Choikhonai Surkh: The Replacement of 'Opium Dens' with Red Teahouses and the Limits of the Soviet Enlightenment Project in Tajikistan," *Central Asian Affairs*, 7, no. 3 (2020): 236–66.
8. Semen Mal't, "V chaikhane," *Komsomolets Vostoka*, June 26, 1934, 4. A brief summary of Mal't's biography is available at "Mal't Semen Adol'fovich," *Sovetskii plakat*, https://tramvaiiskusstv.ru/plakat/spisok-khudozhnikov/item/656-malt-semen-adolfovich-1900-1968.html (accessed May 13, 2024).
9. See, for example, Eugene Schuyler, *Turkistan: Notes of a Journey in Russian Turkistan, Khokand, Bukhara, and Kuldja* (London, 1876), 179–80; Ole Olufsen, *The Emir of Bokhara and His Country: Journeys and Studies in Bokhara (with a Chapter on My Voyage on the Amu Darya to Khiva)* (Copenhagen: Gyldendal Nordisk Forlag, 1911), 305, 336, 436; Ármin Vámbéry, *Sketches of Central Asia: Additional Chapters on My Travels, Adventures, and on the Ethnology of Central Asia* (London: Wm. H. Allen, 1868), 172–73. I am grateful to Yuan Gao for directing me to these travelogues; my understanding of teahouse culture in imperial Turkestan was greatly enriched by her presentation, Yuan Gao, "Tea Trade and Tea Consumption in the Russian Turkestan," Paper presented at Central Eurasian Studies Society Annual Conference, Pittsburgh, PA, October 2018. See also Yuan Gao, "Samovar in Chaikhaneh: Tea Trade, Consumption, and Material Culture in Central Eurasia," in *Silk Roads Papers* (Paris: UNESCO Publishing, 2024). Still, as this survey should indicate, much remains to be learned on the topic. A 1913 album on Central Asia for young Russian speakers noted that teahouses in Turkestan "can't be missed" (*brosaiutsia v glaza*); see Boris Tageev (Rustam-Bek), *Po Azii: Sbornik statei dlia iunoshestva s illiustratsiiami* (Moscow: Pravda, 1903), 46.
10. Olufsen, 305.
11. Ármin Vámbéry, *Sketches*, 172–73.
12. V. P. Nalivkin and Mariia Vladimirovna Nalivkina, *Muslim Women of the Fergana Valley: A Nineteenth-Century Ethnography from Central Asia*, trans. Marianne Kamp and Mariana Markova (Bloomington, IN: Indiana University Press, 2016), 33.
13. Ella Robertson Christie, *Through Khiva to Golden Samarkand; the Remarkable Story of a Woman's Adventurous Journey Alone through the Deserts of Central Asia to the Heart of Turkestan* (London: Seeley, Service, 1925), 127–28.
14. Some teahouses offered food; others served only tea, and patrons brought their own food. Vámbéry, *Sketches*, 172; Schuyler, *Turkistan*, 179.
15. All teahouses provided hot water and dishes; food and tea leaves were frequently but not always provided. Olufsen, *The Emir of Bokhara*, 336; Schuyler, *Turkistan*, 136. There was some geographical variance in the use of opium; in pre-Soviet Central Asia it appears to have been particularly widespread in border regions, and in the Soviet period Afghanistan became the source of much of Soviet Central Asia's opium. On opium consumption in prerevolutionary Bukhara, see Pickett, *Polymaths of Islam*, 170–77. Alisher Latypov suggests that outside of the Pamir region, opium was more often "eaten," or consumed as a tea. See Alisher Latypov, "The Opium War at the 'Root of the World': The 'Elimination' of Addiction in Soviet Badakhshan," *Central Asian Survey*, 32, no. 1 (2013): 22–30.
16. Teahouse musicians are discussed in Olufsen, *The Emir of Bokhara*, 433; Anna Louise Strong, *Red Star in Samarkand* (New York: Coward-McCann, 1929), 30–31; Joshua Kunitz, *Dawn over Samarkand; the Rebirth of Central Asia* (New York: Covici, Friede, 1935), 37–38.
17. Schuyler described *bacha* dances as "by no means indecent, though they were very often lascivious (*Turkistan*, 135). On the Jadid objection to dancing boys, see Khalid, *The Politics of Muslim Cultural Reform*, 145. Adolescent male performers were also present in coffeehouses elsewhere in the Middle East; see Ralph S. Hattox, *Coffee and Coffeehouses: The Origins of a Social Beverage in the Medieval Near East*, University of Washington Press ed. (Seattle: University of Washington

Press, 1988), 109. See also Said Gaziev, "Dancing Boys and Gay Escapades in Fin-de-siécle Tashkent: A Sketch from a Queer History of Central Asia," *SICE Blog, Austrian Academy of Sciences*, https://www.oeaw.ac.at/sice/sice-blog/dancing-boys-and-gay-escapades-in-fin-de-siecle-tashkent-a-sketch-from-a-queer-history-of-central-asia (accessed November 21, 2023). For a discussion of one interpretation of the phenomenon from an outsider's perspective, see Jennifer Wilson, "Queer Harlem, Queer Tashkent: Langston Hughes's 'Boy Dancers of Uzbekistan,'" *Slavic Review*, 76, no. 3 (2017): 637–46.

18. Olufsen, *The Emir of Bokhara*, 336, 436.
19. The available evidence indicates that samovars began to appear in Central Asian teahouses in the nineteenth century, before the Russian conquest and as Russian commerce became more prominent in the region. See Annette M. B. Meakin, *In Russian Turkestan; a Garden of Asia and Its People* (New York: Scribner, 1915), 214.
20. Ella Robertson Christie, *Through Khiva*, 154.
21. Schuyler, *Turkistan*, 179.
22. Vámbéry, *Sketches*, 173.
23. Vambery, *Travels*, 239. The Bukharan Emir was also not alone in attempting to control sociability at these institutions. When coffee and coffeehouses began to appear in the Ottoman Empire, they received a mixed reception with religious authorities, with some muftis issuing *fatwas* against the consumption of coffee—bans that were, however, little heeded. Coffeehouses took seventeenth-century Istanbul by storm.[1] In 1633, Sultan Murad IV made a futile effort to prohibit coffee, even executing some coffee-drinkers. Although the ban was touted as a measure for fire prevention, Lewis suggests, "another purpose may have been to safeguard the government from comment." See Lewis, *Istanbul and the Civilization of the Ottoman Empire*, 132–35. Hattox makes a similar assessment of the early modern Ottoman restrictions; see Hattox, *Coffee and Coffeehouses*, 101–2. Similarly, in late nineteenth-century Tehran, the Qajar Shah was said to have closed most teahouses because they "were supposed to encourage extravagance and idleness, or...evils of a more serious kind." Edward Granville Browne, *A Year amongst the Persians. Impressions as to the Life, Character, and Thought of the People of Persia, Received during Twelve Months' Residence in That Country in the Years 1887–8* (London: A. and C. Black, 1893), 82.
24. Pickett, *Polymaths of Islam*, 218–42; Andreas Wilde, *What Is beyond the River?: Power, Authority, and Social Order in Transoxania 18th–19th Centuries* (Vienna: Verlag der Österreichischen Akademie der Wissenschaften, 2016), 706–11.
25. E. Romanovskaia, "Muzyka v Uzbekistane," *Sovetskaia muzyka*, September 1934 (no. 9), 5. Theodore Levin's post-Soviet informants also allude to restrictions on musical performance under the late Manghit Emirs, not only in teahouses, but throughout their domain; see Theodore Levin, *The Hundred Thousand Fools of God: Musical Travels in Central Asia (and Queens, New York)* (Bloomington: Indiana University Press, 1996), 101. It is, of course, possible that both claims are the result of Soviet-era fabrication.
26. The teahouse appeared in China quite early, possibly as early as the tenth century; see Di Wang, *The Teahouse: Small Business, Everyday Culture, and Public Politics in Chengdu, 1900–1950* (Stanford, Calif.: Stanford University Press, 2008), 13. The precise timing for the appearance of the teahouse in Central Asia is unclear.
27. On the spread of coffee through the Ottoman Empire from the Arab lands during the sixteenth century, see Bernard Lewis, *Istanbul and the Civilization of the Ottoman Empire* (Norman: University of Oklahoma Press, 1963), 132. In Iran by the nineteenth century, the terms "teahouse" and "coffeehouse" were used interchangeably. See L. P. Elwell-Sutton, "Čāy-Ḵẖāna." In parts of Anatolia, coffeehouses were prominent social institutions by the late nineteenth century. See Brian W. Beeley, "The Turkish Village Coffeehouse as a Social Institution," *Geographical Review*, 60, no. 4 (1970): 475–93.
28. Olufsen, *The Emir of Bokhara*, 305.
29. R. D. McChesney, "'Barrier of Heterodoxy'? Rethinking the Ties between Iran and Central Asia in the 17th Century," in *Safavid Persia: The History and Politics of an Islamic Society*, ed. C. Melville (London: Tauris, 1996), 231–67.
30. Indeed, scholars of a range of Eurasian societies have tended to make similar arguments: Wang, for example, argues that the Chengdu teahouse facilitates a kind of "public sphere," albeit not in the strict Habermasian sense; Meeker describes Turkish coffeehouses as facilitating "a form of public life," functioning at times under close state/elite supervision, and at other times more autonomously. Citing Habermas, Rudi Matthee claims that Iranian coffee-/teahouses created a "public sphere by default, one that operated against the grain and in the interstices of officially sanctioned practice." See Di Wang, *The Teahouse under Socialism: The Decline and Renewal of*

Public Life in Chengdu, 1950–2000 (Cornell University Press, 2018), 220; Meeker, *A Nation of Empire*, 342; Rudolph P. Matthee, *The Pursuit of Pleasure: Drugs and Stimulants in Iranian History, 1500–1900* (Princeton.: Princeton University Press, 2005), 296.

31. Serdar Öztürk distinguishes between three types of coffeehouses in early Republican Turkey: village and neighborhood coffeehouses, which served a less elite clientele; and "literary" coffeehouses, which served wealthier and better-educated patrons. See Serdar Öztürk, "The Struggle over Turkish Village Coffeehouses (1923–45)," *Middle Eastern Studies*, 44, no. 3 (2008): 435–54.
32. There were some exceptions in China, especially in the PRC; see Wang, *The Teahouse under Socialism*, 98. In twentieth-century Turkey, "tea gardens" became a gender-inclusive space as opposed to the male-dominated coffeehouses; see Sharon Wohl, "The Turkish Tea Garden: Exploring a 'Third Space' with Cultural Resonances," *Space and Culture*, 20, no. 1 (February 2017): 56–67.
33. Christie, *Through Khiva*, 118.
34. Edward Granville Browne, *The Persian Revolution of 1905–1909* (Cambridge: Cambridge University Press, 1910), 143.
35. Feldman, *On the Threshold of Eurasia*, 47.
36. See Öztürk, "The Struggle over Turkish Village Coffeehouses"; Qin Shao, "Tempest over Teapots: The Vilification of Teahouse Culture in Early Republican China," *The Journal of Asian Studies*, 57, no. 4 (1998): 1009–41.
37. Steven Shapin makes such a provocative suggestion; see Steven Shapin, "At the Amsterdam," *London Review of Books*, Vol. 28, no. 8 (April 20, 2006), https://www.lrb.co.uk/the-paper/v28/n08/steven-shapin/at-the-amsterdam (accessed August 25, 2023).
38. Nataliia Viacheslavovna Apchinskaia, "Khudozhnik Aleksandr Volkov, 'Granatovaia Chaikhana,' 1924 g., Gosudarstvennaia Tret'iakovskaia Galereia," *Art-Reliz.rf*, арт-релиз.рф/2014/08/26/Художник-АЛЕКСАНДР-ВОЛКОВ-ГРАНАТОВА/ (accessed August 14, 2023).
39. Volkov poem, cited in Apchinskaia, "Khudozhnik Aleksandr Volkov."
40. Sigizmund Krzhizhanovskii, "Salyr-Giul'," in *Sobranie sochinenii v piati tomakh*, vol. 3, ed. Vadim Perel'muter (Moscow: Symposium, 2003), 377–78.
41. O'zMDA f. 34, op. 1, d. 1998, l. 33.
42. L. S-v., "Vnimanie krasnym chaikhanam," *Pravda Vostoka*, October 2, 1925, 3.
43. *Qizil Choyxona*, Trans. Rauf Yaqubov (Tashkent: O'rta Osiyo Kasabalar Byurosi, 1927), 3.
44. Spravochnik, "SSSR po raionam: Sredne-Aziatskie respubliki," eds. M. B. Vol'f and G. A. Mebus (Moscow: Gosudarstvennoe izdatel'stvo, 1927), 37n1.
45. In Uzbekistan, it appears Houses of Culture were also called kul'tbazas; see the identical figures for 1933 cited in O'zMDA f. 94, op. 5, d. 1077, l. 3 and O'zMDA f. 94, op. 5, d. 1219, l. 23. Houses of Culture seem to have functioned similarly throughout Central Asia; for further information on their operation, see İğmen, *Speaking Soviet with an Accent*. On worker's clubs in the metropole, see Richard Stites, *Revolutionary Dreams: Utopian Vision and Experimental Life in the Russian Revolution* (New York: Oxford University Press, 1989), 110–12, 203. A high proportion of urban worker's clubs in Uzbekistan were dedicated to members of non-titular nationalities, or for workers in industries dominated by Europeans, such as the railroad. See the 1935 statistics in O'zMDA f. 94, op. 5, d. 1787, ll. 1–36.
46. This is based on the January 1936 survey of Uzbekistan's "club-type institutions," including Red Teahouses, in O'zMDA f. 94, op. 5, d. 1567.
47. For the most thorough exposition of the work of an early Red Teahouse, see the resolution on teahouses in O'zMDA f. 86, op. 1, d. 4106, ll. 34–7.
48. *Qizil Choyxona*, 1927, 8–9.
49. See the description in Abdulla Qahhor's novel: Abdulla Qahhor, *Sarob* (Tashkent: O'zdavnashr, 1937), 99–118.
50. On the periodical press at Red Teahouses, see RGASPI F. 62, op. 2, d. 2445, l. 46 ob.
51. *Qizil Choyxona*, 1927, 10–11. Such markings can still be found in some library editions of early Soviet newspapers.
52. See, for example, the discussion of radio programming in RGASPI f. M-63, op. 1, d. 108, l. 31, August 16, 1931); f. 62, op. 2, d. 2720, ll. 1–21.
53. *Qizil Choyxona*, 1927, 16.
54. Walter Benjamin, *Illuminations*, 265, cited in Benedict Anderson, *Imagined Communities: Reflections on the Origin and Spread of Nationalism* (New York: Verso, 2006), 24.
55. The former two items are composites, but the tax-evading "black" teahouse owner can be found in "Nalogini to'lamagani uchun," *Qizil O'zbekiston*, April 14, 1931, 4.
56. RGASPI f. 62, op. 2, d. 3211, ll. 88–91.

57. Strong, *Red Star in Samarkand*, 145.
58. RGASPI f. 62, op. 2, d. 1957, l. 1; RGASPI f. 62, op. 2, d. 2437, l. 7; "'Boy bo'lingiz' shiori bilan 'kolxozchilarni davlatli qilish' shiori o'rtasida qanday farq bor," *Yosh Leninchi*, June 4, 1934, 2.
59. RGASPI f. 62, op. 2, d. 2482, l. 48 (bulletin for cultural propaganda workers).
60. *Qizil Choyxona*, 1927, 12.
61. Unfortunately, the file with statistics on circles at Red Teahouses and clubs seems to have been trimmed by an overzealous archivist, leaving more than half of the pages without full statistics. In making these claims about the popularity of different types of clubs, I have assumed that the stack of reports that remains intact is representative. See O'zMDA f. 94, op. 5, d. 1567. While musical circles were more common than educational (literacy) circles, the educational circles generally had larger numbers of participants.
62. "Qulub qizil choyxonalar haqida," *Yosh Leninchi*, May 12, 1930, 4.
63. On literary representations of *shefstvo* in 1920s Central Asia, see R. N. Shigabdinov, "Shefskoe dvizhenie v Uzbekistane v literature 20-x godov," *Obshchestvennye nauki v Uzbekistane*, no. 12 (1990): 44–5.
64. A. Khushbekov, *Iz istorii kul'turnogo stroitel'stva v Uzbekistane v gody pervoi piatiletki* (Samarkand: Sredneaziatskii gosudarstvennyi universitet imeni Lenina, 1959), 70.
65. B. Sattor, "Aniqlangan kamchiliklar yo'qotilsin," *Yosh Leninchi*, March 30, 1933, 4.
66. Rasul Karim, "'Yosh Leninchi' ismiga qizil choyxona," *Yosh Leninchi*, April 22, 1932, 2.
67. See, for example, T. Muratov, "Pskent choyxonalari komsomol otaligiga muhtoj," *Yosh Leninchi*, July 9, 1934, 4; J. G., "'Udarnik' sovxoz komsomoli qizil choyxonalardan uzoq," *Yosh Leninchi*, June 22, 1934, 4.
68. RGASPI f. M-63, op.1, d. 257, l. 22 (Komsomol secretariat meeting protocol).
69. "Qizil choyxonalar malakali kadrlar talab qiladi," *Yosh Leninchi*, June 8, 1933, 2.
70. S. Normurzayev, "Namunali choyxona," *Yosh Leninchi*, June 27, 1934, 4; S. Gadoyboyev, Sulaymanov, "Namunali choyxona," *Yosh Leninchi*, July 9, 1934, 4; Abdullo Xalilov, "Namunali choyxona," *Yosh Leninchi*, December 3, 1935; Xoltoy Isaev and Qurbon Oripov. "Madaniy xizmat kuchaytirildi," *Yosh Leninchi*, May 8, 1936, 4.
71. Y. Hamdamov, "Namunali choyxona," *Yosh Leninchi*, November 10, 1935, 4.
72. "Namunali choyxona," *Yosh Leninchi*, November 2, 1937, 4.
73. Vera Dunham, *In Stalin's Time: Middleclass Values in Soviet Fiction* (Durham: Duke University Press, 1990). For a concise description of the concept of "culturedness," see "Kul'turnost'," from *Constructing Russian Culture in the Age of Revolution, 1881–1940*, eds. Catriona Kelly and David Shepherd. Oxford: Oxford University Press, 1998, 293–313.
74. O'zMDA f. 94, op. 5, d. 2701, l. 6a.
75. Ibid., l. 32.
76. Ibid., ll. 7–8.
77. Indeed, it appears that some particularly well-appointed teahouses were "upgraded" to clubs; at least in part, this probably accounts for the reduction in number of Red Teahouses in the late 1930s, while the number of clubs continued to rise. "Eng ozoda va namunali choyxonaga ega bo'laylik," *Yosh Leninchi*, January 5, 1934, 4. See the descriptions of ideal teahouse and club activities in O'zMDA f. 94, op. 5, d. 1785, ll. 7–7 ob.
78. Jurgenev and Kotiboyev, "Butun rayon va shahar maoriflariga," *Madaniy Inqilob*, February 23, 1933, 2.
79. Xaltay Isaev and Qurbon Oripov, "Madaniy xizmat kuchaytirildi," *Yosh Leninchi*, May 8, 1936, 4.
80. Vaxobjon, "Kultbaza mudiri choyxonalar ustidan tomoshabinmi?" *Yosh Leninchi*, January 26, 1934, 4.
81. O'zMDA f. 94, op. 5, d. 1787, ll. 41–5.
82. O'zMDA f. 94, op. 5, d. 1219, l. 19.
83. O'zMDA f. 94, op. 5, d. 2701, l. 36. This inaugurated the ascendancy of the House of Culture as the dominant cultural institution in Central Asia, rather than the teahouse, which eventually reverted to its role as a space for masculine sociability.
84. Although it was couched in Soviet ideological terms, this dynamic reflects the dynamics of authoritarian mass publicity across both liberal and nonliberal contexts. William Mazzarella shows that the logic of state censorship in India depends on an assumption of "immaturity" among the public. At the core of this assumption is a discursive figure whom Mazzarella terms the "pissing man," the type of man that Indian censors insist require censorship in order to maintain their moral continence. The figure of the "pissing man" represents "the attribution to Indian publics of an excessive permeability to affective appeals and its presumed corollary, an underdeveloped political rationality." William Mazzarella, *Censorium: Cinema and the Open Edge of Mass Publicity* (Durham: Duke UP, 2013), 12.

85. On the origins of the workers' correspondent movement in 1920s Russia, and the efforts to reform it in the late 1920s and early 1930s, see Michael S. Gorham, "Tongue-Tied Writers: The Rabsel'kor Movement and the Voice of the 'New Intelligentsia' in Early Soviet Russia," *The Russian Review*, no. 3 (1996): 412–29; Asaoka, "Nikolai Bukharin and the Rabsel'kor movement," from Yasuhiro Matsui, ed., *Obshchestvennost' and Civic Agency*, 82–108. Gorham notes that by the late 1920s, worker correspondents came increasingly under Party supervision. A 1931 Party directive on workers' correspondents called them "commanders of proletarian public opinion" (*komandiry proletarskogo obshchestvennogo mneniia*). The same directive argued that in the past, worker correspondents had primarily focused on critiquing inadequacies in Soviet life, but in the new period of socialist construction, they should turn toward showing "achievements and victories" as well. This part of the directive was little observed in Central Asian teahouse reports, which tended to focus on the negative. See "O perestroike rabsel'korovskogo dvizheniia," from *Direktivy VKP(b) po voprosam prosveshcheniia*, eds. A. Ia. Podzemskii, I. D. Davydov, and I. G. Klabunovskii (Moscow: OGIZ, 1931), 477.
86. "Kruzhok kerak - kruzhok." *Muxbirlar Yo'ldoshi*, 1930 (no.1), last page.
87. These cadres are discussed most extensively in Sergei Abashin's historical ethnography of Oshoba, an Uzbek village in Tajikistan. See S. N. Abashin, *Sovetskii kishlak: Mezhdu kolonializmom i modernizatsiei* (Moskva: Novoe literaturnoe obozrenie, 2015), 265–80.
88. Abashin, *Sovetskii kishlak*, 274.
89. Kassymbekova, *Despite Cultures*, 178.
90. See, for example, Dada Sultoniy, "Ishchi dehqon muxbirlari nohaq hujumdan saqlansin," *Rubilar Yo'ldoshi*, 1930 (no. 5–6), 37–8.
91. Sobir Abdulla, "O'tmas teshalar," *Muxbirlar Yo'ldoshi*, 1930 (no. 5–6), 31–4.
92. In theory, worker's correspondent's reports were supposed to trigger prosecution for crimes, although in many cases such prosecutions did not materialize; see Kassymbekova, *Despite Cultures*, 166–67.
93. In Abdugafurova's analysis, nineteenth-century female poet Anbar Otin reappropriated the term "black," which was usually pejorative. See Donohon Abdugafurova, "'I Was Born in the Wrong Time': The Concept of Selfhood in the Writings of Anbar Otin," *Journal of Islamic and Muslim Studies*, 4, no. 1 (2019): 66–86.
94. For the use of the term "white-boned" in Soviet and post-Soviet Tajikistan, see Roberts, *Old Elites under Communism*, 45. This stratification likely derived from the Mongol-era distinction between "white" nobility and "black" (*qarachu*) commoners. See Christopher Pratt Atwood, *Encyclopedia of Mongolia and the Mongol Empire* (New York: Facts On File, 2004), 505–6.
95. On the often-hidden continuities between pre-Soviet "whites" and Soviet-era "Reds," see Roberts, "Old Elites under Communism."
96. O'zMDA f. 34, op. 1, d. 1998, ll. 32–46.
97. On the tax-exempt status of Red Teahouses by the late 1920s, see O'zMDA f. 86, op. 1, d. 4106, l. 37.
98. *Qizil Choyxona*, 1927, 4.
99. Aminov, "Choyxonalarning vazifasi faqat choy sotish emas," *Yosh Leninchi*, January 26, 1934, 4.
100. Bolg'a, "Savdogar Shamsiev - choyxona mudiri," *Yosh Leninchi*, June 27, 1934, 4.
101. "Qizil choyxona - isropchilar qo'lida," *Yosh Leninchi*, June 24, 1933, 2.
102. "Toshkent qizil choyxonalariga bir nazar," *Madaniy Inqilob*, March 23, 1933, 1.
103. P. Qaynar, "Choyxona mudiri chayqovchi," *Yangi Farg'ona*, October 14, 1935, 4.
104. "Mudirlik qilsinmi, sartaroshlik?" *Yosh Leninchi*, June 8, 1933, 2. On barbers and teahouses in pre-Soviet Central Asia, see Schuyler, *Turkistan*, 180.
105. "Madaniy-maorif markazlari qaytadan qurilish talabiga javob bersin," *Yosh Leninchi*, April 23, 1930, 4.
106. "Faqat choyxo'rliq emas," *Yosh Leninchi*, March 23, 1933, 4.
107. "G'ijduvon choyxonalari gapxonliq makoni bo'lmasin," *Yosh Leninchi*, June 8, 1933, 2.
108. Normat Rajabiy, "Yangi Yo'l choyxonalari talabga javob berarlik emas," *Yosh Leninchi*, June 10, 1934, 4.
109. H. Ermatov, "Men qizil choyxona mudiriman," *Yosh Leninchi*, January 15, 1934, 2.
110. "Qizil choyxona - isropchilar qo'lida," *Yosh Leninchi*, June 24, 1933, 2.
111. Sayohatchi, "Dumda qolgan choyxona," *Yosh Leninchi*, October 28, 1935, 4.
112. "Madaniy bazalarning xizmati joyida bo'lsin," *Yosh Leninchi*, May 9, 1933, 2.
113. Anvarov, "Otalik amalda bo'lsin," *Yosh Leninchi*, June 14, 1934, 4.
114. RGASPI F. 62, op. 2, d. 2913, l. 40.
115. RGASPI F. 62, op. 2, d. 3211, ll. 88–91.
116. RGASPI F. M-1, op. 23, d. 835a, l. 166.

117. For examples, see Begmatov, "Tashlandiq choyxona," *Yosh Leninchi*, June 14, 1934, 4; "Qizil choyxonalar ko'klam xizmatiga," *Yosh Leninchi*, March 6, 1933, 3.
118. Shermatov, "Qo'qon shaharqomi choyxonalar ishi bilan bog'lansin," *Yosh Leninchi*, February 17, 1934, 4.
119. M. Rajabiy, "Gazetalar o'tin o'rniga yoqilmoqda," *Yosh Leninchi*, June 29, 1933, 2.
120. "Toshkent qizil choyxonolariga bir nazar," *Madaniy Inqilob*, March 23, 1933, 1.
121. Ibid.
122. J. Qo'ldashev, "Zararli kayfiyatlar," *Qizil O'zbekiston*, April 10, 1937, 3.
123. RGASPI f. 62, op. 2, d. 3199, l. 114.
124. Ibid., l. 118, 122.
125. Ibid; Farhod Muradov, "Piskentda qizil choyxonalar vazifasi ko'knorixonaliq vazifasiga o'taydi," *Yosh Leninchi*, January 26, 1934, 4; P. Qaynar, "Choyxona mudiri chayqovchi," *Yangi Farg'ona*, October 14, 1935, 4.
126. G'ofurov, "Choyxonami, nashaxonami?" *Yosh Leninchi*, November 28, 1935, 4.
127. P. Qaynar, "Choyxona mudiri chayqovchi," *Yangi Farg'ona*, October 14, 1935, 4. On drug house at teahouses in early Soviet Tajikistan, see Alisher Latypov, "Choikhonai Surkh: The Replacement of 'Opium Dens' with Red Teahouses and the Limits of the Soviet Enlightenment Project in Tajikistan," *Central Asian Affairs*, 7, no. 3 (September 2020): 236–66, https://doi.org/10.30965/22142290-bja10003.
128. Socially smoking tobacco, cannabis, and opium was a widespread practice across Central Asia and Iran in the early modern and modern periods. See Matthee, *The Pursuit of Pleasure*. On teahouses and narcotics in Soviet Central Asia from a public health perspective, see Latypov, "Choikhonai Surkh."
129. *Qizil Choyxona*, 1927, 15–16.
130. "Chilimni qizil choyxonadan chiqarib tashlash qo'rqinchlidir." Ibid., 15.
131. Alcohol consumption was historically widespread in the Islamic world: for example, Rudi Matthee discusses Iranian wine culture in *Pursuit of Pleasure*. However, when they referred to a specific type of alcohol, newspaper reports usually discussed vodka (*aroq*).
132. Shermatov, "Qo'qon shaharqomi choyxonalar ishi bilan bog'lansin," *Yosh Leninchi*, February 17, 1934, 4.
133. M. R., Sh. G, "Akbarovning mehmonxonasiga aylandi," *Yosh Leninchi*, May 24, 1934, 2; Jo'ra Olim, "Nomiga qizil choyxona," *Yosh Leninchi*, May 24, 1934, 2.
134. G'ofurov, "Choyxonami, nashaxonami?" *Yosh Leninchi*, November 28, 1935, 4.
135. T. Boltoyev, "Xorazm choyxonalarida nima gap," *Yosh Leninchi*, March 6, 1933, 3.
136. An interesting example of the Red Teahouse as a site of antireligious agitation in the Nabi Ganiev film *Ramazan* is discussed in Cloé Drieu, *Cinema, Nation, and Empire in Uzbekistan, 1919–1937* (Bloomington: Indiana University Press, 2019), 170–72.
137. "Ro'za va hayitlar, sosializm ishlariga katta to'suqdir," *Qizil O'zbekiston*, January 8, 1931, 4; RGASPI f. M-63, op. 1, d. 106, ll. 1–3.
138. See, for example, the Komsomol and rabfak officials described in Komsomolets, "Ommaviy ish o'rniga choy ichadilar," *Yosh Leninchi*, June 20, 1935, 3.
139. This reflects a common dynamic also in the Middle East, as discussed in Chapter 5; see Amin, *The Making of the Modern Iranian Woman*.
140. As Mazzarella notes with respect to twenty-first-century India, "women are under the care of men and thus, as it were, private even in public." Mazzarella, *Censorium*, 15.
141. Fannina W. Halle, *Women in the Soviet East* (New York: E.P. Dutton, 1938), 193–94. Emphasis original. The precise location of the episode is unclear; it mentions *auls* and "Kirghiz" horses, so it is possible the episode took place in Kyrgyzstan. However, sedentary teahouse culture in Central Asia was fairly uniform across the entire region, so the situation Halle describes applies to Uzbekistan as well.
142. "Qulub qizil choyxonalar haqida," *Yosh Leninchi*, May 12, 1930, 4.
143. A. Muhamatjonov, "Komsomollar qizil choyxona ishidan bir chetda," *Yosh Leninchi*, March 6, 1933, 3; see another report of neglected furniture in "Madaniy-maorif markazlari qaytadan qurulish talabiga javob bersin," *Yosh Leninchi*, April 23, 1930, 4.

Chapter 2

1. "O'zbekiston sovet yozuvchilari soyuzida," *Qizil O'zbekiston*, November 17, 1937, 4.
2. RGALI f. 631, op. 6, d. 246, ll. 95–7.
3. Most primary sources refer to Oydin by her pen name, Oydin, and her male colleagues by their family names (hence Qahhor, not Abdulla); I follow that practice in this chapter.

4. The "shadow public" of the Writers' Union inner circle might productively be compared to Yurchak's concept of the "deterritorialized publics" of late Soviet society, self-organized but existing neither in a relation of "explicit support" or "explicit opposition" to the state. In the case of early Soviet Central Asia, however, we might argue that official discourse had yet to be formulated, let alone ossified in the way that facilitated "deterritorialization." We might thus call the Writers' Union's public a kind of "preterritorialized public," taking shape as official discourse was still under construction. See Yurchak, *Everything Was Forever*, 116–17.
5. Irina Gigova, "In Defense of Native Literature: Writers' Associations, State and the Cult of the Writer in Pre-1945 Bulgaria," *Slavic Review*, 77, no. 2 (2018): 420.
6. Ibid., 417. On "national indifference," see Tara Zahra, "Imagined Noncommunities: National Indifference as a Category of Analysis," *Slavic Review*, 69, no. 1 (2010): 93–119.
7. "O perestroike khudozhestvenno-literaturnykh organizatsii," in *Mezhdu molotom i nakoval'niei: Soiuz sovetskikh pisatelei SSSR. Dokumenty i kommentarii*, Vol. 1, ed. T. M. Goriaeva et al. (Moscow: ROSSPEN, 2010). Unpublished translation by Robert Bird.
8. Ibid.
9. Edward Allworth, *Uzbek Literary Politics* (The Hague: Mouton, 1964), 140.
10. Allworth, *Uzbek Literary Politics*; Naim Karimov, *XX asr adabiyoti manzaralari* (Toshkent: O'zbekiston, 2008); Khalid, *Making Uzbekistan*.
11. For the cleric speaking on behalf of unveiling, see RGASPI f. 62, op. 2, d. 1811, l. 99.
12. Allworth, *Uzbek Literary Politics*, 136.
13. Ingeborg Baldauf, "Educating the Poets and Fostering Uzbek Poetry of the 1910s to Early 1930s," *Cahiers d'Asie Centrale*, no. 24 (2015): 201.
14. Khalid, *Making Uzbekistan*, 380.
15. Alexander Morrison, *Russian Rule in Samarkand* (Oxford: Oxford University Press, 2008), 173–200.
16. For a full description of this episode, see Khalid, *Making Uzbekistan*, 62–5.
17. Bergne, *The Birth of Tajikistan*, 77.
18. On Ayni's role in establishing a Tajik literary canon, see Samuel Hodgkin, "Soviet Persian Anthologies: Transnational, Multinational, International," *Iranian Studies*, 55, no. 3 (July 2022): 631–51.
19. On the cartoonist, see "Khudozhnik-Mikhail Reikh," https://fantlab.ru/art3480 (accessed September 13, 2023).
20. Sheila Fitzpatrick, "Stalin and the Making of a New Elite, 1928–1939," *Slavic Review*, 38, no. 3 (1979): 377–402.
21. I. K. Luppol, M. M. Rozental', and S. M. Tret'iakov, eds., *Pervyi vsesoiuznyi s'ezd sovetskikh pisatelei, 1934: stenograficheskii otchet* (Moscow: Gosudarstvennoe izdatel'stvo "Khudozhestvennaia literatura," 1934), 533.
22. Bruce Grant, *The Captive and the Gift: Cultural Histories of Sovereignty in Russia and the Caucasus* (Cornell University Press, 2016).
23. "Sasanians" is likely an error of transcription or transliteration; Ayni probably said, or meant to say, "Samanids," since the Sasanian Empire predated the Arab conquests of Central Asia.
24. On the formulation of an Iranian national history in the interwar years, see Farzin Vejdani, *Making History in Iran: Education, Nationalism, and Print Culture* (Stanford, CA: Stanford University Press, 2015).
25. Ayni may here be implicitly making a Tajik claim for Bukhara, which was a hotly contested city during the national delimitation.
26. On this topic, see Samuel Hodgkin, *Persianate Verse and the Poetics of Eastern Internationalism* (Cambridge, UK: Cambridge University Press, 2024).
27. On the Persianate cosmopolis, see Pickett, *Polymaths of Islam*.
28. Pickett, *Polymaths of Islam*, 76.
29. See Roberts, "Old Elites under Communism," 290–92.
30. The process of nationalizing and institutionalizing literature exemplified here for Transoxania parallels a broader trajectory in literary politics throughout the Persianate world, which has been traced in the context of Afghanistan, Iran, and Turkey by Alexander Jabbari, *The Making of Persianate Modernity: Language and Literary History between Iran and India*, (Cambridge, UK: Cambridge University Press, 2023); Aria Fani, *Reading across Borders: Afghans, Iranians, and Literary Nationalism* (Austin, TX: University of Texas Press, 2024); Nergis Ertürk, *Grammatology and Literary Modernity in Turkey* (Oxford: Oxford University Press, 2011); Wali Ahmadi, "The Institution of Persian Literature and the Genealogy of Bahar's 'Stylistics,'" *British Journal of Middle Eastern Studies*, 31, no. 2 (2004): 152.

31. Ayni died a natural death in Dushanbe. See K. Hitchins, "'Aynī, Ṣadr-al-dīn," Encyclopedia Iranica, III/2, 144–9; available online at http://www.iranicaonline.org/articles/ayni-sadr-al-din (accessed December 13, 2023).
32. Hodgkin, *Persianate Verse and the Poetics of Eastern Internationalism.*
33. The announcement about the capital transfer, dated August 17, 1930, is held at O'zMDA and has been published by the "Old Tashkent" Telegram channel at https://t.me/oldtashkent_1/905. Unfortunately, I have been unable to access the original archival document.
34. Bergne, *The Birth of Tajikistan*, 49–52. Arne Haugen argues that the decision to allocate Tashkent to Uzbekistan represented a rare central intervention in the otherwise regionally controlled process of national delimitation, and suggests that the decision reflected the central Soviet authorities' concern that the less firmly controlled republic of Uzbekistan, with its pivotal agrarian regions, stay under the strong administrative supervision that was established in Tashkent; see Arne Haugen, *The Establishment of National Republics in Soviet Central Asia* (New York: Palgrave Macmillan, 2003), 200.
35. A significant exception to Uzbekistan's successful appropriation of Tashkent, Bukhara, Samarkand, and Kokand is its transfer of Khujand to Tajikistan; see Bergne, *The Birth of Tajkistan*, 104.
36. Beginning in 1930, many "Tajik" writers had been relocating to Dushanbe, the center of the new-found Tajik literature. See Flora Roberts, "City on Paper: Writing Tajik in Stalinobod (1930–38)," in *Old Elites under Communism*, chapter 5, 290–359. Bergne points out that Dushanbe was considered a "hardship posting," and some of those residents who refused to register as Uzbeks were threatened with deportation to Tajikistan: Bergne, *The Birth of Tajikistan*, 58.
37. Fozil Tojiy. "So'z yosh yozuvchilar ustida." *Yosh Leninchi*, August 27, 1933, 2.
38. This trend seems to have held in the minority sections of the Writers' Union. Thomas Loy points out that the Judeo-Tajik section apologized in its Writers' Union anthology for being overly Tashkent-centric, despite the fact that Judeo-Tajik culture was historically centered in Bukhara. See Thomas Loy. "Rise and Fall: Bukharan Jewish Literature of the 1920s and 1930s," in *Iranian Languages and Literatures of Central Asia: From the Eighteenth Century to the Present*, ed. M. De Chiara (Paris: Peeters, 2015), 307–36, 321.
39. "Vakillar qurultoy minbarida," *Yosh Leninchi*, March 10, 1934, 4; O'zMDA f. 2356, op. 1, d. 4, ll. 24–5; O'zMDA f. 2356, op. 1, d. 5, l. 88.
40. "Tarqalib ketgan tashkilot," *Qizil O'zbekiston*, March 4, 1934, 3.
41. RGALI f. 631, op. 6, d. 199, l. 19. Although this is a purge-era document and must be taken with a grain of salt, this claim is plausible given that, indeed, very few regional submissions made it to central publications during the mid-1930s.
42. Fozil Tojiy, "So'z yosh yozuvchilar ustida," Part II, *Yosh Leninchi*, August 27, 1933, 2.
43. Fozil Tojiy, "So'z yosh yozuvchilar ustida," Part III, *Yosh Leninchi*, August 28, 1933, 2. There was, however, more opportunity for young aspiring writers to publish in regional or non-specialized publications. For example, in an otherwise negative report on her local literary circle, one young woman from Andijan province remarked that she had been able to publish one of her poems in the Ferghana Valley newspaper *The Cotton Front* (*Paxta Fronti*). See "Adabiy to'garaklarga chiniqqan kishilar qo'yilishi kerak," *Yosh Leninchi*, March 9, 1934, 3.
44. O'zMDA f. 2356, op. 1, d. 3.
45. The neglect of Andijan appears to have lasted until 1937, when it was marshaled (spuriously) as evidence of an anti-Soviet conspiracy. See RGALI f. 631, op. 6, d. 199, l. 31.
46. Ismoil Akram, "Samarqand tashkilotini namunali tashkilot qilamiz," *Qizil O'zbekiston*, March 11, 1934, 5.
47. O'zMDA f. 2356, op. 1, d. 19, l. 8.
48. O'zMDA f. 2356, op. 1, d. 19, l. 5.
49. See, for example, the woman poets Nodira and Uvaysiy, both attached to the Khoqand court: Nurten Kılıç-Schubel, "Writing Women: Women's Poetry and Literary Networks in Nineteenth-Century Central Asia," in *Horizons of the World: Festschrift for Isenbike Togan*, ed. Nurten Kılıç-Schubel and Evrim Bimbaş (İstanbul: İthakı, 2011), 405–42.
50. O'zMDA f. 2356, op. 1, d. 5, l. 75. The non-Russian writers included Oydin, Abdulla Qodiriy, Ziyo Said, G'ofur Gulom, Ahmed Okhundiy (Akhundov), A. Saraev, Josur Zokirov, Hamid Olimjon, Pazir Safarov, Husayn Shams, R. Israilov, Giyas Sagatov, Umarjon Ismailov, Hasan Po'lat, Uyg'un, Anqaboy, Komil Yashin, R. Majidiy, Nosir Saidov, Abdullaev, Nigmatullaev, Elbek, Oybek, and Abdulla Qahhor. Six representatives were sent to the organizational committee meeting of the Writers Union in August 1932—including Ayni and Oydin. The other representatives were Alekseev, Majidi, Ismailov, and Ghafur Ghulam.

51. Ishankhodzhaeva argues that these benefits both incentivized cooperation with the Soviet regime's priorities, including whitewashing the repressions, and cultivated authors that made "significant contributions" to Uzbek national literature. See Ishankhodzhaeva, "Ideologizatsiia literatury i iskusstva Uzbekistana i repressii v etoi sfere v 1925–1950," in "Repressivnaia politika," ch. 4, especially 217–70.
52. O'zMDA f. 2356, op. 1, d. 11, l. 24.
53. Likewise, Khalid suggests that many former Jadids survived the 1929–30 purge due to patronage from Xo'jayev. See Khalid, *Making Uzbekistan*, 380.
54. For the rest of the Soviet Union, see John and Carol Garrard, *Inside the Soviet Writers' Union* (New York: Free Press, 1990).
55. The language of "engineers of human souls," which circulated widely during the 1930s as an epithet for Soviet writers, has been attributed to Joseph Stalin, although it may have originated with writer Iuri Olesha. For a foundational citation of the phrase, see A. A. Zhdanov, Speech at the First Congress of the Writers Union, *Pervyi Vsesoiuznyi s'ezd sovetskikh pisatelei, 1934: stenograficheskii otchet*, 4.
56. Abdulla Qahhor, *O'tmishdan Ertaklar* (Tashkent: Yosh Gvardiya, 1976), 129–42.
57. Abdulla Kakhkhar, *Skazki o bylom*, trans. Konstantin Simonov (Moscow: Khudozhestvennaia literatura, 1987), 243.
58. Qahhor's father claimed he had learned to read "in a dream." See Abdulla Qahhor,"Ozgina o'zim haqimda," in Ozod Sharafiddinov, *Abdulla Qahhor. Adabiy va ijodiy faoliyati haqida lavhalar* (Tashkent: Yosh Gvardiya, 1988), 249–55.
59. Ibid.
60. For more detail on the Houses of Knowledge and their activities, see Kamp, *The New Woman*, 2006, pp. 86–8 and p. 293. On Hamza's career in the 1920s, see Khalid, *Making Uzbekistan*, pp. 189–90.
61. I have been unable to determine whether Qahhor ever became a member of Uzbekistan's chapter of APP. For a more extensive discussion of Qahhor's early publications, see N. Iakubov, *Publitsisticheskaia deiatel'nost' Abdully Kakhkhara: avtoreferat dissertatsii* (Tashkent: TashGU, 1970); and V. Smirnova, "Abdulla Kakhkhar iz ferganskoi doliny," *Druzhba Narodov*, no. 7 (1963): 258–68.
62. On the process of land reform in Uzbekistan, see Beatrice Penati, *Rural History of Soviet Central Asia: Land Reform and Agricultural Change in Early Soviet Uzbekistan* (Leiden: Brill, 2025).
63. Kh. B. Begmatov, "K voprosu o roli pechati v osushchestvlenii kul'turnoi revoliutsii v Uzbekistane," in *Trudy Samarkandskogo Gosudarstvennogo Universiteta Im. A. Navoi*, 121st ed. (Samarkand: Izdatel'stvo Samarkandsgogo gos. universiteta, 1963), 60, 50–67. Samarkand, 1963, p. 60.
64. RGASPI f. 62, op. 2, d. 1815, ll. 41–41 ob. For a full account of the "martyrdom" of Hamza, see Khalid, *Making Uzbekistan*, 351–52.
65. My discussion of prerevolutionary *gaps* draws on Khalid, *The Politics of Muslim Cultural Reform*, 96, 132. However, much more remains to be understood about this institution of Central Asian social life, which exists to this day.
66. Flora Roberts describes a *gap* from the same period (called, in her case, a *gashtak*) in Dushanbe, as a site in which men gathered in a home to eat pilaf, drink wine, and socialize. See Roberts, "Old Elites Under Communism," 318–19.
67. *Gapchi* denotes a "discusser" or "debater," or a participant in a *gap*. RGASPI F. 62, op. 2, d. 2199, ll. 2–14. This was not the only *gap* that was shut down at this moment—the employees of Narkompros in Uzbekistan were also said to have sponsored a counter-revolutionary *gap* of their own, named G'ayratlilar Uyushmasi. The "conspiracy" is also discussed in Khalid, *Making Uzbekistan*, 374–78.
68. "O'zbekistondagi butun proletar, sho'ra yozuvchi, adib, shoirlariga va rabochi, batrak, kambag'al kolxozchi muxbirlarga," *Alanga*, 1930, no. 7–8, 8.
69. This view is shared by Khalid; see *Making Uzbekistan*, 374.
70. "O'zbekistondagi butun proletar, sho'ra yozuvchi, adib, shoirlariga va rabochi, batrak, kambag'al kolxozchi muxbirlarga," *Alanga*, 1930, no. 7–8, 4.
71. On anti-colonialism in the early revolutionary years, see Khalid, *Making Uzbekistan*, 102–12.
72. As Adeeb Khalid notes, this purge followed a "script" that played out in most Soviet national republics in the same year. In fact, when it was denounced, Red Pen was explicitly associated with its supposed counterparts in, for example, Belarus (see Aleksandrovich, "Proletariat adabiyotining gegemoniyasi uchun," *Qizil O'zbekiston*, April 12, 1931, 3). There is no reason to believe there was any organized anti-Soviet resistance left in 1930, let alone a fully mobilized conspiracy to overthrow the government. But it is perfectly plausible that, in private, the Brave Debaters did

indeed articulate some of the anti-Soviet sentiments they were accused of harboring: critiques of land reform and the cotton monoculture, or speculations that Moscow was effectively colonizing Central Asia for its cotton revenues. For a more extensive treatment of the Qosimov purge, see Khalid, *Making Uzbekistan*, 373–78.

73. Dilbar Fayzieva, *Husayn Shams: adibning 70 yilligiga* (Tashkent: G'ofur G'ulom nomidagi Adabiyot va san'at nashriyoti, 1973). It is not surprising that one of Central Asia's first "proletarian" writers harkened from the ranks of typographers. Throughout the Russian Empire, typographers were at the forefront of labor organizing in the late imperial years; they were literate in much higher proportions than other industrial workers, and their access to publishing equipment empowered their organizing efforts. As Mark Steinberg has shown, typographers may be considered proletarians, but because they were literate by necessity, they occupied a different social position than other types of workers, such as manual laborers. On the role of printing workers in the development of a Russian revolutionary movement, see Mark Steinberg, *Moral Communities: The Culture of Class Relations in the Russian Printing Industry, 1867–1907* (Berkeley: University of California Press, 1992).
74. Most of the remaining writers described themselves as "white-collar workers" (*sluzhashchii*). The other "workers" were Hasan Po'lat (1911–42), born in the Middle Volga region and therefore likely a Tatar, but raised at an orphanage in Namangan; and G'ayratiy (1902–76), who appears to have been born to the family of a literate artisan and received part of his education at a new-method Jadid school. G'ayratiy's background is therefore more similar to Qahhor's than Shams's, and, like Qahhor, G'ayratiy continued his career into the post-Stalin years. He continues to be read and anthologized today. In contrast, like Shams, Hasan Po'lat has been largely forgotten since his death. See "Khasan Pulat," *Ziyouz*, http://www.ziyouz.uz/ru/uzbekskaya-literatura/55-literatura-sovetskogo-perioda-30-80-kh-xx-veka/878---1911–1942; http://www.ziyouz.com/index.php?option=com_content&task=view&id=103 (accessed December 13, 2023).
75. These works include, but are not limited to, *Radio (hikoya)*. (Tashkent: O'znashr, 1931); *Qurulush* (Tashkent: O'znashr, 1932); *Tanqid (p'esa)* (Tashkent: O'zdavnashr, 1932); *Hikoyalar* (Tashkent: O'zdavnashr, 1933); *Dushman* (Tashkent: O'zdavnashr, 1934); *Haqqoniyat* (Tashkent: O'zdavnashr, 1937).
76. Hamid Olimjon, "Adabiyotimizning tikka ko'tarilish davrida," 2.
77. Rahmat Majidiy, *Literatura Uzbekistana* (Khudozhestvennaia literatura, 1934), 20.
78. Adeeb Khalid identifies a new generation of cultural activists that came to prominence in the late 1920s, a cohort of radical "culture workers" (*madaniyatchi*) who tolerated little dissent. See Khalid, *Making Uzbekistan*, 326.
79. In 1928, TAPP was replaced by a chapter of SAPP, or the Central Asian Association of Proletarian Writers, but this seems to have entailed literal structural or ideological reorganization. See Karimov, *XX asr adabiyoti manzaralari*, 250.
80. Umarjon Ismailov. "Proletariat adabiyoti hegemoniyasi uchun," *Qizil O'zbekiston*, April 13, 1931, 3.
81. N. Karimov, *XX asr adabiyoti manzaralari*, 247. It is likely that the Uzbekistan chapter of Red Pen opened as part of the same initiative, although I have found no direct evidence that Uzbekistan's Red Pen was established under state tutelage. For a discussion of the literary production of Red Pen in Azerbaijan, see Leah Feldman, *On the Threshold of Eurasia: Revolutionary Poetics in the Caucasus* (Ithaca, NY: Cornell University Press, 2018), 176–207. On the Uzbekistan chapter, see Allworth, *Uzbek Literary Politics*, 117–26.
82. The reference is to the critical tone of much Jadid literature, especially prose. The implication is that in an age of socialist construction, critique is not enough: it is imperative also to laud the successes of the revolution.
83. Tohiriy, "Qizil Qalam majmuasi to'grisida." *Maorif va o'qituvchi*, 1929 (no. 9–10), 12–13. The publications of Red Pen are very difficult, if not impossible to access. They appear to have been destroyed after Red Pen was repudiated and are no longer held at most post-Soviet libraries. However, some of the writings of Red Pen were republished elsewhere; see, for example, the satirical poem mocking the refugees from Soviet land reform: "Qochoqlar," *Yosh Leninchi*, October 22, 1930, 4.
84. Khalid, *Making Uzbekistan*, 331–32.
85. Botu, "O'zbek adabiyotining oktabr inqilobidan so'nggi davriga bir qarash," *Alanga*, 1928 (no. 10–11), 3–4.
86. Concerns were raised first in April 1929, and the issue was deferred to a later meeting. In June, a commission of three men with Muslim names was delegated to investigate Qizil Qalam. One is the writer O'razay (in the file designated as Urazaev). The identity of the others is unclear. The APPO as a whole comprised mostly individuals of European background. See RGASPI F. 62, op. 2, d. 2007, ll. 34, 45, 45 ob.

87. Organizational bureau members included Ziyo Said, Uyg'un, Robita Ahmedjonova, Botu, O'razay, Shokir Suleymon, Oltoy, Hamid Olimjon, and Ilhomjon. See RGASPI f. 62, op. 2, d. 2007, l.58 ob.
88. "Adabiyot frontimizning proletar sog'lomligi uchun kurash," *Alanga*, 1930 (no. 7–8), 10–12; N. Muhitdinov, "'Milliy Ittihodchilar'ning madaniy frontdagi ishlari," *Alanga*, 1930 (no. 7–8), 13–21; Otajon, "O'zbek proletariat adabiyoti uchun kurashmoq kerak," *Alanga*, 1930 (no. 7–8), 30–4; Organizing Bureau of the Uzbekistan Association of Proletarian Writers, "O'zbekistondagi butun proletar, sho'ra yozuvchi, adib, shoirlariga va rabochi, batrak, kambag'al kolxozchi mux-birlarga," *Alanga*, 1930 (no. 7–8), 7–9.
89. Organizing Bureau of the Uzbekistan Association of Proletarian Writers, "O'zbekistondagi butun proletar, sho'ra yozuvchi, adib, shoirlariga va rabochi, batrak, kambag'al kolxozchi mux-birlarga," 8.
90. Fayzieva, *Husayn Shams*, 7.
91. Husayn Shams, "Chto nuzhno nachinaiushchemu pisateliu." *Literatura Srednei Azii*, January 16, 1934, 4.
92. For general biographical details, see Kamp, *The New Woman in Uzbekistan*, 101–3; Saidulla Mirzaev, *Oydin: Adabiy portret* (Tashkent: Badiiy adabiyot nashriyoti, 1965); Mashhura Sultonova, *O'zbek sovet adibalari* (Tashkent: "Qizil O'zbekiston," "Pravda Vostoka," and "O'zbekistoni Surkh" birlashgan nashriyoti va bosmaxonasi, 1963), 7–14; Zulfiya, *Oydin Sobirova* (Tashkent: O'zdavnashr, 1953).
93. Kamp, *The New Woman in Uzbekistan*, 101–3.
94. As happened throughout the Soviet Union, but especially in Central Asia, women frequently escaped purges that took their male relatives and colleagues. See Roberts, "Purging the Elite: Politics and Lineage (1931–38)," in *Old Elites*, chapter 4, 232–89.
95. For meeting protocols, see O'zMDA f. 2356, op. 1, d. 2a; O'zMDA f. 2356, op. 1, d. 28; RGALI f. 631, op. 6, d. 118.
96. See Zulfiya, *Oydin Sobirova*, 7–9.
97. For one evening event where Oydin was a lead speaker, see "Katta adabiy kecha o'tkazildi," *Yosh Leninchi*, May 1, 1932.
98. Oydin, "Adolatxonning brigadasi," *Yorqin Turmush*, 1936 (no. 3), 11; Oydin, "Sog'inganda," *Sovet adabiyoti*, 1936 (no. 3), 28; Oydin, "Surma ko'z," *Sovet adabiyoti*, 1935 (no. 3), 20; Oydin, "So'yunchi," *Yorqin Turmush*, 1936 (no. 2), 8–10.
99. Quoted in Zulfiya, *Oydin Sobirova*, 27.
100. RGASPI F. 62, op. 2, d. 2476, ll. 2–3. A literary circle at a girls' school is pictured in *Qurulish*, 1931 (no. 3), 49.
101. "SSSR sovet yozuvchilar soyuzining ustavi," *O'zbekiston sovet adabiyoti*, 1934 (no. 5), 7.
102. The practical work of learning to work in new genres—short stories, newspaper articles—had already been a priority in the late 1920s; see Anqaboy, *Xabar, maqola, she'r, hikoya yozish yo'llari* (Samarqand: O'zbekiston davlat nashriyoti, 1927).
103. "Adabiy to'garaklar uchun programma," *Sovet Adabiyoti*, 1935 (no. 1), 109–14. Prior to 1934, some efforts were made to create curricula, but none were as far-ranging or systematic as the curricula developed beginning in 1934. See, for example, O'zMDA f. 2356, op. 1, d. 7, which critiques an early curriculum by one Abdurahmon Sa'diy. The curriculum covered the eclectic mix of Gor'kii, Serafimovich, and Uyg'un, and the only surviving copy I have been able to find is in Russian. It was apparently distributed for use, but after it was critiqued for ideological inconsistency, it was supposed to be withdrawn from circulation. I have found no full Uzbek-language curricula for literary circles from before 1934.
104. Oydin, "Adabiy to'garaklar uchun qo'llanma," *Sovet Adabiyoti*, 1935 (no. 5), 55–67. The full speech is available in Rahmat Majidi, *Literatura Uzbekistana* (Khudozhestvennaia literatura, 1934).
105. "To'garaklar uchun programma," *Sovet Adabiyoti*, 1936 (no. 4), 84–94.
106. "Adabiy to'garaklar programmasi," *Sovet Adabiyoti*, 1936 (no. 5), 76–81.
107. Samuel Hodgkin, "Soviet Persian Anthologies: Transnational, Multinational, International," *Iranian Studies*, 55, no. 3 (July 2022): 631–51. Postwar Uzbek critics would construct a narrative of Uzbek literature that included nineteenth-century writers from the region, but in the 1930s this would have been too risky to attempt. See Allworth, *Uzbek Literary Politics*, 72. See also Ayni's article on Ferdowsi's *Shahnameh*, published in the same issue as the first program for literary circles: *Shahnameh*: Sadriddin Ayni, "Firdavsiy va uning Shahnamasi to'g'risida," *Sovet Adabiyoti*, 1935 (no. 1), 82–95.
108. Anqaboy, *Xabar, maqola, she'r va hikoya yozish yo'llari* (Samarqand: O'zbekiston davlat nashriyoti, 1927).

109. O'zMDA f. 94, op. 5, d. 1567. This archival file contains the most detailed statistics about cultural circles I have been able to find. However, a sizable chunk of the pages is cut off halfway, meaning that any statistics are provisional and depend on an assumption that the remaining pages are representative of the rest.
110. "Literaturnaia khronika," *Komsomolets vostoka*, May 26, 1934, 4. Some exemplary literary circles are also discussed in "Obraztsovymi kruzhkami vstretim s'ezd pisatelei," December 19, 1933, 3.
111. Khasanbaev, "Govoriat litkruzhkovtsy fabriki im. Khodzhaeva," *Literatura Srednei Azii*, January 16, 1934, 4.
112. RGALI f. 631, op. 6, d. 118, ll. 12–21.
113. The majority of the remainder was in Russian.
114. RGALI f. 631, op. 6, d. 118, ll. 4–11.
115. For the broader context of the Great Terror in Uzbekistan, including the arrests of Fayzulla Xo'jayev and Akmal Ikromov in July 1937, see Khalid, *Making Uzbekistan*, 384–88.
116. Wendy Z. Goldman, *Terror and Democracy in the Age of Stalin: The Social Dynamics of Repression* (New York: Cambridge University Press, 2007).
117. Gail Kligman and Katherine Verdery, *Peasants under Siege: The Collectivization of Romanian Agriculture, 1949–1962* (Princeton, NJ: Princeton University Press, 2011), 256–60.
118. RGALI f. 631, op. 6, d. 200.
119. "Toshkent sovet yozuvchilari yig'ilishi," *Qizil O'zbekiston*, April 12, 1937, 3.
120. RGALI f. 631, op. 6, d. 200, l, 52.
121. O'zMDA f. 2356, op. 1, d. 31.
122. The names of those shot and imprisoned in Uzbekistan and elsewhere in the Soviet Union during the Great Terror have been compiled by the Russian NGO Memorial: "Stalinskie rasstrel'nye spiski," http://stalin.memo.ru/regions/regi74.htm (accessed December 13, 2023).
123. The accusation appeared in a testimony by Umarjon Ismailov. RGALI f. 631, op. 6, d. 198, l. 139. It also seems to have been repeated by others; see O'zMDA f. 2356, op. 1, d. 31, l. 330.
124. O'zMDA f. 2356, op. 1, d. 31, l. 331.
125. She was expelled from the Writers' Union in October 1937 and cleared of the charges against her in March 1938. For her exclusion, see RGALI f. 631, p. 6, d. 198, l. 107. For her reinstatement, see RGALI f. 631, op. 6, d. 246, l. 58.
126. O'zMDA f. 2356, op. 1, d. 28, l. 18.
127. Already in 1933, a group of Party members preparing for the upcoming Convention of Soviet Writers had decried the "groupishness" (*gruppovschina*) of Tashkent's writers, although it is unclear whether they were referring to the Russian or Uzbek-speaking writers. See F. 62, op. 2, d. 3196, ll. 18–20. During the Great Purge, the first such accusation appeared in a letter from Literary Fund Secretary, the Russian Kol'tsov. See RGALI f. 631, op. 6, d. 198, ll. 124–29. The *dom otdykha* seems to have been opened in a town outside Tashkent in mid-1933. See "Adabiy khronika," *Yosh Leninchi*, June 18, 1933, 2.
128. RGALI f. 631, op. 6, d. 198, ll. 124–29.
129. Ibid., l. 124.
130. Ibid., l. 124.
131. Personal correspondence with Marianne Kamp, citing interview with Saodat Shamsieva, September 29, 2017. For further information on Saodat Shamsieva, see Marianne R. Kamp, "Three Lives of Saodat: Communist, Uzbek, Survivor," *The Oral History Review*, 28, no. 2 (2001): 21–58.
132. For one such accusation, see RGALI f. 631, op. 6, d. 198, ll. 131–39.
133. For example, see Shokir Sulaymon's defense in RGALI f. 631, op. 6, d. 199, ll. 43–45.
134. RGALI f. 631, op. 6, d. 199, l. 20.
135. These works include "Bizning Vatan," *Mosholo* 1934, no. 2, p. 15; "Diyorim! (O'zbekiston)," *Guliston*, 1935, no. 3, p. 39; "To'rt Xat," *Guliston*, 1935, no. 5, p. 8. All three works are blatantly patriotic, as if Cho'lpon is desperately trying to prove his loyalty to the regime.
136. RGALI f. 631, op. 6, d. 199, l. 26.
137. In addition to the above, see, for example, *Literatura Srednei Azii* "Obraztsovymi kruzhkami vstretim s'ezd pisatelei," December 18, 1933, 3.
138. "Sovet yozuvchilarining respublika kengashi," *Madaniy Inqilob*, October 17, 1937, p. 2. On Aziz Niallo, a Russian named Stanishevskii who wrote under a pseudonym, see Bakhtiyar M. Babajanov, "'Ulama-Orientalists," in *Reassessing Orientalism: Interlocking Orientologies during the Cold War*, eds. Michael Kemper and Artemy M. Kalinovsky (Abingdon: Routledge: 2015), 114n32.

139. RGALI f. 631, op. 6, d. 198, ll. 116–17; "O'zbekiston sovet yozuvchilari soyuzida," *Qizil O'zbekiston*, November 17, 1937, 4. The precise date of Oydin's exclusion is unclear, but I assume she was excluded in the fall with the others; her reinstatement was documented in March of the following year.
140. These attacks are referenced in O'zMDA f. 2356, op. 1, d. 37, l. 99.
141. The text of the petition and the claims from Sattorzoda are published in Isfandiyār Ādīnah, "Chigūnah Sadr al-Dīn Aynī az tirūr-i Istālīnī jān-i sālim bidar bird?," *BBC Persian*, April 16, 2016, https://www.bbc.com/persian/world/2016/04/160416_u04_how_eini_escaped (accessed February 27, 2025).
142. On the mutilated male body as a trope in socialist realist narrative, see Lilya Kaganovsky, *How the Soviet Man Was Unmade: Cultural Fantasy and Male Subjectivity under Stalin*, Pitt Series in Russian and East European Studies (Pittsburgh: University of Pittsburgh Press, 2008), 19–41.
143. O'zMDA f. 2356, op. 1, d. 37, l. 99.
144. O'zMDA f. 2356, op. 1, d. 37, l 94 (Olimjon and Shams), l. 98 (Oydin); RGALI f. 631, op. 6, d. 246, l. 62.
145. On the "class of '38" in Uzbek politics, see Donald S. Carlisle, "The Uzbek Power Elite: Politburo and Secretariat (1938–83)," *Central Asian Survey* 5, no. 3–4 (January 1986): 91–132.

Chapter 3

1. Fayzulla Xo'jaev, "O'zbekiston mehnatkashlarining turmushidan va ularning SSSR paxta mustaqilligi uchun va O'zbekistonning sosialistik qurilishi uchun kurashidan olingan badiiy asarlarga konkurs e'lon qilish to'g'risida," *Qizil O'zbekiston*, March 28, 1933, 2. The term *basmachi* was a catch-all used by Soviet authorities to refer to a heterogeneous set of armed opposition fighters throughout Central Asia. By the 1930s, the term was being applied to anyone who resisted collectivization. See Adeeb Khalid, *Central Asia: A New History from the Imperial Conquests to the Present* (Princeton: Princeton University Press, 2021), 160–61, 225.
2. Allworth, *Uzbek Literary Politics*; Evgeny Dobrenko, "Hegemony of Brotherhood: The Birth of Soviet Multinational Literature, 1922–1932," *Slavic Review* 81, no. 4 (2022): 869–90.
3. Kristen Fort has argued that Socialist Realism in Uzbekistan was a hybrid form, drawing on Central Asian poetic modes and linking them to Socialist Realist tropes. See Christopher James Fort, "Inhabiting Socialist Realism: Soviet Literature from the Edge of Empire" PhD. diss. (University of Michigan, 2019).
4. Alongside a range of other influences, Sharafiddinov suggests Qahhor may have been imitating *Martin Eden* by Jack London (48–9 of *Abdulla Qahhor*).
5. See O'razay, "Go'zal adabiyot sohasidagi vazifalarimiz haqida," *Alanga*, 1930, no. 1, 11.
6. Igal Halfin, Jochen Hellbeck, and others have shown ego-documents to be important venues for Soviet self-fashioning. When diarist Stepan Podlubny derides himself for his failure to sufficiently excise bad bourgeois habits, for example, Hellbeck argues that he is attempting to sculpt his flawed bourgeois self into a New Soviet Man. Igal Halfin examines the diary as a device for integrating the individual into a collective: "the life story of a singular and autonomous individual needed to be shattered and recreated as the story of a life lived for the sake of the proletarian movement." Thomas Lahusen, meanwhile, has examined one Socialist Realist novel, not as a "finished [aesthetic] product," but as part of a reflection of its author's ongoing process of self-fashioning. "Indeed," concludes Lahusen, quoting Fredric Jameson, "'people formed in a non-market non-consumer-consumptive society do not think like we do.'" According to the adherents of this approach, the entire Soviet system was devoted to creating a New Soviet Person with a new form of "Soviet subjectivity."

   The subjectivity school has offered insights into the experience of Soviet life, the construction of Soviet social categories, and the participatory nature of Soviet mobilization. Other scholars have critiqued the liberal preoccupations that continue to bedevil the adepts of the subjectivity school. Anna Krylova points out that dissimulation (as foregrounded in the totalitarian school) and sincerity (as emphasized by the subjectivity school) are two sides of the same coin, both positing the existence of a "stable and coherent Stalinist subject." Other scholars have gestured to the necessity of new methods that would move beyond liberal notions of subjectivity and more robustly theorize the Soviet collective. By framing my argument in terms of publicity rather than subjectivity, I bracket the questions of sincerity and authenticity, belief and resistance that continue to haunt the study of Soviet culture. If, as subjectivity scholars aver, the ultimate goal was for the subject to become integrated into a collective, then it is imperative that we understand the nature of that collective and how it functioned. See Jochen Hellbeck, *Revolution on My Mind: Writing a Diary under Stalin* (Cambridge, Mass.: Harvard University Press, 2006), especially chapter 4, "Secrets of a Class Enemy: Stepan Podlubny," 165–223. See also Igal Halfin and Jochen Hellbeck, "Rethinking the Stalinist Subject: Stephen Kotkin's 'Magnetic Mountain' and the State of Soviet Historical Studies," *Jahrbücher Für Geschichte Osteuropas*, 44, no. 3 (January 1, 1996): 456–63; Igal Halfin, *Red Autobiographies: Initiating the Bolshevik Self*, Donald W. Treadgold Studies on Russia, East Europe, and Central Asia (Seattle: Herbert J. Ellison Center for Russian, East European, and Central Asian Studies, University of Washington, 2011), 161. For an examination of the novel *Far from Moscow* as an effort to imagine and re-imagine socialism, see Thomas Lahusen, *How Life Writes the Book: Real Socialism and Socialist Realism in Stalin's Russia* (Ithaca, NY: Cornell University Press, 1997), 4. On the legacy of the subjectivity school in Soviet studies, see Sheila Fitzpatrick, "Revisionism in Retrospect: A Personal View," *Slavic Review*, 67, no. 3 (2008): 682–704; Anna Krylova. "The Tenacious Liberal Subject in Soviet Studies," *Kritika: Explorations in Russian and Eurasian History*, 1, no. 1 (2000), 145. On the need to theorize the collective, see Choi Chatterjee and Karen Petrone, "Models of Selfhood and Subjectivity: The Soviet Case in Historical Perspective," *Slavic Review*, no. 4 (2008): 980. See also the exchanges between Adeeb Khalid and Anna Krylova in Goswami, M., Hecht, G., Khalid, A., Krylova, A., Thompson, E. F., Zatlin, J. R., and Zimmerman, A. "AHR Conversation: History after the End of History: Reconceptualizing the Twentieth Century," *American Historical Review*, 121, no. 5 (2016): 1567–1607. For one influential effort to theorize the Soviet collective in Foucauldian terms, see Oleg Kharkhordin, *The Collective and the Individual in Russia: A Study of Practices* (Berkeley: University of California Press, 1999).

7. The classic study on the topic is Katerina Clark, *The Soviet Novel: History as Ritual* (Bloomington, IN: Indiana University Press, 2000).
8. M. M. Bakhtin, "Epic and Novel," in *The Dialogic Imagination*, ed. Michael Holquist, trans. Caryl Emerson and Michael Holquist (Austin: University of Texas Press, 2021), 3–40.
9. Georg Lukàcs, *The Theory of the Novel: A Historico-Philosophical Essay on the Forms of Great Epic Literature*, trans. Anna Bostock (MIT Press, 1971), 88.
10. Georg Lukács, *The Historical Novel*, trans. Hannah and Stanley Mitchell (London: Merlin Press, 1962).
11. Lukács, *The Historical Novel*, 347.
12. Ibid.
13. Clark, *The Soviet Novel*, 33–4.
14. "Rech' sekretaria TsK VKP(b) A. A. Zhdanova," in *Pervyi vsesoiuznyi s'ezd sovetskikh pisatelei, 1934: stenograficheskii otchet* (Moscow: Khudozhestvennaia literatura, 1934), 4.
15. On National Bolshevism, see David Brandenberger, *National Bolshevism: Stalinist Mass Culture and the Formation of Modern Russian National Identity, 1931–1956* (Cambridge, MA: Harvard University Press, 2002). For the defining characteristics of Socialist Realism, see Marina Balina, "Ideinost'—Klassovost'—Partiinost'" and Hans Günther, "Totalitarnaia narodnost' i ee isteki," in *Sotsrealisticheskii kanon*, eds. Hans Günther and Evgenii Dobrenko (St. Petersburg, Russia: Akademicheskii Proekt, 2000), 362–87.
16. "Sho'ra yozuvchilari yig'ilishi," *Qizil O'zbekiston*, April 1, 1933, 4.
17. Indeed, this was a major component in the condemnation of the Jadids; for one example of the "negative" revolutionary aesthetic, see the masterful translation Abdulhamid Sulaymon o'g'li Cho'lpon, *Night and Day*, trans. Christopher Fort (Boston: Academic Studies Press, 2019).
18. Clark pinpoints the first mention of Socialist Realism in a speech delivered on May 17, 1932, but a third of her book on the Socialist Realist novel deals with the period before 1932, and even novels from the 1920s were included in the Socialist Realist canon. See Clark, *The Soviet Novel*, section I, "Socialist Realism before 1932." On model novels as a touchstone for Socialist Realism, see Clark, *The Soviet Novel*, 261–63.
19. Clark, *The Soviet Novel*, 40–41.
20. Djagalov, *From Internationalism to Postcolonialism*, 110–13. See also Kevin M. F. Platt, *Border Conditions: Russian-Speaking Latvians between World Orders* (Ithaca, NY: Cornell University Press, 2024), 19–23.
21. Fredric Jameson, "Third-World Literature in the Era of Multinational Capitalism," *Social Text*, no. 15 (Autumn 1986): 69. Italics original.
22. Ertürk, *Grammatology and Literary Modernity*, x, 5.
23. See, for example, Ertürk's reading of Ahmed Midhat Efendi's *Müşahedat*: Ertürk, *Grammatology and Literary Modernity*, 34–57.
24. Founded in 1918, the leading university in Uzbekistan and in Central Asia was known as Central Asia State University (Sredneaziatskii gosudarstvennyi universitet, or SAGU) from

1923 to 1960. See "Tashkentskii gosudarstvennyi universitet," in *Bol'shaia rossiiskaia entsiklopediia*, electronic version, https://old.bigenc.ru/education/text/4184263 (accessed December 15, 2023).

25. Abdulla Qahhor, *Sarob* (Tashkent: O'zdavnashr, 1937), 11.
26. Among other commendations of Qahhor as a prose stylist, see Hamid Olimjon, "Adabiyotimizning tikka ko'tarilish davrida," *Yosh Leninchi*, March 6, 1934, 3.
27. For one discussion of Qahhor's dialogue with the Jadid legacy, see Christopher James Fort, "Inhabiting Socialist Realism: Soviet Literature from the Edge of Empire" (University of Michigan, 2019), 32–45.
28. Georg Lukács, "Narrate or Describe?," in *Writer and Critic, and Other Essays*, ed. Arthur Kahn (London: Merlin Press, 1970), 110–48. The text was also published in Russian: Georg Lukács, "Rasskaz ili opisanie," *Literaturnyi Kritik*, no. 8 (1936): 44–67.
29. Lukács, "Narrate or Describe?," 136.
30. The novel was initially published between early 1932 and spring 1935 in the official journal of the Uzbekistan Writers' Union.
31. O'zMDA f. 2356, op. 1, d. 56, l. 43.
32. Although the counterrevolutionary group remains unnamed, Ozod Sharafiddinov identifies it as the group Milly Istiqlol. Sharafiddinov, *Abdulla Qahhor*, 50. *Sarob*, 1937, 290–91.
33. Habib Musaev, "'Sarob' qanday roman?" *Yosh Leninchi*, January 30, 1939, 3–4.
34. Yusuf Sultonov, "*Sarob* haqida," *Qizil O'zbekiston*, November 17, 1937, 3.
35. As Christopher Fort argues, the novel is profoundly intertextual, directly responding in its emphasis on dreamworlds to Jadid author Abdulhamid Cho'lpon and his work on *xayol*, or fantasy. See Fort, *Inhabiting Socialist Realism*, 92–145.
36. Qahhor, *Sarob* (1937), 57–8.
37. Qahhor, *Sarob* (1937), 33.
38. Green apricots (g'o'ra/dovcha) are frequently eaten as a snack during the spring in Central Asia.
39. See for example, the Timurid gardens described in Lisa Golombek, "The Gardens of Timur: New Perspectives," *Muqarnas* 12 (1995): 137–47.
40. Sharafiddinov, *Abdulla Qahhor*, 78–9.
41. Qahhor, *Sarob* (1937), 365.
42. Eric Naiman, *Sex in Public* (Princeton University Press, 1997), 124–47.
43. Most such officers had a Turkish national and modernist bent that aligned with that of Central Asia's Jadids. See Khalid, *Making Uzbekistan*, 79–81. Due to their Turkist orientation, by the time of Qahhor's writing these officers had become *personae non gratae* from the perspective of the Soviet state.
44. Qahhor, *Sarob* (1937), 46.
45. Ibid., 45.
46. Ibid., 188.
47. Ibid., 75.
48. Ibid., 43, 278.
49. Ibid., 139.
50. Ibid., 364.
51. Ibid., 222.
52. O'zMDA f. 2356, op. 1, d. 56, ll. 103–6.
53. Saidg'ani Valiev, "Abdulla Qahhor to'g'risida," *O'zbekiston sovet adabiyoti*, 1935 (no. 6), 47–54.
54. O'zMDA f. 2356, op. 1, d. 9, ll. 11–12.
55. Qahhor, *Sarob* (1937), 81–8 (chapter 15). The obstruction of aspiring Saidiy's work, as discussed in the previous chapter, likely echoes the experience of many young writers during the mid-1930s; the 1937 addition of a conspiracy to explain the young writer's failure is also characteristic of the moment of the Terror.
56. Qahhor, *Sarob* (1937), 96–9 (chapter 18).
57. Qahhor, *Sarob* (1937), 325.
58. RGALI f. 631, op. 6, d. 281, l. 8.
59. A full summary of the revisions can be found in Rahmon Qo'chqorov, "Uch 'Sarob.'"
60. The 1937 edition encountered a series of delays: while the manuscript was sent for typesetting in 1936, printing was delayed for 14 months, likely due to the chaos instigated by Terror. Qahhor wrote a petition in April 1938 asking for it to be printed, and the book finally appeared in spring 1938 even though the date still said 1937 (Sharafiddinov, *Abdulla Qahhor*, 51–2).
61. Qo'chqorov, "Uch Sarob"; Otabek Jo'raboyev, "'Ikkinchi Cho'qqi'ning matnosti sirlari (So'ngso'z)," in Qahhor, *Tanlangan Asarlar*, vol. 3, 415–16.

62. R. Amonov describes the geographical scope of Ayni's works as spanning "from Badakhshan to Turkmenistan and from Turkestan to Iran and Afghanistan." See R. Amonov, "Geografiiai osori badeii ustod Ainī," in *Jashnnomai Aini*, vol. 5 (Dushanbe: Nashriëti Akademiiai fanhoi RSS Tojikiston, 1963), 16.
63. On the slave trade in Central Asia, see Jeff Eden, *Slavery and Empire in Central Asia* (New York: Cambridge University Press, 2018); Scott C. Levi, "Hindus beyond the Hindu Kush: Indians in the Central Asian Slave Trade," *Journal of the Royal Asiatic Society* 12, no. 3 (2002): 277–88.
64. Although Book 2 is set in the Russian imperial period, its main antagonists are the local administrators—aqsaqals, amlakdors, begs—rather than Russian colonial administrators. This likely corresponded to the experience of landless farmers in Central Asia, most of whose interactions with the tsarist state would have gone through local intermediaries.
65. In highlighting the Persianate dimension of Soviet internationalism, I follow the work of Sam Hodgkin; see Hodgkin, "Revolutionary Springtimes"; Hodgkin, *Persianate Verse and the Poetics of Eastern Internationalism.*
66. Hodgkin, "Revolutionary Springtimes," 284.
67. Ayni, *Qullar* (1935), 59.
68. Ibid., 88.
69. "Suvoqar" literally means "that which through water flows."
70. Although the vast majority of Persian love poetry presumed a male speaker, it is important to note that it did not always entail a female addressee. Much ink has been spilled on the homoerotic undertones of Persianate lyric poetry; for a useful summary, see Encyclopedia Iranica, "Homosexuality iii. In Persian Literature," *Encyclopædia Iranica*, XII/4, 445–48 and XII/5, 449–54, http://www.iranicaonline.org/articles/homosexuality-iii (accessed December 15, 2023). Ayni both creates a place for a female speaker and firmly situates the Persianate lyric in a heterosexual context.
71. Sadriddin Ayni, *Raby: roman*, trans. Sergei Borodin (Dushanbe: Irfon, 1977).
72. Qulmurod is referring to the fact that Muslim clergy were the most prominent educated class in pre-Soviet Central Asia; "mullah" is shorthand for a highly educated person.
73. "Fuqaro" is a technical term for a citizen, implying the rights and responsibilities of a participant in representative democracy. "Hamshahri," or "fellow city-dweller," is less technical, implying shared residence but no specific political theory; it was the term most commonly used to describe Iranian migrants on the periphery of the Russian Empire in the nineteenth to twentieth centuries. By making this shift in vocabulary, Qulmurod casts aspersions on Shokir's claim that the Ottoman and Iranian governments are really better for the common people than that of Manghit Bukhara. Touraj Atabaki has argued that the major factors driving Iranian migration to the Russian Empire, primarily the Caucasus and Central Asia, were economic transformation and famine, but the cultural and communal loyalties between Iranians (particularly Iranian Azeris) and Turkic citizens of the Russian Empire cemented their choice of destination. See Touraj Atabaki, "Disgruntled Guests: Iranian Subaltern on the Margins of the Tsarist Empire," *International Review of Social History*, 48, no. 3 (December 2003): 401–26.
74. H. Tursunova, *Tadqiqi Muqoisavii Frazeologizmhoi Paralleli Zabonhoi Tojiki va Uzbeki (dar Asosi Asari S. Ainii Ghulomon/Qullar)* (Dushanbe: Donish, 1979), 25.
75. In later years, Ayni was christened the father of Tajik literature, and his contribution to the formation of Uzbek literature was correspondingly downplayed. When Soviet scholars noted this aspect of his work, they cited it as evidence of the Uzbeks and Tajiks as "brother nations." For example, this aspect of Ayni's work is the subject of Matiakub Koshchanov, "Pisatel' dvukh literatur," in *Shchedrost′ talanta: stat′i ob uzbekskoĭ literature* (Moskva: Sovetskii pisatel′, 1980), 51–71.
76. Arabic vocabulary is also an important component of the Uzbek language, but in this case, it is difficult to disaggregate from Persian vocabulary, since most Arabic vocabulary would be shared between Uzbek and Tajik/Persian. It is worth noting, however, that Ayni downplays both religious themes and religious language, minimizing the proportion of Arabic-origin vocabulary in the text.
77. "Turkmen" meant very different things in early-nineteenth-century Turkestan, in which Part I of *Slaves* is set, and in 1930s Uzbekistan. This is a reality of which Ayni was surely aware, but a large portion of his desired readership would not have grasped the distinction. Although Ayni uses footnotes liberally, he chose not to clarify the definition of "Turkmen" here, which suggests that he did not consider it important. On Soviet attitudes toward nomadism and the formation of the Soviet Turkmen nation, see *Tribal Nation.*
78. Qahhor, *Qullar* (1935), p. 79.

79. In contrast to Ayni's reductive representation, many nomadic pastoralists practiced a combination of agriculture and herding, cultivating seasonal crops such as millet, and migrating between summer pastures (*yaylov*) and winter pastures (*qishlaq*). On the varieties of Eurasian nomadism, see Anatoly M. Khazanov, *Nomads and the Outside World* (Madison: University of Wisconsin Press, 1994).
80. Sarah Cameron. *The Hungry Steppe: Famine, Violence, and the Making of Soviet Kazakhstan* (Ithaca, NY: Cornell University Press, 2018), 45–69.
81. Ayni, *Qullar* (1935), 412.
82. The term "qutb" has an extensive history in astronomy and science, as well as in Sufi thought, where the *qutb* is a figure toward which the mystical search is directed. See "ḳuṭb,", in: P. J. Bearman, Th. Banquis, C. E. Bowworth, E. van Donzel, and W. P. Heinrichs Bowworth (eds.), *Encyclopaedia of Islam*, Second Edition. Leiden: Brill, 1960–2005. http://dx.doi.org.yale.idm.oclc.org/10.1163/1573-3912_ei2glos_SIM_gi_02573 (accessed December 15, 2023).
83. The woman as "witch and temptress" was a common trope in early Socialist Realist texts; see Clark, *The Soviet Novel*, p. 185.
84. Ayni, *Qullar* (1935), 394.
85. Ibid., 476.
86. Ibid.
87. One Soviet critic described *Slaves* "as if three large novels were encompassed in a single narration (Rus. *povestvovanie*)." A. Rakhmatullaev, *Proza Aini* (Dushanbe: Irfon, 1970), 56.
88. As a result of the checkered publication history of *The Law*, there is no authoritative manuscript of the novel. The one held by the Alisher Navoiy Literary Museum archive in Tashkent (hereafter ANLM), which is the only extant copy from Shams's own lifetime that I have been able to find, is missing pages and, in many portions, illegible due to Shams's own markings. The only published version, from a 1958 collected works, is not a critical edition; it appears merely to reproduce most of the legible portions of the ANLM copy, with very little editorial effort. See *Huquq*, from Husayn Shams, *Tanlangan asarlar* (Tashkent: O'zSSR Davlat Badiiy Adabiyot Nashriyoti, 1959), 271–481. Whenever possible, I have checked quotes and facts against the earliest version from the ANLM. Citations to the 1959 edition are the only available copies of the given passage. I have cited page number (rather than archival leaf number) when referring to the archival copy of *The Law*.
89. There are still many gaps in our understanding of the Kokand Autonomy, but a concise English-language discussion can be found in Khalid, *Making Uzbekistan*, 72–83; see also Dilorom Alimova and R. Ia. Radzhapova, eds., *Turkestan v nachale XX veka: k istorii istokov natsional′noi nezavisimosti* (Tashkent: Sharq, 2000), 80–112.
90. On the Soviet historiography of the 1916 uprising, see the editors' introduction in Alexander Morrison, Cloé Drieu, and Aminat Chokobaeva, eds., *The Central Asian Revolt of 1916: A Collapsing Empire in the Age of War and Revolution* (Manchester University Press, 2019), 3–7.
91. On Soviet historical revisionism more broadly, see Kevin M. F. Platt and David Brandenberger (eds.), *Epic Revisionism: Russian History and Literature as Stalinist Propaganda* (Madison: University of Wisconsin Press, 2006).
92. What appears to be the last chapter of the novel, entitled "The Bolsheviks Come out on Top," was published in a paperback brochure marketed to "beginning readers," a series which I discuss below. The chapter concludes with a Bolshevik flag being hung on Sodiq's factory, and all the workers of the factory waving red ribbons with joy. See Husayn Shams, *Haqqoniyat* (Tashkent: O'zSSR Davlat Nashriyoti, 1937), 65–75.
93. For Qahhor, *The Life of Klim Samgin* is the closest analogue, while Ayni's *Slaves* has been compared to *The Artamonov Business*; see Qo'shjonov, *Ayniy badiiyatining evolyutsiyasi*, 76.
94. Frederick C. Corney, *Telling October: Memory and the Making of the Bolshevik Revolution* (Ithaca, NY: Cornell University Press, 2004).
95. OzMDA f. 2356, op. 1, d. 9, ll. 12–13.
96. ANLM, Shams fond, d. 15, l. 32.
97. *Xola* is not a name but a title. It means "aunt" but is used to refer to any woman of the speaker's parents' generation.
98. For a discussion of female honor in Central Asia and how it was negotiated under new Soviet policies, with special reference to woman writers, see Kamp, *The New Woman in Uzbekistan*, especially pp. 119–22. In the early Turkish Republic, gender-related policies entailed strikingly similar negotiations around *nomus*; see three articles by A. Holly Shissler, "Beauty Is Nothing to Be Ashamed Of: Beauty Contests as Tools of Women's Liberation in Early Republican Turkey,"

Comparative Studies of South Asia, Africa and the Middle East, no. 1 (2004): 107; Ada Holland Shissler, "'If You Ask Me': Sabiha Sertel's Advice Column, Gender Equity, and Social Engineering in the Early Turkish Republic," *Journal of Middle East Women's Studies*, no. 2 (2007): 1; Ada Holland Shissler, "Womanhood Is Not for Sale: Sabiha Zekeriya Sertel against Prostitution and for Women's Employment," *Journal of Middle East Women's Studies*, no. 3 (2008): 12.

99. See, for example, Leila Ahmed, *Women and Gender in Islam: Historical Roots of a Modern Debate* (New Haven: Yale University Press, 1992); Lila Abu-Lughod, *Do Muslim Women Need Saving?* (Cambridge: Harvard University Press, 2013); Saba Mahmood, *Politics of Piety: The Islamic Revival and the Feminist Subject* (Princeton: Princeton University Press, 2012). For a broader analysis of western feminism as a colonial discourse, see Antoinette Burton, *Burdens of History: British Feminists, Indian Women, and Imperial Culture, 1865–1915* (Chapel Hill: UNC Press, 1994). In the Central Asian context, historian Douglas Northrop has developed this argument most trenchantly, while philosopher Madina Tlostanova presents a birds-eye critique of western feminist approaches to the study of Eurasia, although not without methodological weaknesses; see Northrop, *Veiled Empire*, 42–6; Madina V. Tlostanova, *Gender Epistemologies and Eurasian Borderlands* Basingstoke: Palgrave Macmillan, 2010).
100. For examples of such narratives beyond the Soviet Union, see Naiman, *Sex in Public*.
101. Shams, *Huquq* (1959), 279.
102. The quote is "Musurmonchani [sic] suv qilib ichib yuborgan edi." ANLM, Shams fond, d. 15, l. 23. With "speaking Muslim," Shams here probably refers to vernacular Turkic.
103. ANLM, Shams fond, d. 15, l. 25.
104. ANLM, Shams fond, d. 16, 113. The 1959 edition simply summarizes all these hints in an epithet: Faxri "the Tajik." See *Huquq* 1959, 321.
105. In this respect, Shams's proletarian masculinity mirrors a pattern Eliot Borenstein has observed in Russian literature of the 1920s; see Eliot Borenstein, *Men without Women: Masculinity and Revolution in Russian Fiction, 1917–1929* (Durham, NC: Duke University Press, 2001).
106. On prostitution in colonial Central Asia, see Malika Zekhni, "Invisible Bodies: Civilising Mission, Sexuality, and Prostitution in Fin de Siècle Russian Turkestan," *Cultural and Social History*, 19, no. 2 (2022): 141–59.
107. ANLM, Shams fond, d. 15, l. 29.
108. For a slightly overstated, but influential argument on this point, see Massell, *The Surrogate Proletariat: Moslem Women and Revolutionary Strategies in Soviet Central Asia, 1919–1929* (Princeton, N.J: Princeton University Press, 1974).
109. ANLM, Shams fond, d. 16, p. 157.
110. ANLM, Shams fond, d. 16, p. 158.
111. Shams, *The Law* (1959), 351.
112. ANLM, Shams fond, d. 17, 219.
113. The phrase is "nomusiga chidolmay, qizini olib, qishloqqa qochib ketganmish." ANLM, Shams fond, d. 15, l. 32.
114. This passage comes from pages that are now missing from the archival version. See Shams, *Huquq* (1959), 310.
115. "nomus, ruz-qiyomat azobim," ANLM, Shams fond, d. 16, l. 100.
116. Cheprunov had also submitted a novel, *Junayd Khan*, to the novel competition, but his novel was rejected on account of its "idealization of the Jadids of Khorezm." See O'zMDA f. 2356, op. 1, d. 9, l. 13.
117. Ibid., l. 7.
118. This review can be found in ANLM, Shams fond, d. 231. Based on Shams's overview of the novel's publication history in ANLM, Shams fond, d. 259, I conjecture this is Boris Cheprunov's 1937 review of the novel. The archival version is a typewritten document and appears to be intended for internal use within the Writers' Union. I have found no published version.
119. To be sure, many of these "errors" were actually failures properly to apply a Bolshevik teleological reading to the events Shams had personally witnessed: in 1917, it would certainly have been difficult to distinguish a "February Revolution" or an "SR" in Kokand's political setting.
120. ANLM, Shams fond, d. 230, l.7. This review is undated, but internal evidence suggests it was written around the same time as Cheprunov's review; certainly, no earlier than January 1937, because it refers to the 1936 edition of *The Law*.
121. RGALI f. 631, op. 6, d. 198, ll. 24–8.
122. Ibid., l. 26.
123. Ibid., l. 27.
124. Brandenberger, *National Bolshevism*.

125. A similar argument has been made by Gregory Massell with reference to early Soviet policy in Central Asia write large. Massell argues that, in the absence of any significant proletariat in the technical sense, women formed a "surrogate proletariat" for purposes of Soviet policy in the 1920s. See Massell, *The Surrogate Proletariat.*
126. On the "zoological" as a critique commonly leveled during the formulation of Socialist Realism in 1933–34, see Clark, *The Soviet Novel*, 183.ANLM, Shams fond, d. 231, l. 5.
127. RGALI f. 631, op. 6, d. 198, l. 76.
128. ANLM, Shams fond, d. 258.

Chapter 4

1. Zulfiya Isroilova, "Har Tebranish Bir Sur'at," *Yangi Yo'l* (July 1932), 12.
2. For a useful study of temporality as a category of postcolonial analysis, see Keya Ganguly, "Temporality and Postcolonial Critique," in *The Cambridge Companion to Postcolonial Literary Studies* (Cambridge: Cambridge University Press, 2004), 162–79.
3. Akmal Ikramov, *Osnovnye voprosy kul'turnogo stroitel'stva v uzbekistane* (Tashkent: UzGIZ, 1932), 11.
4. Ibid., 22. Fayzulla Xo'jayev followed suit, arguing that certain *maqom* modes reflected "hard labor and a superfluous life," even when combined with lyrics about "the Young Pioneers, the emancipated woman, the Red Army"; see Faizulla Khodzhaev, "Perestroit' radiofront: rech' na soveshchanii rabotnikov radio," in Fayzulla Khodzhaev, *Izbrannye trudy*, vol. 3 (Tashkent: Fan, 1973), 467.
5. Khodzhaev, "Perestroit' radiofront," 467.
6. See Robert A. Rothstein, "Homeland, Home Town, and Battlefield," in *Culture and Entertainment in Wartime Russia*, ed. Richard Stites (Bloomington: Indiana University Press, 1995), 77–107. On the gathering of "folklore" more broadly, see Margaret Ziolkowski, *Soviet Heroic Poetry in Context: Folklore or Fakelore* (Newark: University of Delaware Press, 2013).
7. Malte Rolf, *Soviet Mass Festivals, 1917–1991*, (Pittsburgh: University of Pittsburgh Press, 2013); Brandenberger, *National Bolshevism.*
8. Exceptions include Grant, *In the Soviet House of Culture*; Ali F. İğmen, *Speaking Soviet with an Accent*ş Isabelle R. Kaplan, "Comrades in Arts: The Soviet Dekada of National Art and the Friendship of Peoples," *RUDN Journal of Russian History*, 19, no. 1 (December 1, 2020): 78–94.
9. Hamit Zübeyr, "Halk terbiyesi vasıtaları," *Ülkü*, 1933 (no. 3), 152. See also Zübeyr's book-length treatise, *Cultivating the People*, which included sections on Hungarians, Czechs, Finns, "Fascists," Germans, the English, and America, in addition to Turkey: Hamit Zübeyr, *Halk terbiyesi* (Ankara: Köy Hocası Matbaası, 1931).
10. On the broader music scene in prerevolutionary Bukhara and elsewhere in Transoxania, see Theodore Levin, Saida Daukeeva, and Elmira Köchümkülova, eds., *The Music of Central Asia* (Bloomington, IN: Indiana University Press, 2016), 317–43, 435–60.
11. Ibid, 438–45; see also Tanya Merchant, *Women Musicians of Uzbekistan from Courtyard to Conservatory* (Urbana, IL: University of Illinois Press, 2015), 4–8.
12. For example, see Maria Eva Subtelny, "Art and Politics in Early 16th Century Central Asia," *Central Asiatic Journal*, 27 (1983): 121–48; Maria Eva Subtelny, "The Poetic Circle at the Court of the Timurid, Sultan Husain Baiqara, and Its Political Significance" (Ph.D. Diss., Harvard University, 1979).
13. Aftandil Erkinov, "Striving for Cultural Perfection at the Khivan Royal Court under Muhammad Rahim Khan II as a Means of Resistance to the Russian Protectorate Regime," in *Proceedings of the International Conference: Reassessing the Heritage of Khoja Ahmet Yasawi*, ed. Ashirbek Muminov and Nurlan Dukenbaev (Istanbul: Research Centre for Islamic History, Art and Culture, 2024), 171–73.
14. Vyzgo and Karomatov term this "professional music of oral tradition." See T. S. Vyzgo, I.N. Karelova, and F. M. Karomatov, eds., *Istoriia uzbekskoi sovetskoi muzyki*, vol. 1, 2 vols. (Tashkent: G'ofur G'ulom nomidagi Adabiyot va san'at nashriyoti, 1972), 24.
15. Levin, *The Hundred Thousand Fools*, 101.
16. E. Romanovskaia, "Muzyka v Uzbekistane."
17. This account seems plausible but must still be taken with a grain of skepticism because there was a strong bias against the Emir both among Jadids and among the Soviet activists who took their place. Theodore Levin argues that the emir's attitude toward music was "mercurial," and that the *maqom* was performed primarily outside his court—a description that is corroborated here. See Levin, *The Hundred Thousand Fools*, 101–4. According to Levin, the term for a musician under the patronage of the Emir was *râstaxâr*, though it was still presumed that the beneficiary would have some form of (non-musical) outside employment; the musician Levin describes worked as a cobbler and a caterer for large events.

18. The most thorough and concise available summary of the *maqom*, from which this description is derived, can be found in Will Sumits and Theodore Levin, "*Maqom* Traditions of the Tajiks and Uzbeks," in *The Music of Central Asia*, 320–43.
19. Ibid., 321.
20. Ibid., 320–21.
21. Romanovskaia, "Muzyka v Uzbekistane," 5.
22. For a summary of the work of *bachas*, see Levin, *The Hundred Thousand Fools*, 298n13. Unsurprisingly, bachas were a sensational sight for European travelers and were discussed at length in many travelogues; see Olufsen, 436–39. See also Jennifer Wilson, "Queer Harlem, Queer Tashkent." For a brief discussion of the Jadid critique of this practice, see Khalid, *The Politics of Muslim Cultural Reform*, 145–46.
23. Levin, *The Hundred Thousand Fools*, 102; Alexander Djumaev, "Power Structures, Culture Policy, and Traditional Music in Soviet Central Asia," *Yearbook for Traditional Music*, 25 (1993), 43.
24. Avgust Eikhgorn, *Muzykal'naia fol'kloristika v Uzbekistane*, ed. V. M. Beliaev (Tashkent: Akademiia nauk uzbekskoi SSR, 1963), 119–21.
25. Ibid., 103.
26. V. M. Beliaev, *Central Asian Music: Essays in the History of the Music of the Peoples of the USSR*, ed. Mark Slobin, trans. Mark and Greta Slobin (Middletown, CT: Wesleyan University Press, 1975), 284.
27. See Ravshan Yunusov, "Qo'shiqmi yo ashula?" *Guliston*, 1997 (no. 2), 26–8.
28. Levin, *The Hundred Thousand Fools*, 101.
29. According to Levin, later stories circulated that the Emir had threatened to cut off Babakhanov's head because he consented to be recorded, and that Babakhanov's subsequent move to Samarkand was an attempt to flee the Emir's ire. Babakhanov's descendants deny these stories, but it is clear that the emir resisted recording even the most accomplished performers.
30. Otanazar Matyakubov and Harold Powers, "Nineteenth Century Khorezmian Tanbur Notation: Fixing Music in an Oral Tradition," *Yearbook for Traditional Music* 22 (1990), 29.
31. Ibid., 32.
32. The earliest known transcriptions of songs using Khorezmian notation appear to date to 1887; for a longer history of the transcription of Uzbek music, see F. Karomatov, "O'zbek muzika folklorining yozilishi tarixidan," *Sharq Yulduzi* 1956 (no. 12), 103–10.
33. O'zRFASI, unnumbered archival file (timeline of Qori-Yoqubov's life), l. 611.
34. For further discussion of Hamza's early activity in the Ferghana Valley, see Shavkatjon Xursanalievich Xonqulov, "Farg'ona vodiysida jadidchilik harakatida Hamza Hakimzoda Niyoziyning o'rni" (Ph.D. Diss., Ferghana, Ferghana State University, 2021).
35. See Khalid, *The Politics of Muslim Cultural Reform*, 129–32, 153–54.
36. It is unclear precisely what buildings Jadid performances were held in. Allworth describes the location of the premiere of Behbudiy's *Parricide* (*Padarkush*) as a "370-seat house" in Samarkand. Prerevolutionary Jadid theater performances were also held in Kokand and Tashkent. See Edward Allworth, "The Beginnings of the Modern Turkestanian Theater," *Slavic Review* 23, no. 4 (1964): 684.
37. O'zRFASI, T(M) M34 No. 218 t. IV, l. 22.
38. Hamza Hakimzoda Niyoziy, *To'la asarlar to'plami*, vol. 2 (Tashkent: Fan, 1988), 24.
39. Ibid., 25.
40. Ibid, 48.
41. This scene is described in the reminiscences of actor Mannon Uyg'ur, excerpts of which are published in Russian translation in L. A. Avdeeva, *Mukhitdin Kari-Iakubov: dokumental'naia monografiia* (Tashkent: G'ofur G'ulom, 1984), 34–6.
42. Niyoziy, *To'la asarlar to'plami*, 160–61.
43. Ibid., 41–2.
44. Ibid., 34–6.
45. On the death of Qori-Yoqubov's father, see Bahrom Irzayev, "O'zbek Shalyapini," *Milliy Tiklanish*, June 6, 2024, https://mtgazeta.uz/news/editors-choice/ozbek-shalyapini-.htm. It is impossible to verify Irzayev's sources, but the date and place are plausible. Unless otherwise noted, the basic outlines of Qori-Yoqubov's biography are drawn from Avdeeva, *Mukhitdin Kari-Iakubov*, 11–27, and E. Kari-Iakubova, *Mukhitdin Kari-Iakubov: ocherk Zhizni i Tvorchestva* (Tashkent: Izdatel'stvo khudozhestvennoi literatury im. Gafura Guliama, 1968).
46. The precise timeline here comes from O'zRFASI, unnumbered archival file (timeline of Qori-Yoqubov's life), l. 611–12.

47. The biography below is derived from Charles D. Shaw, "The Many Nationalities of Tamara Khanum: Friendship of the Peoples at Home, Abroad, and Within," *The Russian Review*, 82, no. 3 (2023), 437–42.
48. In the rest of the Soviet Union and the worldwide stage, Tamara Khanum nevertheless became representative of the "emancipation" of all Central Asia's women. For example, Langston Hughes, who met Tamara Khanum during his travel in Central Asia, described her as being representative of all the region's women. See Langston Hughes, "Tamara Khanum: Soviet Asia's Greatest Dancer," *Theatre Arts Monthly*, 18, no. 11 (November 1934): 829–35.
49. Boram Shin describes the project of the 1920s as one of "modernizing the national form." See Boram Shin, "National Form and Socialist Content: Soviet Modernization and Making of Uzbek National Opera between the 1920s and 1930s," *Interventions*, 19, no. 3 (April 3, 2017): 416–33.
50. See Abdurrauf Fitrat, *O'zbek klassik musiqasi va uning tarixi* (Tashkent: Fan, 1993); V. A. Uspenskii, *Shest' muzykal'nykh poem (makom) zapisannykh V.A. Uspenskim v Bukhare* (Bukhara: Narodnyi nazarat prosvescheniia Bukhrespubliki, 1924).

    In the course of the 1920s, Uspenskii proceeded to conduct extensive studies of folk and classical music throughout Uzbekistan. See Vyzgo, Karelova, and Karomatov, *Istoriia uzbekskoi sovetskoi muzyki*, 52–3.
51. Djumaev, "Power Structures," 47–8.
52. Djumaev, "Power Structures," 48. This episode is also discussed in Levin, *The Hundred Thousand Fools*, 90.
53. Abdurrauf Fitrat, "O'zbek musiqasi to'g'risida." *Alanga*, 1928 (no. 2), 14. In later years, once the Uzbek nation could be taken for granted as existing a priori, scholars acknowledged the regional diversity in Uzbekistan's performance practices; for a discussion of the "four basic local groups" of musical performance practice, see Vyzgo, Karelova, and Karomatov, *Istoriia Uzbekskoi Sovetskoi Muzyki*, vol. 1, 26–31. This text names the four groups as Khorezm, Bukhara (and Samarkand), Surxondaryo (and Qashqadaryo), and Ferghana-Tashkent.
54. Vyzgo, Karelova, and Karomatov, *Istoriia Uzbekskoi Sovetskoi Muzyki*, vol. 1, 110.
55. O'zRFASI, T(M) M34 No. 218 t. IV, ll. 49–50.
56. Some of these institutions were renamed *tekhnikum* in the late 1920s and later became known as *uchilishche*. For a full discussion of the musical institutions opened during the 1920s, see Vyzgo, Karelova, and Karomatov, *Istoriia Uzbekskoi Sovetskoi Muzyki*, vol. 1, 103–12. This treatment does not emphasize the involvement of Jadids in the institutionalization of Uzbek music, and the authors are particularly interested in identifying when western instruments, such as the piano, began to be taught. Consequently, little distinction is made between institutions of "national" origin and institutions oriented toward Europeans. Nevertheless, it remains the most thorough summary of musical institutions in early Central Asia.
57. On the Samarkand institute, see F. Rahmon. "O'zbek musiqiy tekshirish instituti." *Alanga*, 1928 (no. 9), 13. A detailed description of the Institute's curricular and research plans for the following three years can be found in Nikolai Mironov, "O'zbekistonning klassik va xalq musiqasini o'rganish faniy tadqiqot instituti," *Alanga*, 1930 (no. 5–6), 41–6. Among other subjects, the curriculum included music theory, instruction in a variety of Central Asian and European instruments, orchestral performance, and music history, including Indian, Chinese, and "primitive people's" (*yovoyyi xalq*) musical traditions. It also called for students to learn the songs of a "variety of nations," including Japanese, Tuvan, Khakas, Mordvinian, and "Great Russian."
58. Bakjon Rahmon o'g'li. "O'zbek notasi," *Alanga*, 1928 (no. 3–4), 13–14.
59. *Khanaqas* and *qalandar-khanas* are types of Sufi lodges. Djumaev, "Power Structures," 44.
60. Djumaev, "Power Structures," p. 43.
61. *barmak* means "finger"; the term is a reference to the fact that the metric feet can be counted on one's fingers. Fitrat, *O'zbek klassik musiqasi*, 10.
62. Fitrat, *O'zbek Klassik Musiqasi*, 51.
63. N. Muhitdinov, "'Milliy Ittihodchilar'ning madaniy frontdagi ishlari" *Alanga*, July–August 1930 (no. 7–8), 19.
64. In Uzbek, the phrase is "*mehnatkash o'zbek dehqonlarning turmushidan hozirgi zamon kuylari.*"
65. Tamara Khanum discusses the couple's time in Paris in an undated interview: O'zRFASI, T(M) K23 N. 433/23, ll. 19–28.
66. O'zRFASI, T(M) M34 No. 218 vol. II (part 2), l. 15.
67. Komil Aliyev, "Bazm," *Qizil O'zbekiston*, March 25, 1927, 4.

68. Iupatova was almost certainly "Prekrasnaia Elena," a performer at the for-profit pre-revolutionary Iupatov Circus. See "Tsirk Filippa Iupatova," *Tashkent*, https://m.ok.ru/tashkent.zvezda.vostoka/topic/69943172606778 (accessed April 18, 2025).
69. Eric Naiman, *Sex in Public*.
70. M. Rasul, "Yana davlat etnografik truppasi haqida," *Qizil O'zbekiston*, March 26, 1927, 4.
71. "40000 na prazdnike," *Komsomolets Vostoka*, June 18, 1934, 1; "Fanfary vozvestili otkrytie," *Komsomolets Vostoka*, June 18, 1934, 1. The precise capacity of Tashkent's Dinamo stadium is unclear, but it is highly unlikely it could fit a full 40,000 people. The estimate of "up to 20,000" in the SATASS press release is probably more realistic. See RGASPI f. M-63, op. 1, d. 260, ll. 22–3. The newspaper's attendance figures probably included revelers from both the park and the stadium and was undoubtedly a generous estimate. The opening date for the Musical-Artistic Olympiad and the Conference on Culture and Everyday Life was June 17.
72. O'zRFASI, T(M) M34 No. 218 t. IV, l. 81–2.
73. RGASPI f. M-63, op. 1, d. 258, ll. 3–4.
74. Coverage of the opening day was extensive, including multiple articles in *Pravda Vostoka* on June 17. Examples include "Uchastnikam sredneaziatskoi muzykal'no-khudozhestvennoi olimpiady privet!" *Pravda Vostoka*, June 17, 1934, 2; "Segodnia otkrytie olimpiady i konferentsii," *Komsomolets Vostoka*, June 17, 1934, 1.
75. "Nodir talantlar bayrami," *Yosh Leninchi*, June 17, 1934, 1.
76. TENK, "Kolonial'noe proshloe kanulo v vechnost'," *Komsomolets Vostoka*, June 17, 1934, 2. The section heading, with evocatively placed scare quotes, expressed the tone of casual neo-Orientalism in the Russian-language press: "Their 'culture' is at the brink of standstill." This tone is quite distinct from that of the Uzbek-language press, which was less reflexively critical of the pre-Soviet popular performance traditions of the region.
77. See the 1936 figures available in O'zMDA f. 94, op. 5, d. 1567. The figures are incomplete and some pages have been cropped off, but there is no reason to believe the available statistics are significantly skewed.
78. RGASPI f. M-63, op. 1, d. 260, l. 35.
79. For performances at factories, see RGASPI f. M-63, op. 1, d. 260, l. 40. The schedule was published in "Konferensiya va olimpiada kunlarida nimalar bo'lajak." *Yosh Leninchi*, June 18, 1934, 2.
80. RGASPI f. M-63, op.1, d. 260, l. 36.
81. "San'atimizga, san'atkorlarimizga ko'ruk," *Yosh Leninchi*, June 21, 1934, 4.
82. The examples from the above paragraph appeared in a press release, apparently from SATASS, which is reproduced in RGASPI f. M-63, op. 1, d. 260, ll. 25–7.
83. In this respect, the Olympiad participants might be described as "performing" their nationality, as opposed to representing some internalized national subjectivity or primordial national identity. For an analysis of Soviet nationality that foregrounds this performative dimension, see Brigid O'Keeffe, *New Soviet Gypsies: Nationality, Performance, and Selfhood in the Early Soviet Union* (Toronto: University of Toronto Press, 2013).
84. "Zal slushaet Nurisari: Tov. Saklatvala voskhishchen molodymi darovaniiami." *Komsomolets Vostoka*, June 21, 1934, 1.
85. Unless otherwise noted, all statistics derive from RGASPI f. M-63, op. 1, d. 260, l. 35.
86. Halima Nosirova, *Solntse nad vostokom* (Moscow: Molodaia Gvardiia, 1962), 150.
87. At the Kokand Olympiad, for example, only eight amateur circles from collective farms participated, as opposed to twenty-five from the city itself. RGASPI F. M-63, op. 1, d. 259, l. 2.
88. According to the 1939 census, Uzbeks comprised 65.1% of the total population of Uzbekistan. The other 35% include other Central Asian nationalities as well as Russians. Figures come from Martin, *The Affirmative Action Empire*, 381.
89. RGASPI f. M-63, op. 1, d. 260, l. 65.
90. On Tashkent's most active amateur music groups in the 1920s and 1930s, see Vyzgo, Karelova, and Karomatov, 71–5.
91. The below examples are found in RGASPI f. M-63, op. 1, d. 259, l. 56.
92. Romanovskaia, "Muzyka v Uzbekistane," 5.
93. N. Rahimiy, "Kuchli bir san'atkorimiz," *Alanga*, 1930 (no. 8–9), 27.
94. G'ulom Zafariy (1889–1938), a composer and participant in the transcription of the *maqom*, was affiliated with the Jadids in the prerevolutionary period, and was shot along with many other such intellectuals on December 4, 1938. See "G'ulom Zafariy (1889–1938)." Ziyouz.com. http://www.ziyouz.com/index.php?option=com_content&task=view&id=97&Itemid=210 (accessed January 29, 2019). Zafariy also composed one of the first Uzbek "operas"; see Shin, "National Form," 423.

95. RGASPI f. M-63, op. 1, d. 260, 26.
96. Levin, *The Hundred Thousand Fools of God*, 56–9.
97. It is impossible to reconstruct the identity of this musician, Sadir Khan, and where or how the recordings of him were made. Ma'ruf Xo'ja's story represents an interesting combination between face-to-face and modern, mediated forms of musical transmission. Although he heard Sadir Khan first in person, Ma'ruf Xo'ja did not have the opportunity to learn from him directly because he soon died. Instead, Ma'ruf Xo'ja learned to play from recordings that he obtained from Sadir Khan's students. The fact that Ma'ruf Xo'ja learned from recordings evinces the changing landscape of musical transmission. Nevertheless, it is still significant that Ma'ruf Xo'ja first learned music not by reading notes, but by improvising based on listening.
98. Levin, *The Hundred Thousand Fools of God*, p. 39.
99. Roberts, "Old Elites under Communism", especially chapter 3, "The Culture of Cotton Farms (1930s–1960s)," pp. 175–231.
100. The case study of Uzbekistan might effectively be compared to those of Armenia and Kazakhstan, analyzed in Knar Abrahamyan, "Opera as Statecraft in Soviet Armenia and Kazakhstan" (Ph.D. Diss., Yale University, 2022).
101. Viktor Beliaev, *Muzykal'nye instrumenty Uzbekistana* (Moscow: Gosudarstvennoe muzykal'noe izdatel'stvo, 1933), 122–23.
102. "Rohat beraturgan kuy," 107. The balalaika also received a similar treatment, and enormous bass balalaikas, albeit rare, still appear on Russian stages to this day.
103. On these experimental efforts with musical instruments, see Xotam Qirg'iz, "Yangi sozlar," *Guliston*, no. 6 (1935), 32.
104. A. Novosel'skii. "K voprosu ob organizatsii massovogo proizvodstva muzykal'nykh instrumentov." *Sovetskaia muzyka*, May 1934 (no. 5), 43–50. The factory was probably never actually built.
105. Beliaev, *Muzykal'nye instrumenty Uzbekistana*, 125.
106. Ibid., 122.
107. O'zMDA f. 737, op. 1, d. 1717, ll. 52–53. The names of the Uzbek melodies were Usmanya, Kashgarcha, Mirzodavlat, and "Signal." Kashgarcha is a piece from the maqom. The sources for Usmanya and Mirzodavlat are unclear, but their names suggest prerevolutionary provenance and link them to a Turkic, Islamic world. Usmanya shares a root with "Ottoman," while "Mirzo" is a noble title, roughly corresponding to "prince." These melodies are also mentioned in N. Lomakin, "Pobednyi itog." *Komsomolets Vostoka*, June 30, 1934, 3.
108. "San'atimizga, san'atkorlarimizga ko'ruk." *Yosh Leninchi*, June 21, 1934, 4.
109. I. Akbarov, *Tukhtasyn Dzhalilov* (Moscow: Sovetskii kompozitor, 1974), 4–6.
110. Ibid., 8.
111. Ashrafii, *Muzyka v moiei zhizni*: *sbornik statei* (Tashkent: Izdatel'stvo literatury i iskusstva im. Gafura Guliama, 1975), 86.
112. Ashrafiy, *Muzyka v moei zhizni*, 87. A choral recording of "Signal" was also made: Mukarama Turgunbaeva, *Signal*, arr. Jalilov, with the Orchestra and Choir of the Uzbek Musical Theater, on *Signal*, Gramplasttrest GRK 465-UZRK 567, 1935, https://russian-records.com/details.php?image_id=28087 (accessed December 15, 2023).
113. Akbarov, *Dzhalilov*, 28–9.
114. Interview with Ahmadjon Umurzakov, O'RFASI, T(M) M34 No. 218 t. IV, l. 77. The original melody can be heard here: "Mushkuloti dugox Farg'ona—Toshkent makom ijro yo'laridan. Sozanda Shamsiddin Nuriddinov ijrosi," posted March 25, 2023, by Shamsiddin Nuriddinov, YouTube, 7:58, https://www.youtube.com/watch?v=Dujaic6qMzg&list=RDDujaic6qMzg&start_radio=1.
115. *Signal*, Gramplasttrest, 1935.
116. On the corresponding project in Russia, see Richard Stites, *Russian Popular Culture: Entertainment and Society since 1900* (Cambridge: Cambridge University Press, 1992), 48. Muxtor Ashrafiy lists the names of several performers from whom musicologists transcribed *maqom* and popular melodies; see Ashrafii, *Muzyka v moei zhizni*.
117. Ziolkowski, *Soviet Heroic Poetry in Context*, 91–122 offers a detailed account of how this process worked in a few exemplary cases. For an older, though less archivally informed account, see Frank J. Miller, *Folklore for Stalin: Russian Folklore and Pseudofolklore of the Stalin Era* (Armonk, N.Y.: M.E. Sharpe, 1990).
118. The most notorious case is that of Jambyl Jabaev. See Konstantin Bogdanov, ed., *Dzhambul Dzhabaev*: *Prikliucheniia kazakhskogo akyna v sovetskoi strane* (Moskva: Novoe literaturnoe obozrenie, 2013).
119. In Uzbekistan, for example, the prominent woman poet Oydin was involved in the gathering of folklore. The collector of the works I discuss below is unknown.

120. The expedition is described in E. E. Romanovskaia, *Stat'i i doklady. Zapisi muzykal'nogo folk'lora*, eds. T. S. Vyzgo, F. M. Karamatov, and M. S. Kovbas (Tashkent: Khudozhestvennaia literatura, 1957), 16, 63–72.
121. Hamidulla Akbarov, "Lutfixonim qo'shiqlari," *Ma'rifat*, https://www.ziyouz.com/portal-haqida/xarita/madaniyat-va-san-at/lutfixonim-qo-shiqlari (accessed August 18, 2023).
122. Romanovskaia, *Stat'i i doklady*, 64.
123. Romanovskaia's team collected twenty-four songs from Sarimsoqova, more than from any other source in Andijon. Romanovskaia, *Stat'i i doklady*, 64.
124. E. Romanovskaia, "Muzyka v Uzbekistane," 7.
125. Marina Frolova-Walker, "'National in Form, Socialist in Content': Musical Nation-Building in the Soviet Republics." *Journal of the American Musicological Society*, 51, no. 2 (1998): 348.
126. Romanovskaia, "Muzyka v Uzbekistane," 7.
127. Elena Romanovskaia, *O'zbek ashulalari* (Moscow: OGIZ-Muzgiz, 1934); Xafiyaxon Muhamedova and Ilyos Akbarov, *O'zbek ashulalari* (Moscow: OGIZ-Muzgiz, 1934).
128. "O'rtaosiyo yoshlarining madaniy-maishiy konferensiyalari va musika san'at olimpiadasining yakunlari to'g'risida." *Yosh Leninchi*, July 14, 1934, p. 3. A more extensive discussion of the work undertaken to create a national, harmonized repertoire can be found in "Obrabotka narodnykh melodii," from Vyzgo et al., *Istoriia uzbekskoi sovetskoi muzyki*, 57–67.
129. RGALI f. 631, op. 6, d. 118, l. 3.
130. Mahmud Ahmedov, *Yunus Rajabiy* (Tashkent: O'qituvchi, 1967), 25.
131. "Ro'molim," *Uzbekskie narodnye pesni*, Vol. II (Tashkent, 1929, in Uzbek), reproduced in Beliaev, *Central Asian Music*, trans. Slobin, 272. The song also appeared in E. E. Romanovskaia and Ilyos Akbarov, eds., *O'zbek xalq qo'shiqlari*, vol. 2 (Tashkent: O'zdavfimnashr, 1939), 63–5.
132. Tamara Khanum, *Ro'molim*, arr. Safo Mugani, with Safo Mugani (accordion) and M. Otajonov (doira) on *Signal*, Gramplasttrest, 965, 1935.
133. The performance at the Ferghana Canal is described, albeit tendentiously, in "RTdan va'z: Ro'molim qo'shig'i," *Eltuz*, https://eltuz.com/lat/video/220469/ (accessed December 15, 2023).
134. Arrangements were also made by Yunus Rajabiy and Ilyos Akbarov; see Romanovskaia and Akbarov, *O'zbek xalq qo'shiqlari*, vol. 1, 22–3.
135. Ashrafi, *Muzyka v moei zhizni*, 84.
136. Ulug'bek Haydarov, "Gulnoraxon, bo'ylaringdan, gulyor," O'zbekiston Erk Demokratik Partiyasi, https://www.uzerk.org/%d0%b3%d1%83%d0%bb%d0%bd%d0%be%d1%80%d0%b0%d1%85%d0%be%d0%bd-%d0%b1%d1%9e%d0%b9%d0%bb%d0%be%d1%80%d0%b8%d0%bd%d0%b3%d0%b4%d0%b0%d0%bd-%d0%b3%d1%83%d0%bb%d0%bd%d0%be%d1%80.html (accessed September 8, 2023).
137. Akbarov, "Lutfixonim qo'shiqlari."
138. On dekadas, see Kaplan, "Comrades in Arts."
139. A full transcription of the song's melody and lyrics can be found in Beliaev, *Central Asian Music*, trans. Slobin, 318–20. A more complete text can be found in Hamza, *To'la asarlar to'plami*, vol. 2, 160–1.
140. Naim Karimov cites *Atir Gul* by way of Sotti Husayn as the first publication in which the text appeared but does not seem to have accessed that text for himself and expresses doubt about the precise content of that original publication. I have not been able to find any copies of *Atir Gul* myself. See Hamza, *To'la asarlar to'plami*, vol. 2, 503.
141. Hamza, *To'la asarlar toplami*, vol. 2, 160.
142. Avdeeva, *Mukhitdin Kari-Iakubov*, 14–15.
143. Ibid., 35.
144. Reminiscences of M. Rahmanov, in Avdeeva, *Mukhitdin Kari-Iakubov*, 15–16.
145. O'zMDA f. 2454, op. 1, d. 299, l. 62. I am grateful to Bahrom Irzayev for providing the citation and scan for this file.
146. Hamza, *To'la asarlar to'plami*, vol. 2, 155.
147. For one such suggestion that Qori-Yoqubov preferred "Turan," see, for example, Abduqodir Hayitmetov, "Yasha Turon," Ziyouz, November 2, 2013, https://n.ziyouz.com/portal-haqida/xarita/uzbek-nasri/abduqodir-hayitmetov-1926-2005/abduqodir-hayitmetov-yasha-turon-hikoya. This memoir/story is somewhat unreliable: although Qori-Yoqubov appears in the story, it is set in the mid-1960s (well after Qori-Yoqubov's death).
148. O'zRFASI, T(M) K23 No. 433/23, l. 25.

Chapter 5

1. RGALI f. 631, op. 6, d. 86, l. 8. To'rayeva joined many other Stakhanovites and shock workers who descended upon Moscow in November and December 1935 for a series of events focused on hyper-production.

2. *Yosh Leninchi*, December 24, 1935, 2. This speech follows a general paradigm in Stakhanovite peasants' speeches; see Sheila Fitzpatrick, *Stalin's Peasants: Resistance and Survival in the Russian Village after Collectivization* (New York: Oxford University Press, 1994), 274–79.
3. By "political affect," I mean "the domain of feeling that comes before or beyond its narration as emotion," a domain that is "intersubjective" rather than rooted in individual subjectivity. See Mateusz Laszczkowski and Madeleine Reeves, eds., *Affective States: Entanglements, Suspensions, Suspicions*, Studies in Social Analysis 5 (New York: Berghahn, 2018), 4–5. I argue below, particularly in the last section, that textiles produced affective resonances that were not—in fact, could not be—articulated explicitly as emotions. Following William Mazzarella, I am interested not only in the political mobilization of affect, but also the emergent affective currents that arose around Stalin-era attempts to mobilize affect through luxury textiles. Luxury textiles both mobilized women for cotton production and generated more unpredictable lateral affective ties that went beyond the Stalinist "hierarchies of consumption." See Elena Aleksandrovna Osokina, *Ierarkhiia potrebleniia: o zhizni liudei v usloviiakh stalinskogo snabzheniia, 1928–1935 gg.* (Moscow: MGOU, 1993); Mazzarella, *Censorium*.
4. Here I draw on the argument by Leora Auslander, writing on textiles and dress in revolutionary Europe and America, that "the aesthetics of everyday life [...are] crucially important in the constitution of national identities, or personal affinities or group consciousness." Leora Auslander, *Cultural Revolutions: Everyday Life and Politics in Britain, North America, and France* (University of California Press, 2009), 2.
5. For a discussion of the representation of textiles in the Soviet media outside Uzbekistan, see Emma Widdis, "Sew Yourself Soviet: The Pleasures of Textile in the Machine Age," in *Petrified Utopia: Happiness Soviet Style*, edited by Marina Balina and E. A. Dobrenko (London: Anthem Press, 2009), 115–32. Widdis concludes that tactile pleasure should be considered a major element of the "happiness" that Soviet discourse prioritized in the 1930s. My discussion below extends such an analysis to the Soviet periphery, arguing for the importance of sensory experience in grafting Uzbek women into an all-Soviet public.
6. Yılmaz, *Becoming Turkish*, 87–93.
7. Davron, "Tuyg'un Oy," *Yangi Yo'l*, 1927 (no. 6), 11. The author's name is given in quotation marks, suggesting it is a pseudonym.
8. Ibid.
9. Gullar ichida bir gul, ul qayrilaman dedi./ Bizdan nogunoh o'tdi, yor ayrilaman dedi./ Essizgina o'rtog'im, yordan ayrilib qoldi./ Shirin turmushdan kechib, ul sotilaman dedi. (Ibid., 10). Written in a figural but colloquial register, the meter of this verse roughly corresponds to that of a traditional *ruboiy* quatrain. A footnote in the story also indicates that the first two lines come from a "folk song" (*xalq ashulasi*). The two last lines, presumably written by Davron himself, fixate the meaning of the folk source as referring to specific concerns of the Hujum: forced child-marriage and bride-price. The use of the *ruboiy* form and the folk attribution serve to stake a claim for the classical Turco-Persian lyric as capable of containing "socialist content." Meanwhile, the inclusion of this form in the decidedly non-native form of the short story also stakes a claim for the short story as a national Uzbek form—a claim that retains its power for the remainder of Soviet Uzbek literary history.
10. A. A. Seyed-Gohrab, ed., *Metaphor and Imagery in Persian Poetry*, Iran Studies, v. 6 (Leiden: Brill, 2012), 133.
11. Davron, "Tuyg'un Oy," 11.
12. Ibid., 12. "Uzoq, qorong'i burchak."
13. Ibid., 11. "Kun kech bo'lib, dunyo qorong'ulashgan sayin, Tuyg'unning ko'ngli undan battar qorong'ulasha borar edi."
14. Oydin, "Ochilgan Lolalar," *Yangi Yo'l*, 1930 (no. 2–3), 13.
15. Ibid., ll. 9–10. "Ochilgandir lolalarning/ Bugun amal yuzlari."
16. Ibid., l. 15. "Fabrik, sovxoz, kolxozlarda."
17. Common topics also included colonial India, Germany, China, and the United States. See, for instance, A. Ts., "Emma (Oqsoch): shanxai yavropalilarning uyida xizmat qiluvchi xitoy oq soch xotinlar turmushidan olingan hikoya / Emma (The White-Haired): A Story of the Life of the White-Haired Servant Women in Shanghai's European Homes," trans. N. Baykova from German to Russian; trans. Mahbuba Rahim Qizi from Russian to Uzbek, *Yangi Yo'l*, 1932 (no. 5), 14–16.; Author Unknown, "Bombay," *Yangi Yo'l*, 1933 (no. 3–4), 48; about Kashgar, see G'ayratiy, "Onamga Xat," *Yangi Yo'l*, 1933 (no. 6), 18–21; Lohutiy, "Eron Qizi," *Yangi Yo'l*, 1933 (no. 6), 21. For representations of the oppressive "past," see Jalol Mashrabiy, "So'roqsiz Hukum," *Yangi Yo'l*, 1930 (no. 6), 12; Jalol Mashrabiy, "O'tmishdan Bir Varaq," *Yangi Yo'l*, 1930 (no. 7), 9; Emin Umarii, "Lenin Avlodi," *Yangi Yo'l*, 1933 (no. 11–12), 13; Qurbon Bedil, "To'xta Bibi," *Yangi Yo'l*, 1934 (no. 1), 18–19.

18. "Mendan, 'Qanday qilib birinchi terimda 115–120 Kilo paxta terasan?' deb so'raydilar, men javob beraman." *Yangi Yo'l*, 1933 (no. 11–12), 14.
19. Uzb., "Yuz o'n besh-yigirma / kilo bo'ladur."
20. On the role of the senses in Socialist Realism, see Emma Widdis, *Socialist Senses: Film, Feeling, and the Soviet Subject, 1917–1940* (Bloomington, Indiana: Indiana University Press, 2017).
21. Uzb., "gard va tuproq."
22. Uzb., "tungi bir posbondir."
23. Uzb., "sochlar."
24. Uzb., "Nozlatib/ kuldirib/ tarayman!"
25. Uzb., "Yangi tug'ulgan qizni / yuvintirib so'ng / ko'ylaklar kiygizib / yo'rgaklayman! / va kech-qurun / tortib ko'raman! / Qizning / og'irligi qancha keladi? / Men ona / U-meni yaxshi biladir / Og'irligi / yuz o'nbesh-yigirma / kilo bo'ladir!"
26. The majority of the description of colonial-era Central Asian dress in the following paragraph is adapted from the information given by M. A. Bikzhanova, who drew on fieldwork among Tashkent women; O. A. Sukhareva, who aggregated data from throughout Uzbekistan; and an ethnography written by the Nalivkins based on their observations in the Ferghana Valley during the late 1870s and 1880s. See M. A. Bikzhanova, "Odezhda uzbechek tashkenta XIX-nachala XX v.," in *Kostium narodov Srednei Azii: istoriko-etnograficheskie ocherki*, ed. O. A. Sukhareva (Moscow: Nauka, 1979), 133–50; V. P. Nalivkin and Mariia Vladimirovna Nalivkina, *Muslim Women*, 89–102; O. A. Sukhareva, *Istoriia sredneaziatskogo kostiuma (2-ia polovina XIX-nachalo XX v.)* (Moscow: Nauka, 1982).
27. Sukhareva, *Istoriia sredneaziatskogo kostiuma*, 25.
28. Nalivkin and Nalivkina, *Muslim Women*, 97; Sukhareva, *Istoriia sredneaziatskogo kostiuma*, 25.
29. Nalivkin and Nalivkina, *Muslim Women*, 100; Susan Meller et al., *Russian Textiles: Printed Cloth for the Bazaars of Central Asia* (New York: Harry N. Abrams, 2007).
30. The *paranji* was most commonly gray or white with blue stripes, but young women could also wear red *paranjis* (Kamp, *The New Woman in Uzbekistan*, 136). On the red *paranji*, see Bikzhanova, "Odezhda uzbechek," 142.
31. Kamp suggests that rural women who worked in the fields did not veil (Kamp, *The New Woman in Uzbekistan*, 135).
32. Nalivkin and Nalivkina, *Muslim Women*, 163–64.
33. The Nalivkins report in the late nineteenth century that a shirt (*ko'ylak*) made of native cotton fabrics cost under two rubles; Russian-made chintz was more expensive, while the most "festive and dressy" fabrics, silk and *adras* semisilk, cost as much as six or seven rubles. Nalivkin and Nalivkina, *Muslim Women*, 99.
34. Willem Floor, "*Kel'at*," in *Encyclopædia Iranica XVI/3* (2017), 226–29, http://www.iranicaonline.org/articles/kelat-gifts (accessed December 15, 2023); G. Minault, "The Emperor's Old Clothes: Robing and Sovereignty in Late Mughal and Early British India," in *Robes of Honour: Khil'at in Pre-Colonial and Colonial India*, ed. Stewart Gordon (New Delhi: Oxford University Press, 2003), 125–39.
35. For further examples of the reactivation of the *khil'at* ritual with reference to Soviet Central Asia, see Hodgkin, *Persianate Verse*, 118–24.
36. Veiling was never a universal practice in Central Asia and was most widespread in the sedentary urban areas where the Bolsheviks first gained their foothold. Women who did cover their faces began doing so once they were seen as having reached maturity, between the ages of nine and sixteen. Rural women who worked in the fields probably did not always wear a veil (Kamp, *The New Woman*, 135). More extensive discussions of veiling practices can be found in Northrop, *Veiled Empire*, 43–6; Kamp, *The New Woman*, 134–44; Nalivkin and Nalivkina, *Muslim Women*, 95.
37. Throughout the Islamic world, the meaning and extent of women's veiling, and the female seclusion that accompanied it, had long been the subject of heated debate. In the late nineteenth and early twentieth century in particular, Muslim women and men had experimented with various styles of veiling and unveiling, with a view toward forging a mode of femininity that was both Muslim and modern. As had been the case throughout Islamic history, some women saw no conflict between being unveiled and being Muslim. Others proposed decoupling the veil as an article of clothing from the system of women's seclusion with which it was associated, arguing that veiling had not always entailed women's subordination. This range of views was represented in Central Asian society as well. For one example from within the Russian Empire, in which measures for women's equality, including unveiling, were framed in terms of Sharia law, see Marianne

Kamp, "Debating Sharia: The 1917 Muslim Women's Congress in Russia," *Journal of Women's History* 27, no. 4 (2015): 13–37. On Central Asian ideas about veiling and unveiling before the Hujum, see Kamp, *The New Woman*, 123–49. In the few cases when religious authorities openly argued that unveiling was licit according to Islamic law, this led to much more widespread unveiling than when nonreligious or openly atheist activists tried to persuade women to unveil. See the case of a pro-unveiling mullah in RGASPI f. 62, op. 2, d. 1811, l. 99. This episode is also discussed in RGASPI f. 62, op. 2, d. 2064, l. 18.

38. This argument is put forward by Northrop (Northrop, *Veiled Empire*, 320).
39. Northrop, *Veiled Empire*, 69–101.
40. Douglas Northrop adduces further examples of this complaint (Northrop, *Veiled Empire*, 131–34). Similar dynamics affected state sartorial reforms in Turkey; see Yılmaz, *Becoming Turkish*, 97.
41. RGASPI f. 62, op. 2, d. 1811, l. 140.
42. Anne Anlin Cheng terms Ornamentalism "a theory about the profound imbrication of things and persons." See Anne Anlin Cheng, *Ornamentalism* (Oxford: Oxford University Press, 2019), 152. Drawing on close readings of legal, cinematic, photographic, and literary representations of Asian women, Cheng argues that in Euro-American culture, Asiatic femininity became closely linked with inanimate materials, such as porcelain, sumptuous furniture, and luxury textiles. Encrusted with these "prosthetic extensions," Asian women's bodies receded to the margins, rendering them at once less-than-corporeal and extracorporeal. For Cheng, Asian women's "fusion between thingness and personhood" contributed to their legal and political marginalization, but at the same time offered opportunities for a new kind of relationship between the political and the aesthetic. If, on the one hand, Ornamentalism objectified Asian women, it also animated the objects to which they were attached, opening up new modes of being in the world and new kinds of relations between objects and persons. Following Cheng, I argue that the imbrication of Central Asian femininity with textiles had ambivalent results, both subordinating Central Asian women to violent state agendas and articulating new modes of solidarity and ways of being in public. In this respect, "Ornamentalism" offers a key to understanding the implications for Central Asians of the transposition of modernist aesthetics to the Soviet "Orient"; see Nariman Skakov, "Eisenstein in Fergana: From Avant-Garde to National Form," *Studies in Russian & Soviet Cinema*, 15, no. 1 (March 2021): 23–38.
43. Of course, not all textiles were attached to nationality; Russian-made chintz, for example, was associated with foreignness more than local nationality. However, during the Soviet period, Central Asian-made silk fabrics became a key visual component in the pageantry of national performance. *Atlas* silk became attached to Central Asian nationhood in the early Soviet period, and remains a major symbol of Uzbek, Tajik, and Kyrgyz nationality until the present day. As Julia Obertreis points out, in the early Soviet period, "economic functions and characteristics merged with folkloristic features of the republic in the image of the female statue, wearing the national dress and holding the twig of a cotton plant." Obertreis, *Imperial Desert Dreams*, 242. The "national dress" itself was usually made of silk. One prominent early example of this linkage between silk fabric and Central Asian nationhood appears in the color film of the 1939 *Youth in Bloom* physical culture parade, in which the female marchers from Uzbekistan wear *atlas* silk pantaloons in bright yellow, green, red, and white. Their yellow shirts are adorned with cotton blossoms, and on their heads, they wear embroidered skullcaps. The women's costumes are more overtly "national" than the men's—some men wear white dress shirts and white slacks with light blue ties, a few march only in tan pantaloons and skullcaps (*do'ppi*), and others wear bright-pink athletic shorts, exhibiting their sculpted physiques. See "Tsvetushchaia Iunost'," dir. Alexander Medvedkin and Vladimir Feinberg (1939), YouTube video, 17:18, https://www.youtube.com/watch?v=xtMSvRuSkTE&list=RDxtMSvRuSkTE&start_radio=1 For a useful analysis of the imbrication of nation, gender, and the politics of dress in contemporary Central Asia, see Mohira Suyarkulova, "Fashioning the Nation: Gender and Politics of Dress in Contemporary Kyrgyzstan," *Nationalities Papers*, 44, no. 2 (March 2016): 247–65.
44. In Uzbek, *ko'ylak*, the word Ikromov uses here, means "dress" for women and "shirt" for men; it could perhaps more accurately be translated as "tunic." "19-dekabrda O'zbekiston, Qozog'iston, va Qoraqalpog'iston ilg'or kolxozchilarining kengashida o'rtoq Akmal Ikromov so'zi," *Yangi Farg'ona*, December 22, 1935, 3–4.
45. The language of "congealment" derives from Marx's discussion of the commodity as a vessel of congealed labor. Karl Marx, *Capital: A Critique of Political Economy* (London: Penguin, 2004), 130.

46. Skallerup indicates that women did not generally work in the shops where silk fabric was produced as a final product; however, it is clear that women were significantly involved in silk production. Thomas Mark Skallerup, "Artisans between Guilds and Cooperatives: A History of Social and Economic Change in Russian Turkestan and Soviet Central Asia 1865–1928" (Ph.D Diss., Indiana University, 1990), 61, 97.
47. "G'alabani mustahkamlashga!" *Yosh Leninchi*, March 8, 1932, 1.
48. Incongruously, given the previous statistic from *Yosh Leninchi*, the note also recommended increasing the proportion of women in sewing to 75%. See O'zMDA f. 86, op. 10, d. 207, l. 142.
49. For example, one of the slogans put forward by the Central Asian Bureau's Agitprop Division in 1930 was "Toward fulfilling the cotton and silk program, and toward a full engagement of the textile and silk-producing industry of the Union with Soviet raw material!" See RGASPI f. 62, op. 2, d. 2437, l. 7.
50. There was a reference to textile production in almost every issue of the women's magazine; a few examples among many include Yo'ldosh, "Atlaschi qizlar," *Yorqin Hayot*, 1938 (no. 2), 18; Mo'minov, "Buxoro ipak fabrikasi millionlar shartnomasini bajarishda namuna bo'lsin," *Yangi Yo'l*, 1933 (no. 1), 37; "Ipakchilik sanoati yangi vazifalar oldida," *Yangi Yo'l*, 1934 (no. 1), 5–7.
51. Skallerup, *Artisans*, 58.
52. Ibid., 194–95.
53. Sukhareva, *Istoriia sredneaziatskogo kostiuma*, 26.
54. Skallerup's description of prerevolutionary garment-making suggests that artisans produced mostly robes (*khalat*), hats, coats, and belts, not dresses; we can assume these were mostly made at home and by hand. With respect to the 1920s, Skallerup notes that urban dressmakers often made dresses according to European fashions, but rural dressmakers sewed according to local styles (Skallerup, *Artisans*, 67, 195). More research is needed to understand the proportion of clothing that was made at home versus by professional dressmakers, although I suspect that many women sewed their own clothing in this period. On the banning of dressmaking in Russia, see Sheila Fitzpatrick, *Everyday Stalinism Ordinary Life in Extraordinary Times: Soviet Russia in the 1930s* (New York: Oxford University Press, 1999), 44.
55. Kassymbekova, *Despite Cultures*, 1, 205n1. Similarly, in Sadriddin Ayni's *Slaves*, a wealthy man, or *boi*, is rewarded with a silk mattress for agreeing to cooperate with Soviet authorities (Ayni, *Qullar*, 252–60).
56. See, for example, RGASPI f. 62, op. 2, d. 1811 l. 111.
57. Prizes of textiles and clothing were given to Stakhanovites elsewhere in the Soviet Union, but nowhere but Central Asia do silk and velvet seem to have figured so prominently in the discourse of Stakhanovism: Siegelbaum, *Stakhanovism*, 229–32; Fitzpatrick, *Stalin's Peasants*, 274–79.
58. Tamara Kondrat´eva, *Kormit´ i pravit´: O vlasti v Rossii XVI–XX vv.* (Moskva: ROSSPEN, 2006).
59. Osokina, *Ierarkhiia potrebleniia.*
60. Examples include Mahbuba, "Ish maydoniga 17 nafar madaniyat armiyasi," *Yangi Yo'l*, 1933 (no. 6), l. 33; Ergash Niyoziy, "8-nchi martda mukofotlandilar," *Yangi Yo'l*, 1933 (no. 3–4), 51.
61. "Mirzacho'l zarbdor xotin-qizlari sosial mehnat qo'ynida," *Yangi Yo'l*, 1931 (no. 10–11), 11–12. For another example from the early 1930s, this time portrayed in a poem, see Zohira Tohirova, "Terim xotiralari," *Yangi Yo'l*, 1932 (no. 3–4), 14.
62. "Chem premiruiutsia brigady," *Pravda Vostoka*, January 4, 1934, 4.
63. See the reports on the March 8 festivities in RGASPI f. 112, op. 61, d. 76 and f. 112, op. 61, d. 77.
64. RGASPI f. 112, op. 61, d. 77, l. 56.
65. Interview with Maryam Yoqubova, 1956, in O'zRFASI T(M) M34 No. 218 t. II, 17.
66. On the particularly harsh famine of 1933, see Marianne Kamp, "Hunger and Potatoes: The 1933 Famine in Uzbekistan and Changing Foodways," *Kritika: Explorations in Russian & Eurasian History*, 20, no. 2 (2019): 237–67.
67. RGASPI f. 112, op. 61, d. 78, ll. 9-26; the prize is mentioned on l. 11. In addition to twelve positive nominations, the collection also includes two negative evaluations. It is impossible to tell the nationality of the subjects of the nominations by name alone, especially since in this period, national categories were in flux. All the nominations are written in Russian. However, only one nominee, Beliaeva (l. 11), has a Russian-sounding name; the others have Muslim names, and one is identified as an Uzbek. Some authors do not identify their location, and for others, the geographical reference is unclear. Because the prize was intended for a cotton farmer, we can conjecture that the letters came from Uzbekistan or the cotton-growing regions of Tajikistan, Turkmenistan, or Kyrgyzstan. In cases where I have been able to identify the locations, they are all in Uzbekistan, for example Bukhara and New Chirchiq. The MTS political division was an ephemeral bureaucratic entity, functioning only in 1933–34. A. N. Nuritov, "Rabota Politotdelov MTS Uzbekistana Sredi Sel'skoi Molodezhi (1933–1934 Gody)," *Nauchnye Trudy (TashGU)*, no. 281 (1966): 97–103.

68. The autobiographies thus roughly follow a format that will be familiar to most scholars of early Soviet culture from the work of Igal Halfin, *Red Autobiographies*.
69. The most accomplished woman, who became a Party candidate in 1928 and studied abroad in Baku before becoming a literacy teacher and collective farm activist, does not offer any evidence of a difficult background. Instead, her letter reads like a resume, describing the woman's many educational and professional accomplishments. Among the biographies of this length—hers is a full single-spaced page long—this is a remarkable omission. It suggests that the author believed her background to be a liability. This woman composed her biography in excellent Russian despite apparently not being a native speaker; it is also, of course, possible that the biography was ghostwritten. See RGASPI f. 112, op. 61, d. 78, l. 17.
70. Orphanhood not only served as a useful plot point in a narrative of salvation by the Party; it also deprived women of paternal guardianship, which offered social protections that many women were unwilling to sacrifice in order to become a Party activist. Examples include ibid., ll. 25, 26. One woman reported living with her parents for only seven years before moving to Kokand. She does not give further detail, but this too suggests a difficult background. See ibid., l. 20.
71. This is an autobiography composed in good Russian with some grammatical and spelling errors. RGASPI f. 112, op. 61, d. 78, l. 10.
72. Some authors mention other evidence of prosperity, including cows, blankets, food, etc. Clothing is nevertheless the most frequently mentioned item.
73. Ibid., ll. 12, 26.
74. Ibid., l. 25.
75. Ibid., l. 10.
76. Nortoji Abdullayeva, "Ipak ko'ynagim," *O'zbek sovet adabiyoti*, 1935 (no. 6), 53.
77. Kamp, *The New Woman*, 162.
78. On shimmering as a deflection of the invasive Orientalizing gaze, see Cheng, *Ornamentalism*, 61–85.
79. The uses of "silk and velvet" in official discourse in the 1930s should be understood within the broader context of Soviet efforts to cultivate the senses through tactile experience and the representation thereof. In her analysis of the role of the senses in early Soviet film, Emma Widdis has argued that the "primitive East" served as the locus for an embodied, premodern sensuality—one that had the potential to be appropriated in constructing socialist senses. By the mid-1930s, Widdis argues, the "primitive" had receded as a resource for Soviet sensuality, in favor of representations of the "East" as a backward space in need of modernization (Widdis, *Socialist Senses*, 165–202, 265–96). Here, I suggest that some Central Asian women's poetry articulated a vision of the "national" as a resource for a refashioned Soviet sensorium, but rejecting, or at least reimagining the Orientalist assumptions of the all-Soviet discourse about "backwardness." My analysis of textiles and textile-texts can also be brought into conversation with Christina Kiaer's analysis of the early Soviet Constructivist effort to create a new relation between the human person and the material world under the conditions of socialism. As Kiaer notes, artist and theorist Alexander Rodchenko imagined that the "the new relation to person, to woman, to things" was the "light from the East." Christina Kiaer, *Imagine No Possessions: The Socialist Objects of Russian Constructivism* (Cambridge, Mass: MIT Press, 2005). Writing from Paris, Rodchenko likely meant to refer to the Soviet Union at large. But the role of Russia's "East" (including Central Asia) in constructions of Soviet aesthetics is still underexplored. For one promising analysis of the afterlives of the Russian avant-garde in Central Asia, see Nariman Skakov, *Reorientalism: From Avant-Garde to Soviet National Form* (Columbia University Press, 2025).
80. "Tursunoy," *Yorqin Turmush*, August 1936 (no. 2), 15.
81. Shodieva was a great deal more prominent than To'rayeva, whose speech opened this chapter.
82. "Aka" is an honorific term for an older brother or any older man. "Akam" means "my brother," and emphasizes the speaker's personal relationship to him (though it is still impossible to assume he is a blood relation).
83. This is the Turkic version of a Persian epithet, *māh-chihr*, meaning "face bright as the moon." Francis Joseph Steingass, *A Comprehensive Persian-English dictionary, including the Arabic words and phrases to be met with in Persian literature* (London: Routledge & K. Paul, 1892), 1146.
84. "Tojixon," *Yorqin Turmush*, 1936 (no. 3), 9.
85. Oydin, "Adolatxonning brigadasi," *Yorqin Turmush*, 1936, no. 3, 11.
86. Compare to the argument about Iranian women's submission to the patriarchal state after their "emancipation" from the patriarchal family in Amin, *The Making of the Modern Iranian Woman*.

Chapter 6

1. On the comparability of Soviet systems of mass publicity with western ones, see Stephen Kotkin, "Modern Times: The Soviet Union and the Interwar Conjuncture," *Kritika: Explorations in Russian*

and Eurasian History, no. 1 (2001): 111–64; David L. Hoffmann, *Cultivating the Masses: Modern State Practices and Soviet Socialism, 1914–1939* (Ithaca, NY: Cornell University Press, 2011).

2. Fred Inglis, *A Short History of Celebrity* (Princeton: Princeton University Press, 2010), 9; Chris Rojek, *Celebrity* (London: Reaktion Books, 2004), 103–6.
3. Inglis, *A Short History of Celebrity*, 5, 9.
4. Rojek, *Celebrity*, 29.
5. On the 1916 revolt, see Morrison et al., eds., *The Central Asian Revolt of 1916*.
6. Even in this respect, Shodieva's celebrity is not as different from western celebrity in the interwar period as one might expect. As Löwenthal notes, interwar popular biographies—an early form of celebrity culture—focused primarily on heroes of business and the arts. It was only in the postwar period that celebrity as an icon of consumption came to the fore. See Löwenthal, "The Triumph of Mass Idols."
7. Shissler, "Beauty Is Nothing to Be Ashamed Of," 107–22.
8. Farzin Vejdani, "The Women's Movement, the Press, and Exemplary Biographies," in *Making History in Iran: Education, Nationalism, and Print Culture* (Stanford: Stanford University Press, 2015), 97–116.
9. Marilyn Booth, *May Her Likes Be Multiplied: Biography and Gender Politics in Egypt* (Berkeley: University of California Press, 2001).
10. Beth Baron, "Mother of the Egyptians," in *Egypt as a Woman: Nationalism, Gender, and Politics* (Berkeley: University of California Press, 2005), 135–61.
11. Inglis, *Celebrity*, 11–12.
12. Unless otherwise noted, the facts of Shodieva's life in the following description come from Kamp, *The New Woman*, 105–6; "Tojixon Shodieva," *Uzbekskaia Sovetskaia Entsiklopediia*. Tashkent: Fan, 1979, 87; I. Finkel'shtein, "V trude i bor'be," in *Probuzhdennye velikim oktiabrem* (Tashkent: GosIzdat Uzbekskoi SSR, 1961), 211–15; Madirim Mahmudov, *Barhayot siymolar: qatag'on qurbonlari haqida lavhalar* (Tashkent: O'zbekiston, 1991), 157–65; Strong, *Red Star in Samarkand*; Halle, *Women in the Soviet East*, 310–15.
13. Stories of forced childhood marriage and abuse against girls were common propaganda narratives during the Hujum, so it is likely that some components of the story were exaggerated. Unveiling was contextual; it is likely that Shodieva, like many other Uzbek women, continued wearing a veil in some contexts. Although unreliable, Halle's account of Shodieva's life indicates that her husband required her to re-veil on the train back to Tashkent after she unveiled before Natalia Krupskaya.
14. "Shodievaning qisqacha tarjima-i holi," *Yangi Yo'l*, no. 10–11 (1927), 28. Her first teacher was likely an *otin*, or female in-home instructor . On *otins*, see Kamp, *The New Woman in Uzbekistan*, 77–83.
15. The record of Shodieva's 1929 (re-)appointment as editor of *New Way* can be found in RGASPI f. 62, op. 2, d. 2007, l. 83.
16. For the speech, see RGASPI f. M-1, op. 23, d. 835a 1928, ll. 125–33. Shodieva applied in 1929 to study in Moscow but was rejected; she did manage to go in 1931. See RGASPI f. 17, op. 27, d. 22, ll. 53, 67. Another speech by Shodieva, discussing the relative merits of different varieties of cotton, can be found in "Rech' Tadzhikhan Shadievoi," *Pravda*, December 22, 1935, 2. On the Communist University of the Toilers of the East during Shodieva's tenure, see Masha Kirasirova, "The 'East' as a Category of Bolshevik Ideology and Comintern Administration: The Arab Section of the Communist University of the Toilers of the East," *Kritika: Explorations in Russian and Eurasian History* 18, no. 1 (2017): 7–34.
17. Gerasimova notes this request from Shodieva with admiration, suggesting that Shodieva was too ambitious to be limited merely to "women's work." The point thus exemplifies the general assumption in Soviet society that work among women was less important than work among the general population (i.e., men). See the Uzbek and Russian versions of Gerasimova's article: "Mukofot," *O'zbek Sovet Adabiyoti*, 1934, no. 6 (June), 52–4; Valeriia Gerasimova, "Nagrada," *Pravda*, no. 156 (June 8, 1934), 4.
18. The Machine-Tractor Station Political Divisions were a short-lived, but significant institution, existing only from 1933 to 1934. They were intended to ease the transition from regionally oriented administration to "production"-oriented administration, that is, to a bureaucracy oriented toward supporting collective farms. MTS Political Divisions ran literacy courses, seminars, agitation meetings, shock-worker events, and local newspapers. For more detail on the works of MTS Political Divisions in Uzbekistan, see Nuritov, "Partiino-massovaia rabota politotdelov MTS Uzbekistana (1933–34 gg)," in *Sbornik rabot aspirantov TashGU: Istoriia KPSS. Istoriia*, ed. Iu. I. Ibragimov and V. P. Kharin (V. I. Lenin nomidagi Toshkent davlat universiteti, 1964), 164–72.

19. Her participation in dekulakization is supported by archival evidence, although the numbers are unverifiable. The figure of 563 comes from Gerasimova, "Mukofot" and "Nagrada." RGASPI f. 112, op. 61, d. 22 contains an undated MTS file showing Tojixon Shodieva's appraisal of the case of a couple, the Muhammedjanovs, who are accused of unsavory class connections; Shodieva recommends Muhammedjanov be removed from his official post.
20. On Tojixon Shodieva's purging and rehabilitation, see Mahmudov, *Barhayot Siymolar*, 157–65. A facsimile of the NKVD decree condemning Shodieva to exile can be found in Rustambek Shamsutdinov et al., eds., *Repressiia. 1937–1938 gody. Dokumenty i materialy* (Tashkent: Shark, 2005), 223.
21. B. Aziziy, "Tojixon," *Guliston*, 1935, no. 3, 8–9.
22. For examples of Hujum-era narratives about women's "emancipation" in the press see Kamp, *The New Woman*, 109–12.
23. Blindness was a frequent trope in Soviet representations of pre-Soviet life in Central Asia; see, for example, the repeated images of blind people in Vertov's *Three Songs of Lenin*, punctuated with intertitles like "Blind was my life..." Blind activists in the Soviet Union objected to representations of blindness as disqualifying from Soviet labor; see Maria Cristina Galmarini, "Turning Defects to Advantages: The Discourse of Labour in the Autobiographies of Soviet Blinded Second World War Veterans," *European History Quarterly*, 44, no. 4 (October 2014): 651–77.
24. Northrop, *Veiled Empire*, pp. 62–6. The sallow face was also a common trope in Persianate representations of abject lovers.
25. Here, the astronomical metaphor evokes the discourse of enlightenment that was ubiquitous in the mid-1930s. The Revolution brings enlightenment literally, in the form of electrification. But electrification also implies scientific progress, and brings with it education, hygiene, and sanitation, and the modernization of everyday life.
26. Shodieva was a delegate to the 5th Congress of the Turkestan Komsomol in 1924, the Sixth All-Soviet Congress of the Komsomol in 1925 (discussed above); see Mahmudov, *Barhayot Siymolar*, 158.
27. Béla Balázs, *Béla Balázs: Early Film Theory*, ed. Erica Carter, trans. Rodney Livingstone (New York: Berghahn Books, 2011), 109.
28. Some women activists, such as Jahon Obidova and Oydin (Manzura Sobirova), did dress in menswear such as blazers and button-down shirts; I have identified no one, however, who consistently wore the *gimnasterka* like Shodieva. See the photographs in Halle, *Women of the Soviet East*, and the portrait of Jahon Obidova in Marianne Kamp, "Jahon Obidova (1900–1967)," in *Russia's People of Empire: Life Stories from Eurasia, 1500 to the Present*, ed. Stephen M. Norris and Willard Sunderland (Bloomington: Indiana University Press, 2012), 309–16. On the gimnasterka, see R. M. Kirsanova, "Gimnasterka," in *Kostium v russkoi khudozhestvennoi kul'ture 18-pervoi poloviny 20 v.v.*, ed. T. G. Morozova and V. D. Siniukova (Moscow: Bol'shaia rossisskaia entsiklopediia, 1995), 79.
29. This concern was not specific to Tojixon; as Samuel Hodgkin argues, the question of whether literary representatives must resemble those they claim to represent was at issue throughout Persianate literary culture in Central Asia and beyond; see Hodgkin, *Persianate Verse and the Poetics of Eastern Internationalism*, 47–54.
30. The Russian *bogatyr'* emerges from the same Turkic root.
31. Ikromov, "Tojixon Shodievalar o'sayotir," *Yosh Leninchi*, May 20, 1936, 2. The full speech can be found in O'zMDA f. 86, op. 10, d. 634, ll. 198–204. The speech was apparently delivered in Uzbek, but this archival copy is in Russian. For other examples of Tojixon's use as a model, see "Madaniy turmush uchun musobaqa boshlangiz!" *Yosh Leninchi*, December 8, 1935, 1; "Bizning vazifalar," *Yorqin Turmush*, July 1936 (no. 1), 1; Zulfiya, "Qizlar kuylaydi," *Yorqin Hayot* 1938 (no. 2), 23.
32. Oydin, "Tabrigim sizga," *O'zbekiston Sovet Adabiyoti*, June 1934 (no. 6), 55–6.
33. Oydin's frame narrative suggests that she was sensitive to the challenges inherent in creating a sense of "time-discipline" among Uzbek women, unaccustomed to the norms of industrial production. For the classic discussion of this process among the English working class, see E. P. Thompson, "Time, Work-Discipline, and Industrial Capitalism," *Past & Present*, no. 38 (1967): 56–97.
34. Qiziqishib: "gazet" deya/Qichqirishar nechalar.
35. Emphasis mine.
36. Balázs, *Béla Balázs*, 39.
37. The "pomegranate-faced" and the "flower-faced" woman were common tropes in Uzbek poetry, and drew on classical Persianate conventions for describing women's faces. In the post-Hujum era, these tropes took on a new meaning.

38. For a more extensive discussion of the term *nomus* with relation to women's sexual honor, see Chapter 3, "Novels."
39. Like *nomus*, *sharaf* and *shon* also distinctly reference religious piety. On *uyat* in contemporary Kazakhstan with historical context, see Nari Shelekpayev, "Govorit' so stisnutymi zubami: styd, vlast' i zhenskoe telo v sovremennom Kazakhstane," *Novoe literaturnoe obozrenie*, no. 161 (1/2020), 157–74. Shelekpayev attributes the increasing prominence of *uyat* in Kazakhstan to the post-colonial condition; Oydin's poem represents an early mobilization of the category as a colonial discourse.
40. The project was spearheaded by prominent filmmaker Aleksandr Medvedkin, but by the time *Tadzhikhan Shadieva* was produced, he had left the project; the film was directed by Liudmila Snezhinskaia. On the Film Train under Medvedkin's direction, see Emma Widdis, *Alexander Medvedkin* (London: I.B. Tauris, 2005), 22–34. See also Alexander Medvedkin, "The Kino-Train: 294 Days on Wheels," in *The Alexander Medvedkin Reader*, ed. and trans. Jay Leyda, and N. M. Lary (Chicago: University of Chicago Press, 2016), 27–95.
41. Ia. Krasutskii, A. Shablitskii, and S. Fridman, eds., *12 udarnykh reisov* (Kokand: Izdanie kinofabriki poezda imeni K. E. Voroshilova, Soiuzkinokhroniki i TsOPKADR NKPS, 1934), 9.
42. Widdis, "The Film Train," 34.
43. A. Medvedkin, "Chto takoe kinopoezd?" in *Iz istorii kino*, vol. 11 (Moscow: Iskusstvo, 1985), 30.
44. The script of the Snezhinskaia film is so similar to the Gerasimova article, in fact, that it is quite clear that Snezhinskaia used Gerasimova as a source.
45. The soundtrack included early recordings of Soviet popular songs, including, for example, Orkestr i khor Uzbekskogo muzykal'nogo teatra, "Ak Altun," arr. To'xtasin Jalilov, lyrics Sobir Abdulla, Gramplasttrest 953, 1935. https://russian-records.com/details.php?image_id=28086 (accessed September 5, 2023).
46. *12 udarnykh reisov*, 30. The Film Train organized 163 film screenings while in Central Asia, but the pamphlet produced on the project indicates that only previously made films, rather than the locally produced ones, were screened in Central Asia due to delays in production. The film does seem to have been accessible at least to some Central Asian audiences; for example, S. Normatov's 1966 biography of Shodieva (discussed below) includes a number of still shots from the film among its photo plates. See Normatov, *Tadzhikhon*, photo inserts.
47. *12 udarnykh reisov*, 29. Translation in Emma Widdis, *Alexander Medvedkin*, 34.
48. The medals appear to be an Order of the Red Flag and a Lenin Prize. In May 1934, Shodieva was among 110 Politotdel directors awarded the Order of Lenin. See "O nagrazhdenii nachal'nikov politotdelov i direktorov MTS i sovkhozov," *Pravda*, no. 127 (8013), May 10, 1934, 1.
49. This is likely to be an exaggeration: polygamy, while tolerated in Central Asia before the Revolution, was limited by Islamic law to four wives.
50. The similarity in these lines with those reported in Gerasimova's account cannot be an accident. It is unclear, however, whether Snezhinskaia derived the lines from Gerasimova or vice versa. It is also possible that these lines were part of a story that Shodieva told about herself, or that both Snezhinskaia and Gerasimova had access to another source that is unavailable to me.
51. Cf. the transition from patriarchal to state authority described in Amin, *The Making of the Modern Iranian Woman*.
52. It is unclear whether the speech was pre-recorded in the 1920s or recorded by Snezhinskaia herself. Certainly, its text seems more characteristic of the Hujum era than the mid-1930s. But even for the late 1920s, the speech clearly conveys a sense of ownership and control in the Soviet project.
53. This scene can also be understood as a moment of queering: while heteronormative companionate marriage is becoming the norm in Central Asia, Shodieva stands aloof from the new romantic norms. Although apparently Shodieva remarried after escaping her marriage with the *rais*, her husband rarely appears in representations of her.

Conclusion

1. For his discussion of hybridity, see İğmen, *Speaking Soviet with an Accent*, 6.
2. See Kassymbekova, *Despite Cultures*; Botakoz Kassymbekova and Aminat Chokobaeva. "On Writing Soviet History of Central Asia: Frameworks, Challenges, Prospects," *Central Asian Survey*, 40, no. 4 (2021): 483–503.
3. William Mazzarella, "Against Contextualization: An Ethics of Encounter," *Comparative Studies of South Asia, Africa and the Middle East*, 42, no. 1 (2022): 262.
4. Adeeb Khalid, "The Historiography of Modern Central Asia Today," *Kritika: Explorations in Russian and Eurasian History*, 26, no. 1 (2025): 107. For a useful summary of the debate, see Nari

Shelekpayev, "Thinking beyond Soviet Teleologies: Perspectives for the Study of Central Asia," *Kritika: Explorations in Russian and Eurasian History*, 26, no. 1 (2025): 133–59. Key stances in this far-reaching debate include Kassymbekova and Chokobaeva, "On Writing Soviet History of Central Asia"; Alexander Morrison, "After the War: Central Asia without Russia," *SICE Blog* (blog), October 24, 2022, http://www.oeaw.ac.at/sice/sice-blog/after-the-war-central-asia-without-russia. For a Russophone intervention that has been particularly influential in Central Asia, see Madina Tlostanova, *Dekolonial'nost' bytiia, znaniia i oshchushcheniia: sbornik statei* (Almaty: Tselinnyi, 2020).

5. Vicente L. Rafael, *Contracting Colonialism: Translation and Christian Conversion in Tagalog Society under Early Spanish Rule* (Durham, NC: Duke University Press, 2005, 21.
6. This is not to say that the study of resistance is a dead end; in fact, I believe it is a promising and hitherto underdeveloped avenue for future research on Soviet Central Asia. However, it requires identifying new sources, formulating new theoretical approaches, and developing new methodologies for working with official sources.
7. Soviet Central Asians' adaptations of Socialist Realism might thus be seen as analogous to colonial American interpretations of the Latin Classics; see Erika Valdivieso, "Searching for Dido in the Latin Epics of Colonial Mexico," *TAPA*, 154, no. 2 (2024): 537–76; Erika Valdivieso, "The Inca Garcilaso in Dialogue with Neoplatonism," *Bulletin of Latin American Research*, 37 (2018): 74–85.
8. Kassymbekova, *Despite Cultures*, 8, emphasis original. For influential critiques of liberal subjectivity and the reification of "Bolshevik" as a category, see Krylova, "The Tenacious Liberal Subject," and Krylova, "Soviet Modernity."
9. Zulfiya, *Oydin Sobirova.*
10. Fayzieva, *Husayn Shams.*
11. On Qori-Yoqubov's indictment and death, see Bahrom Irzayev, "Sobiq masjid qorisi, jahon yulduzi—Muhiddin qori Yoqubov nima uchun sho'ro hukumatiga dushmanlikda ayblangan?" *Oyina* (July 5, 2023), https://oyina.uz/uz/article/1752 (accessed March 21, 2025). See also Saodat Nazarova, "XX asrning 20–30 yillaridagi o'zbek sahna san'ati rivojida Muhiddin Qori Yoqubovning o'rni," *O'zMU Xabarlari*, special issue (2013), 97–9.
12. Shaw, "The Many Nationalities of Tamara Khanum."
13. See Gulsanam Halmuradova, "The Eternal Muse of Eastern Dance," *Elle Uzbekistan*, July 3, 2024, https://elleuzbekistan.com/en/the-eternal-muse-of-eastern-dance/ (accessed March 21, 2025).
14. The document condemning Shodieva to exile can be found in Shamsutdinov et al. *Repressiia*, 223.
15. Evgeniia Ginzburg, *Krutoi marshrut: khronika vremen kul'ta lichnosti* (Moscow: Sovetskii pisatel', 1990).
16. Quoted in Kamp, "Three Lives of Saodat," 40–1. Kamp notes that this oral history, conducted in 1991, differs profoundly from Shamsieva's triumphal 1961 account of her participation in carrying out a purge.
17. Gerasimova repeats the old tropes about unveiling exposing Tojixon to the media: "Cameras clicked, and the cinematographer's lights shone, as Tojixon removed her *chachvan*." Valeriia Gerasimova, "Ozarennye litsa," *Pravda*, March 8, 1963, 4.
18. Normatov, *Tadzhikhan*. This version is a translation from the Uzbek, but I have so far been unable to locate the Uzbek original.

Bibliography

Archives

ANDAMA (Alisher Navoiy davlat adabiyot muzeyi arxivi), the Alisher Navoiy State Literature Museum Archive.

O'zMDA (O'zbekiston respublikasi markaziy davlat arxivi, known since 2019 as O'zbekiston Milliy arxivi), the Central State Archive of the Republic of Uzbekistan, Tashkent.

O'zRFASI (O'zbekiston Respublikasi Fanlar Akademiyasi San'atshunoslik Instituti Arxivi), the Republic of Uzbekistan Academy of Sciences Archive of the Institute for the Study of the Arts, Tashkent.

RGALI (Rossiiskii gosudarstvennyi arkhiv literatury i iskusstva), the Russian State Archive of Literature and the Arts, Moscow.

RGASPI (Rossiiskii gosudarstvennyi arkhiv sotsial'no-politicheskoi istorii), the Russian State Archive of Socio-Political History, Moscow.

Periodicals

Alanga
Izvestiia
Kambag'al dehqon
  Renamed *Kolxoz yo'li* (from 1931)
Kommunist vostoka
Komsomolets vostoka
Literatura srednei azii
Madaniy inqilob
Maorif va o'qitg'uvchi
Mushtum
Muxbirlar yo'ldoshi
Ogonek
O'zbekiston fizkulturachisi
Pravda
Pravda vostoka
Qizil O'zbekiston
Qurilish (1931–32)
  Renamed *O'zbekiston sho'ro adabiyoti* (1932–34)
  Renamed *O'zbekiston sovet adabiyoti* (1934)
  Renamed *Sovet adabiyoti* (1935–37)
  Renamed *O'zbekiston adabiyoti va san'ati* (1937–41)
  Renamed *Sharq Yulduzi* (1946–present)
Sovetskaia muzyka
Uzbekistanskaia pravda
Ülkü
Xudosizlar
Yangi Farg'ona
Yangi yo'l (1926–34)
  Renamed *Yorqin turmush* (1936–37)
  Renamed *Yorqin hayot* (1938–41)
  Renamed *O'zbekiston xotin-qizlari* (1950–66)

Renamed *Saodat* (1966 onward)
Yer yuzi (1925–34)
Renamed *Guliston* (1934–41)
Yosh kuch
Yosh leninchi
Za partiiu
Zvezda vostoka

Reference Works

Encyclop ædia Iranica, edited by Ehsan Yarshater. London: Routledge & Kegan Paul, 1983; and online edition. New York, 1996-present. iranicaonline.org.
Encyclopedia of Islam, 2nd ed, edited by P. J. Bearman et al. Leiden: Brill, 1960–2005.

Selected Published Primary Sources

Adabiyot darsligi: o'rta maktablarning VI sinfi uchun. Tashkent: O'quv-pedagogik davlat nashriyoti, 1937.
Adabiyot xrestomatiyasi—o'rta maktablarning VI sinfi uchun. Tashkent: O'zdavnashr, 1936.
Aini, Sadriddin. *Raby: roman*. Translated by Sergei Borodin. Dushanbe: Irfon, 1977.
Aini, Sadriddin. *The Sands of Oxus: Boyhood Reminiscences of Sadriddin Aini*. Translated by John R. Perry and Rachel Lehr. Costa Mesa, CA: Mazda, 2012.
Akbarov, Ilyos, and X. Rasulov, eds. *O'zbek xalq ashulalari*. 2 vols. Tashkent: O'zdavnashr, 1937.
Alimova, Dilorom. *Tragediia sredneaziatskogo kishlaka: kollektivizatsiia, raskulachivanie, ssylka, 1929–1955 gg.: dokumenty i materialy*. Tashkent: Shark, 2006.
Arkhangel'skii, S. F., and P. K. Lutsenko. *10 let bor'by za khlopok v uzbekistane*. Tashkent: O'zdavnashr, 1935.
Mukhtar Ashrafii. *Muzyka v moei zhizni: sbornik statei*. Tashkent: Izdatel'stvo literatury i iskusstva im. Gafura Guliama, 1975.
'Ayni, Sadr al-Dīn. *Namuna-'i adabiyāt-i Tājīk*. Moscow: Nashrīyāt-i markazī-i khalq-i Ittiḥād-i Jamāhīr-i Shūravī-i Sūsiyālīstī, 1926.
Ayniy, Sadriddin. *Qullar*. Tashkent: O'zdavnashr, 1935.
Ainii, Sadriddin. *Raby*. Translated by Sergei Borodin. Moscow: Sovetskii Pisatel', 1950.
Bakhtin, Mikhail. *The Dialogic Imagination: Four Essays*. Edited by Michael Holquist. Translated by Caryl Emerson and Michael Holquist. Austin, TX: University of Texas Press, 1981.
Balázs, Béla. *Béla Balázs: Early Film Theory*. Edited by Erica Carter. Translated by Rodney Livingstone. New York: Berghahn Books, 2011.
Behbudiy, Mahmudxo'ja. *Tanlangan Asarlar*. Edited by Begali Qosimov. Tashkent: Ma'naviyat, 1999.
Burnes, Alexander. *Travels into Bokhara: Being the Account of a Journey from India to Cabool, Tartary and Persia. Also, Narrative of a Voyage on the Indus, from the Sea to Lahore. Performed under the Orders of the Supreme Government of India in 1831, 1832, 1833*. Philadelphia: E. L. Carey & A. Hart, 1835.
Christie, Ella Robertson. *Through Khiva to Golden Samarkand; the Remarkable Story of a Woman's Adventurous Journey Alone through the Deserts of Central Asia to the Heart of Turkestan*. London: Seeley, Service & Co. Limited, 1925.
Cho'lpon, Abdulhamid Sulaymon o'g'li. *Night and Day*. Translated by Christopher Fort. Academic Studies Press, 2019.
Eikhgorn, Avgust. *Muzykal'naia fol'kloristika v Uzbekistane*. Edited by V. M. Beliaev. Tashkent: Izdatel'stvo akademii nauk uzbekskoi SSR, 1963.
Engels, Frederic. *Anti-Dühring*. In *Marx and Engels Collected Works*, vol. 25. London: Lawrence & Wishart, 1987, 5–312.
Fitrat, Abdurrauf. *Eng eski turk adabiyoti namunalari*. Tashkent: O'zbekiston davlat nashriyoti, 1927.
Fitrat, Abdurrauf. *O'zbek klassik musiqasi va uning tarixi*. Tashkent: Fan, 1993.

Gavrilov, Mikhail, trans. *Risolia sartovskikh remeslennikov.* Tashkent: Tipografiia pri kantseliarii general-gubernatora, 1912.
Ginzburg, Evgeniia Semenovna. *Krutoi marshrut: khronika vremen kul'ta lichnosti.* Moscow: Sovetskii pisatel', 1990.
Halle, Fannina W. *Women in the Soviet East.* New York: E.P. Dutton & Co., Inc., 1938.
Hughes, Langston. "Tamara Khanum: Soviet Asia's Greatest Dancer," *Theatre Arts Monthly*, 18, no. 11 (November 1934): 829–35.
Ikramov, Akmal. *Osnovnye voprosy kul'turnogo stroitel'stva v uzbekistane.* Tashkent: Gosudarstvennoe izdatel'stvo Uzbekskoi SSR, 1932.
Kakhkhar, Abdulla. *Skazki o bylom: povesti i rasskazy.* Translated by Konstantin Simonov. Moscow: Khudozhestvennaia literatura, 1987.
Khodzhaev, Faizulla. *Izbrannye Trudy.* Vol. 3. Tashkent: Fan, 1973.
Kommunisticheskaia partiia sovetskogo soiuza. *Kommunisticheskaia partiia sovetskogo soiuza v rezoliutsiiakh i resheniiakh s'ezdov, konferentsii i plenumov TsK. 1898–1953.* Moscow: Gosudarstvennoe izdatel'stvo politicheskoi literatury, 1953.
Krasutskii, Ia, A. Shablitskii, and S. Fridman, eds. *12 udarnykh reisov.* Kokand: Izdanie kino-fabriki poezda imeni K. E. Voroshilova, Soiuzkinokhroniki i TsOPKADR NKPS, 1934.
Krzhizhanovskii, Sigizmund. "Salyr-Giul." In *Sobranie sochinenii v piati tomakh*, vol. 3. Ed. Vadim Perel'muter. Moscow: Symposium, 2003.
Kunitz, Joshua. *Dawn over Samarkand; the Rebirth of Central Asia.* New York: Covici, Friede, 1935.
Lenin, V. I. "Gosudarstvo i revoliutsiia." In *Sobranie sochinenii*, vol. 14, no. 2, *Burzhuaznaia revoliutsiia 1917 g.* Moscow: Gosudarstvennoe izdatel'stvo, 1923, 308–13.
Lukács, György. *The Historical Novel.* Translated by Hannah and Stanley Mitchell. London: Merlin Press, 1962.
Lukàcs, Georg. "Rasskaz ili opisanie," *Literaturnyi Kritik*, no. 8 (1936): 44–67.
Lukàcs, Georg. "Narrate or Describe?" In *Writer and Critic, and Other Essays*, edited by Arthur Kahn. London: Merlin Press, 1970.
Lukàcs, Georg. *The Theory of the Novel: A Historico-Philosophical Essay on the Forms of Great Epic Literature.* Translated by Anna Bostock. Cambridge, MA: MIT Press, 1971.
Luppol, I. K., M. M. Rozental', and S. M. Tret'iakov, eds. *Pervyi vsesoiuznyi s'ezd sovetskikh pisatelei, 1934: stenograficheskii otchet.* Moscow: Gosudarstvennoe izdatel'stvo "Khudozhestvennaia literatura," 1934.
Maillart, Ella. *Turkestan Solo: One Woman's Expedition from the Tien Shan to the Kizil Kum.* London: W. Heinemann, 1938.
Majidiy, Rahmat. *Literatura Uzbekistana.* Moscow: Khudozhestvennaia literatura, 1934.
Majidiy, Rahmat. "Sarob to'g'risida," *O'zbekiston adabiyoti va san'ati*, no. 5 (1941).
Mannin, Ethel. *South to Samarkand.* New York: E. P. Dutton and Company, Incorporated, 1937.
McGuire, Gabriel, Chris Fort, Naomi Caffee, Emily Laskin, Samuel Hodgkin, and Ali F. İğmen, eds. *Tulips in Bloom: An Anthology of Modern Central Asian Literature.* Singapore: Palgrave Macmillan, 2024.
Mironov, Nikolai *Pesni Fergany, Bukhary, i Khivy.* Tashkent: UzGIZ, 1931.
Muhamedova, Xafiyaxon, and Ilyos Akbarov. *O'zbek ashullalari.* Moscow: Muzgiz, 1934.
Niyoziy, Hamza Hakimzoda. *To'la asarlar to'plami.* Edited by Naim Karimov, Yusuf Sultonov, et. al. Tashkent: Fan, 1988.
Normatov, S. *Tadzhikhon.* Tashkent: Uzbekistan, 1966.
Olufsen, Ole. *The Emir of Bokhara and His Country: Journeys and Studies in Bokhara (with a Chapter on My Voyage on the Amu Darya to Khiva).* Copenhagen: Gyldendal, Nordisk Forlag, 1911.
O'zbekiston kommunistik partiyasi. *Rezoliutsii i resheniia s'ezdov Kommunisticheskoi partii Uzbekistana.* Tashkent: Gosudarstvennoe izdatel'stvo uzbekskoi SSR, 1957.
O'zSSR MXK Boshlang'ich va o'rta maktab boshqarmasi. *Adabiyot programmasi: O'rta maktablarning V-VI va VII sinflari uchun.* Tashkent: O'zdavnashr, 1935.

O'zSSR MXK Sirtqi Pedbilim Yurtlari Sektori, ed. *Sirtqi pedbilim yurtlari uchun Adabiyot programmasi va metodik ko'rsatma*. Tashkent: O'zSSR Maorif Xalq komisarligi, 1939.

Pekhovich, L. *Komsomol uzbekistana v bor'be za khlopok: k IX vsesoiuznomu s'ezdu VLKSM*. Moscow: OGIZ - Molodaia Gvardiia, 1931.

Qahhor, Abdulla. *Dardakdan chiqqan qahramon*. Tashkent: O'zdavnashr, 1942.

Qahhor, Abdulla. *Hikoyalar*. O'zdavnashr, 1935.

Qahhor, Abdulla. *Hikoyalar*. Boshlang'ich kitobxonlar uchun. O'zdavnashr, 1938.

Qahhor, Abdulla. *Hikoyalar*. O'zOGIZ - Nafis Adabiyot Nashriyoti, 1939.

Qahhor, Abdulla. *Olam yasharadir*. Tashkent: O'znashr, 1933.

Qahhor, Abdulla. *O'tmishdan ertaklar*. Tashkent: Yosh gvardiia, 1976.

Qahhor, Abdulla. *Qishloq hukm ostida*. Tashkent: O'znashr, 1932.

Qahhor, Abdulla. *Qotilning tug'ilishi*. Tashkent: O'zdavnashr, 1933.

Qahhor, Abdulla. *Qo'zg'olish: "Sarob" romanidan parchalar*. Boshlang'ich kitobxonlar uchun. Tashkent: O'zdavnashr, 1936.

Qahhor, Abdulla. *Qanotsiz chittak*. Tashkent: O'zdavnashr, 1937.

Qahhor, Abdulla. *Sarimsoqnoma ("Sarob" romanidan parchalar)*. Tashkent: O'zSSR Davlat Nashriyoti, 1937.

Qahhor, Abdulla. *Sarob*. Tashkent: O'zdavnashr, 1937.

Qahhor, Abdulla. *Tanlangan Asarlar*. Edited by Nodira Jalolova, Otabek Jo'raboyev, et al. 3 vols. Tashkent: Yangi Asr Avlodi, 2015.

Ramazanov, S. *O'zbek muziqa to'plami: Xorazm, Farg'ona kuylari*. Tashkent: O'zdavnashr, 1933.

Rasulov, X., and Ilyos Akbarov, eds. *O'zbek xalq ashulalari*. Tashkent: O'zbekiston davlat nashriyoti, 1937.

Rimskii, I. M., ed. *Uzbekskaia muzyka v grammofonnoi zapisi*. Moscow: Gramplasttrest, 1937.

Romanovskaia, Elena, and Ilyos Akbarov, eds. *O'zbek xalq qo'shiqlari*. 2 vols. Tashkent: O'zdavfimnashr, 1939.

Schuyler, Eugene. *Turkistan: Notes of a Journey in Russian Turkistan, Khokand, Bukhara, and Kuldja*. London: S. Low, Marston, Searle & Rivington, 1876.

Shamsutdinov, Rustambek, et al., eds. *Repressiia. Dokumenty i materialy*. Tashkent: Shark, 2005.

Sobirova, Oydin. *Chaqaloqqa Chakmancha*. Tashkent: O'zdavnashr, 1939.

Sobirova, Oydin. *Chechan qo'llar (dostonlar)*. Tashkent: O'znashr, 1932.

Sobirova, Oydin. *Tong qo'shig'i*. Tashkent: O'znashr, 1931.

Shams, Husayn. *Dushman*. Tashkent: O'zdavnashr, 1934.

Shams, Husayn. *Haqqoniyat*. Tashkent: O'zSSR Davlat Nashriyoti, 1937.

Shams, Husayn. *Hikoyalar*. Tashkent: O'zdavnashr, 1933.

Shams, Husayn. *Qurulush*. Tashkent: O'znashr, 1932.

Shams, Husayn. *Radio (hikoya)*. Ishchilar kutubxonasi. Tashkent: O'znashr, 1931.

Shams, Husayn. *Tanlangan asarlar*. Tashkent: O'zSSR Davlat Badiiy Adabiyot Nashriyoti, 1959.

Shams, Husayn. *Tanqid (p'esa)*. Tashkent: O'zdavnashr, 1932.

Stalin, Joseph. *Marksizm i natsional'no-kolonial'nyi vopros: sbornik izbrannykh statei i rechei*. Moscow: Partiinoe izdatel'stvo, 1934.

Strong, Anna Louise. *Red Star in Samarkand*. New York: Coward-McCann, 1929.

Tchokaieff, M. A., "Fifteen Years of Bolshevik Rule in Turkistan," *Journal of the Royal Central Asian Society*, vol. 20 (1933), 351–59.

Teichman, Eric. *Journey to Turkistan*. London: Hodder and Stoughton, 1937.

Uspenskii, Viktor A. *Shest' muzykal'nykh poem (makom) zapisannykh V.A. Uspenskim v Bukhare*. Bukhara: Izdanie narodnogo nazarata prosveshcheniia Bukhrespubliki, 1924.

Vámbéry, Ármin. *Travels in Central Asia: Being the Account of a Journey from Teheran across the Turkoman Desert on the Eastern Shore of the Caspian to Khiva, Bokhara, and Samarcand; Performed in the Year 1863*. New York: Harper & Brothers, 1865.

Vohidov, Erkin, G. Nurullaeva, and N. Komilov. "Abdulla Qahhor zamondoshlari xotirasida," *Sharq Yulduzi*, no. 9 (1987): 165.

Zübeyr, Hamit. *Halk terbiyesi*. Ankara: Köy Hocası Matbaası, 1931.

Zulfiya. *Dugonalar bilan suhbat*. Tashkent: O'zdavnashr, 1953.

Zulfiya. *Oydin Sobirova.* Tashkent: O'zdavnashr, 1953.
Zulfiya. *Qizlar qo'shig'i.* Tashkent: O'zdavnashr, 1939.

Selected Secondary Sources

Abashin, Sergei. "The 'Fierce Fight' at Oshoba: A Microhistory of the Conquest of the Khoqand Khanate." *Central Asian Survey* 33, no. 2 (2014): 215–31.

Abashin, Sergei. *Sovetskii kishlak: Mezhdu kolonializmom i modernizatsiei.* Biblioteka zhurnala "Neprikosnovennyi zapas," Moscow: Novoe literaturnoe obozrenie, 2015.

Abdugafurova, Donohon. "'I Was Born in the Wrong Time': The Concept of Selfhood in the Writings of Anbar Otin," *Journal of Islamic and Muslim Studies*, 4, no. 1 (2019): 66–86.

Abdukadyrov, Nurzhigit, Tolkyn Mukhazhanova, and Gulmira Sabdenova. "Ottoman Subjects and Prisoners of War in the Semirechye Oblast during the First World War." *International Journal of Asian Studies* 21, no. 2 (2024): 272–83.

Abdusamatov, Hofiz. *Abdulla Qahhor hayoti va ijodi haqida ocherk.* Tashkent: O'zSSR Davlat Badiiy Adabiyot Nashriyoti, 1960.

Abu-Lughod, Lila. *Do Muslim Women Need Saving?* Cambridge, MA: Harvard University Press, 2013.

Abykayeva-Tiesenhausen, Aliya. *Central Asia in Art: From Soviet Orientalism to the New Republics.* London: I.B. Tauris, 2016.

Ahmadi, Wali. "The Institution of Persian Literature and the Genealogy of Bahar's 'Stylistics.'" *British Journal of Middle Eastern Studies* 31, no. 2 (2004): 141–52.

Ahmedov, Mahmud. *Yunus Rajabiy.* Tashkent: O'qituvchi, 1967.

Aini, Kholida, and Iurii Stepanovich Mal'tsev. *Zhizn' Sadriddina Aini: kratkii khronologicheskii ocherk.* Dushanbe: Donish, 1982.

Akbarov, Adham. *Qalb kuychisi.* Tashkent: O'zbekiston KP MKning nashriyoti, 1965.

Akilov, K. A., and M. A. Guliamova. *Sovetskaia intelligentsiia Uzbekistana.* Tashkent: Fan, 1978.

Alimova, D. A., and R. Ia. Radzhapova, eds. *Turkestan v nachale XX veka: k istorii istokov natsional'noi nezavisimosti.* Tashkent: Shark, 2000.

Alimova, Markhamat Nasyrovna. "'Saodat'ning tarixiga bir nazar," *Muxbir*, no. 11 (1975): 10–11.

Alimova, Markhamat Nasyrovna. "Yangi Hayot ijodkorlarining kuychisi," *Muxbir*, no. 11 (1979): 36–7.

Alimova, Markhamat Nasyrovna. *Ular birinchilardan edilar.* Tashkent: O'zbekiston, 1983.

Alimuhamedov, A. "Abdulla Qahhor hikoyalarida psixologik tasvir," *Sharq Yulduzi*, no. 2–3 (1947).

Allworth, Edward. *Uzbek Literary Politics.* The Hague: Mouton, 1964.

Allworth, Edward. *Central Asian Publishing and the Rise of Nationalism; an Essay and a List of Publications in the New York Public Library.* New York: New York Public Library, 1965.

Allworth, Edward. *Nationalities of the Soviet East: Publications and Writing Systems. A Bibliographical Directory and Transliteration Tables for Iranian- and Turkic-Language Publications, 1818–1945, Located in U.S. Libraries.* New York: Columbia University Press, 1971.

Allworth, Edward. *Soviet Asia, Bibliographies: A Compilation of Social Science and Humanities Sources on the Iranian, Mongolian, and Turkic Nationalities, with an Essay on the Soviet-Asian Controversy.* New York: Praeger, 1975.

Allworth, Edward. *The Preoccupations of 'Abdalrauf Fitrat, Bukharan Nonconformist: An Analysis and List of His Writings.* Berlin: Das Arabische Buch, 2000.

Allworth, Edward. *Evading Reality: The Devices of 'Abdalrauf Fitrat, Modern Central Asian Reformist.* Leiden: Brill, 2002.

Aminova, R. Kh. *Pobeda kolkhoznogo stroia v Uzbekistane: 1933–1941 gg.* Tashkent: Fan, 1981.

Amonov, R. "Geografiyai osori Badeii ustod Aini," in *Jashnnomai Aini*, Vol. 5. Edited by M. Shukurov and L. Demidchik. Dushanbe: Donish, 1978, 13–23.

Anderson, Benedict. *Imagined Communities: Reflections on the Origin and Spread of Nationalism.* New York: Verso, 2006.

Andronikashvili, Zaal. "National Form: The Evolution of Georgian Socialist Realism." *Slavic Review* 81, no. 4 (2022): 914–35.

Arbuthnot, Mollie. "Heritage Modernism: Museums and Craft Revival in Early Soviet Tashkent." *Kritika: Explorations in Russian and Eurasian History* 26, no. 1 (2025): 5–34.

Atabaki, Touraj. "Disgruntled Guests: Iranian Subaltern on the Margins of the Tsarist Empire." *International Review of Social History* 48, no. 3 (2003): 401–26.

Atabaki, Touraj and Erik Jan Zürcher. *Men of Order: Authoritarian Modernization under Atatürk and Reza Shah.* London: I.B. Tauris, 2004.

Atnashev, Timur, Mikhail Velizhev, and Tatiana Vaizer, eds. *Nesovershennaia publichnaia sfera: istoriia rezhimov publichnosti v Rossii.* Moscow: Novoe literaturnoe obozrenie, 2021.

Attwood, Lynne. *Creating the New Soviet Woman: Women's Magazines as Engineers of Female Identity, 1922–53.* New York: St. Martin's Press, 1999.

Auslander, Leora. *Cultural Revolutions: Everyday Life and Politics in Britain, North America, and France.* Berkeley: University of California Press, 2009.

Avdeeva, L. A. *Mukhitdin Kari-Iakubov: dokumental'naia monografiia.* Tashkent: Izdatel'stvo literatury i iskusstva im. Gafura Guliama, 1984.

Baldauf, Ingeborg. "Educating the Poets and Fostering Uzbek Poetry of the 1910s to Early 1930s." *Cahiers d'Asie Centrale* 24 (March 2015): 183–211.

Baron, Beth. *Egypt As a Woman: Nationalism, Gender, and Politics.* Berkeley: University of California Press, 2005.

Bečka, Jiří. *Sadriddin Ayni: Father of Modern Tajik Culture.* Vol. 5. Naples: Istituto universitario orientale, Seminario di studi asiatici, 1980.

Beeley, Brian W. "The Turkish Village Coffeehouse as a Social Institution." *Geographical Review* 60, no. 4 (1970): 475–93.

Begmatov, Kh. B. "K voprosu o roli pechati v osushchestvlenii kul'turnoi revoliutsii v Uzbekistane." *Trudy Samarkandskogo gosudarstvennogo universiteta im. A. Navoi* 121 (1963), 50–67.

Beliaev, Viktor. *Central Asian Music: Essays in the History of the Music of the Peoples of the USSR.* Edited by Mark Slobin. Translated by Mark and Greta Slobin. Middletown, CT: Wesleyan University Press, 1975.

Bellér-Hann, Ildikó. "Crafts, Entrepreneurship and Gendered Economic Relations in Southern Xinjiang in the Era of 'socialist Commodity Economy.'" *Central Asian Survey* 17, no. 4 (1998): 701–18.

Bergne, Paul. *The Birth of Tajikistan: National Identity and the Origins of the Republic.* London: I. B. Tauris, 2007.

Bird, Robert. "The Poetics of Peat in Soviet Literary and Visual Culture, 1918–1959." *Slavic Review* 70, no. 3 (2011): 591–614.

Blitstein, Peter A. "Cultural Diversity and the Interwar Conjuncture: Soviet Nationality Policy in Its Comparative Context." *Slavic Review* 65, no. 2 (2006): 273–93.

Bogdanov, Konstantin, ed. *Dzhambul Dzhambaev : prikliucheniia kazakhskogo akyna v sovetskoi strane.* Moscow: Novoe literaturnoe obozrenie, 2013.

Booth, Marilyn. *May Her Likes Be Multiplied: Biography and Gender Politics in Egypt.* Berkeley: University of California Press, 2001.

Borolina, I. V. *Abdulla Kakhkhar: ocherk tvorchestva.* Tashkent: Gosudarsvennoe izdatel'stvo khudozhestvennoi literatury, 1957.

Bradley, Joseph. "Subjects into Citizens: Societies, Civil Society, and Autocracy in Tsarist Russia." *The American Historical Review* 107, no. 4 (2002): 1094–1123.

Braginskii, Iosif Samoilovich. *Problemy tvorchestva Sadriddina Aini.* Dushanbe: Irfon, 1974.

Braginskii, Iosif Samoilovich. *Sadriddin Aini: Zhizn' i tvorchestvo.* Moscow: Sovetskii pisatel', 1978.

Brandenberger, David. *National Bolshevism: Stalinist Mass Culture and the Formation of Modern Russian National Identity, 1931–1956.* Cambridge, MA: Harvard University Press, 2002.

Brandenberger, David. *Propaganda State in Crisis: Soviet Ideology, Indoctrination, and Terror under Stalin, 1927–1941.* New Haven: Yale University Press, 2011.

Brooks, Jeffrey. "Socialist Realism in Pravda: Read All about It!" *Slavic Review* 53, no. 4 (1994): 973–91.
Brooks, Jeffrey. *Thank You, Comrade Stalin!: Soviet Public Culture from Revolution to Cold War.* Princeton, NJ: Princeton University Press, 2000.
Brooks, Jeffrey. *When Russia Learned to Read: Literacy and Popular Literature, 1861–1917.* Evanston, IL: Northwestern University Press, 2003.
Brophy, David. *Uyghur Nation.* Cambridge, MA: Harvard University Press, 2016.
Buck-Morss, Susan. *Dreamworld and Catastrophe: The Passing of Mass Utopia in East and West.* Cambridge, MA: MIT Press, 2000.
Buckley, Mary. *Mobilizing Soviet Peasants: Heroines and Heroes of Stalin's Fields.* Lanham, MD: Rowman & Littlefield, 2006.
Bustanov, Alfrid K. "Muslim Literature in the Atheist State: Zainap Maksudova between Soviet Modernity and Tradition." *Journal of Islamic Manuscripts* 9, no. 1 (January 1, 2018): 1–31.
Bustanov, Alfrid K. "A Space for the Subject: Tracing Garden Culture in Muslim Russia." *Journal of the Economic and Social History of the Orient* 65, no. 1–2 (2022): 74–125.
Caffee, Naomi. "How Tatiana's Voice Rang across the Steppe: Russian Literature in the Life and Legend of Abai." *Journal of Eurasian Studies* 9, no. 1 (2018): 12–19.
Calhoun, Craig. "Civil Society and the Public Sphere." In *The Oxford Handbook of Civil Society,* Edited by Michael Edwards. Oxford: Oxford University Press, 2012.
Calhoun, Craig J. *Habermas and the Public Sphere.* Cambridge, Mass: The MIT Press, 1992.
Cameron, Sarah. *The Hungry Steppe: Famine, Violence, and the Making of Soviet Kazakhstan.* Ithaca, NY: Cornell University Press, 2018.
Cameron, Sarah. "New Directions in the Study of Modern Central Asian History." *Kritika: Explorations in Russian and Eurasian History* 26, no. 1 (2025): 161–76.
Carey, James W. "Technology and Ideology: The Case of the Telegraph." *Prospects* 8, no. 10 (1983): 303–25.
Carlisle, Donald S. "The Uzbek Power Elite: Politburo and Secretariat (1938–83)." *Central Asian Survey* 5, no. 3/4 (1986): 91.
Carrère d'Encausse, Hélène. *Islam and the Russian Empire: Reform and Revolution in Central Asia.* London: I.B. Tauris, 2009.
Castillo, Greg. "Peoples at an Exhibition: Soviet Architecture and the National Question." *South Atlantic Quarterly* 94, no. 3 (1995): 715.
Çeçen, Anıl. *Halk evleri: Atatürk'ün kültür kurumu.* Ankara: Gündoğan Yayınları, 1990.
Charles, Guy-Uriel and Luis Fuentes-Rohwer. "Habermas, the Public Sphere, and the Creation of a Racial Counterpublic." *Michigan Journal of Race & Law* 21, no. 1 (Fall 2015): 1–21.
Chatterjee, Partha. *The Nation and Its Fragments: Colonial and Postcolonial Histories.* Princeton, NJ: Princeton University Press, 2020.
Cheng, Anne Anlin. *Ornamentalism.* Oxford: Oxford University Press, 2019.
Clark, Katerina. *Moscow, the Fourth Rome: Stalinism, Cosmopolitanism, and the Evolution of Soviet Culture, 1931–1941.* Cambridge, MA: Harvard University Press, 2011.
Clark, Katerina. *The Soviet Novel: History as Ritual.* Bloomington, IN: Indiana University Press, 2000.
Clement, Victoria. *Learning to Become Turkmen: Literacy, Language, and Power, 1914–2014.* Pittsburgh, PA: University of Pittsburgh Press, 2018.
Corney, Frederick C. *Telling October: Memory and the Making of the Bolshevik Revolution.* Ithaca, NY: Cornell University Press, 2004.
Crews, Robert D. *For Prophet and Tsar: Islam and Empire in Russia and Central Asia.* Cambridge, MA: Harvard University Press, 2006.
David-Fox, Michael. "Review: *Obshchestvennye organizatsii Rossii v 1920-e gody.*" *Kritika: Explorations in Russian and Eurasian History* 3, no. 1 (2002): 173–81.
David-Fox, Michael. *Crossing Borders: Modernity, Ideology, and Culture in Russia and the Soviet Union.* Pittsburgh, PA: University of Pittsburgh Press, 2015.

David-Fox, Michael. "The Intelligentsia, the Masses, and the West." In *Crossing Borders: Modernity, Ideology, and Culture in Russia and the Soviet Union*, 48–74. Pittsburgh, PA: University of Pittsburgh Press, 2015.

Djagalov, Rossen. *From Internationalism to Postcolonialism: Literature and Cinema between the Second and the Third Worlds.* Montreal: McGill-Queen's University Press, 2020.

Djumaev, Alexander. "Power Structures, Culture Policy, and Traditional Music in Soviet Central Asia." *Yearbook for Traditional Music* 25 (1993): 43–50.

Djumaev, Alexander. "Abdurauf Fitrat i ego sovremenniki na 'muzykal'nom fronte' Uzbekistana (20–30e gody)." *CA&C Press AB* (Accessed July 10, 2023). https://ca-c.org.ru/journal/1997/07-1997/st_21_gumaev.shtml.

Dobrenko, Evgeny *Political Economy of Socialist Realism.* New Haven: Yale University Press, 2007.

Dobrenko, Evgeny. "Hegemony of Brotherhood: The Birth of Soviet Multinational Literature, 1922–1932." *Slavic Review* 81, no. 4 (2022): 869–90.

Drieu, Cloé. *Cinema, Nation, and Empire in Uzbekistan, 1919–1937.* Bloomington, IN: Indiana University Press, 2019.

Dunham, Vera Sandomirsky. *In Stalin's Time: Middleclass Values in Soviet Fiction.* Durham: Duke University Press, 1990.

Eden, Jeff. "Beyond the Bazaars: Geographies of the Slave Trade in Central Asia." *Modern Asian Studies* 51, no. 4 (2017): 919.

Edgar, Adrienne. "Emancipation of the Unveiled: Turkmen Women under Soviet Rule, 1924–29." *Russian Review* 62, no. 1 (2003): 132–49.

Edgar, Adrienne. "Bolshevism, Patriarchy, and the Nation: The Soviet 'Emancipation' of Muslim Women in Pan-Islamic Perspective." *Slavic Review* 65, no. 2 (2006): 252–72.

Edgar, Adrienne Lynn. *Tribal Nation: The Making of Soviet Turkmenistan.* Princeton, NJ: Princeton University Press, 2004.

Edgar, Adrienne Lynn. *Intermarriage and the Friendship of Peoples : Ethnic Mixing in Soviet Central Asia.* Ithaca, NY: Cornell University Press, 2022.

Emami, Farshid. "Coffee Houses, Urban Spaces, and the Formation of a Public Sphere in Safavid Isfahan." *Muqarnas* 33 (2016): 177–220.

Engelstein, Laura. "The Dream of Civil Society in Tsarist Russia: Law, State, and Religion." In *Civil Society before Democracy: Lessons from Nineteenth-Century Europe.* Edited by Nancy Bermeo and Philip Nord. New York: Rowman & Littlefield, 2000.

Erdman, Michael J. "Vehicularizing the Vernacular: Using the Periodical Press to Popularize Vernacular Languages in Soviet Turkic Communities." *Central Asian Survey* 42, no. 3 (2023): 1–19.

Erkinov, Aftandil. "How Muhammad Rahīm Khān II of Khiva (1864–1910) Cultivated His Court Library as a Means of Resistance against the Russian Empire." *Journal of Islamic Manuscripts* 2 (2011): 36–49.

Erkinov, Aftandil. "Striving for Cultural Perfection at the Khivan Royal Court under Muhammad Rahim Khan II as a Means of Resistance to the Russian Protectorate Regime." In *Proceedings of the International Conference: Reassessing the Heritage of Khoja Ahmet Yasawi.* Edited by Ashirbek Muminov and Nurlan Dukenbaev. Istanbul: Research Centre for Islamic History, Art and Culture, 2024, 163–94.

Ernazarov, T. E., and A. I. Akbarov. *Istoriia pechati Uzbekistana.* Tashkent: O'qituvchi, 1977.

Ertürk, Nergis. *Grammatology and Literary Modernity in Turkey.* Oxford: Oxford University Press, 2011.

Fairclough, Pauline. "Was Soviet Music Middlebrow? Shostakovich's Fifth Symphony, Socialist Realism, and the Mass Listener in the 1930s," *Journal of Musicology*, 35, no. 3 (2018): 336–67.

Fani, Aria. "Disciplining Persian Literature in Twentieth-Century Afghanistan." *Iranian Studies* 55, no. 3 (2022): 675–95.

Fani, Aria. *Reading across Borders: Afghans, Iranians, and Literary Nationalism.* Austin, TX: University of Texas Press, 2024.

Fayzieva, Dilbar. *Husayn Shams: adibning 70 yilligiga*. Tashkent: G'ofur G'ulom nomidagi adabiyot va san'at nashriyoti, 1973.

Feldman, Leah. *On the Threshold of Eurasia: Revolutionary Poetics in the Caucasus*. Ithaca, NY: Cornell University Press, 2018.

Fine, Robert. "Civil Society Theory, Enlightenment and Critique." *Democratization* 4, no. 1 (1997): 7–28.

Finkel, Stuart. *On the Ideological Front: The Russian Intelligentsia and the Making of the Soviet Public Sphere*. New Haven: Yale University Press, 2007.

Fitzpatrick, Sheila. "Cultural Revolution in Russia 1928–32." *Journal of Contemporary History* 9, no. 1 (1974): 33–52.

Fitzpatrick, Sheila. *Education and Social Mobility in the Soviet Union, 1921–1934*. Cambridge, UK: Cambridge University Press, 1979.

Fitzpatrick, Sheila. "Stalin and the Making of a New Elite, 1928–1939." *Slavic Review* 38, no. 3 (1979): 377–402.

Fitzpatrick, Sheila. *The Cultural Front: Power and Culture in Revolutionary Russia*. Ithaca, NY: Cornell University Press, 1992.

Fitzpatrick, Sheila. "Ascribing Class: The Construction of Social Identity in Soviet Russia." *Journal of Modern History* 65, no. 4 (1993): 745–70.

Fitzpatrick, Sheila. *Stalin's Peasants: Resistance and Survival in the Russian Village after Collectivization*. New York: Oxford University Press, 1994.

Fitzpatrick, Sheila. *Everyday Stalinism Ordinary Life in Extraordinary Times: Soviet Russia in the 1930s*. New York: Oxford University Press, 1999.

Florin, Moritz. "Beyond Colonialism? Agency, Power, and the Making of Soviet Central Asia." *Kritika: Explorations in Russian & Eurasian History* 18, no. 4 (2017): 827–38.

Fort, Christopher James. "Inhabiting Socialist Realism: Soviet Literature from the Edge of Empire." Ph.D. Diss. University of Michigan, 2019.

Fraser, Nancy. "Rethinking the Public Sphere: A Contribution to the Critique of Actually Existing Democracy." *Social Text*, no. 25/26 (1990): 56.

Fraser, Nancy, and Kate Nash. *Transnationalizing the Public Sphere*. Cambridge: Polity Press, 2014.

Frolova-Walker, Marina. "'National in Form, Socialist in Content': Musical Nation-Building in the Soviet Republics." *Journal of the American Musicological Society* 51, no. 2 (1998): 331–71.

Garrard, John Gordon and Carol Garrard. *Inside the Soviet Writers' Union*. New York: Free Press, 1990.

Getty, J. Arch. *Practicing Stalinism: Bolsheviks, Boyars, and the Persistence of Tradition*. New Haven: Yale University Press, 2013.

Gigova, Irina. "In Defense of Native Literature: Writers' Associations, State and the Cult of the Writer in Pre-1945 Bulgaria." *Slavic Review* 77, no. 2 (2018): 417–40.

Goff, Krista A. *Nested Nationalism: Making and Unmaking Nations in the Soviet Caucasus*. Ithaca, NY: Cornell University Press, 2021.

Goldman, Wendy Z. *Terror and Democracy in the Age of Stalin: The Social Dynamics of Repression*. New York: Cambridge University Press, 2007.

Golombek, Lisa. "The Gardens of Timur: New Perspectives." *Muqarnas* 12 (1995): 137–47.

Gordon, Stewart, ed. *Robes of Honour: Khil'at in Pre-Colonial and Colonial India*. New Delhi: Oxford University Press, 2003.

Gorham, Michael S. "Tongue-Tied Writers: The Rabsel'kor Movement and the Voice of the 'New Intelligentsia' in Early Soviet Russia." *The Russian Review*, no. 3 (1996): 412–29.

Grant, Bruce. *In the Soviet House of Culture: A Century of Perestroikas*. Princeton, NJ: Princeton University Press, 1995.

Grant, Bruce. *The Captive and the Gift: Cultural Histories of Sovereignty in Russia and the Caucasus*. Ithaca, NY: Cornell University Press, 2016.

Günther, Hans, and Evgenii Dobrenko, eds. *Sotsrealisticheskii kanon*. Akademicheskii Proekt, 2000.

Habermas, Jürgen. *The Structural Transformation of the Public Sphere: An Inquiry into a Category of Bourgeois Society*. Cambridge, MA.: The MIT Press, 1991.

Halfin, Igal. *Red Autobiographies: Initiating the Bolshevik Self*. Seattle: University of Washington Press, 2011.

Halfin, Igal, and Jochen Hellbeck. "Rethinking the Stalinist Subject: Stephen Kotkin's 'Magnetic Mountain' and the State of Soviet Historical Studies," *Jahrbücher Für Geschichte Osteuropas*, 44, no. 3 (1996): 456–63.

Hall, Stuart, Dorothy Hobson, Andrew Lowe, and Paul Willis, eds. *Culture, Media, Language: Working Papers in Cultural Studies, 1972–79*. London: Routledge, 1991.

Hattox, Ralph S. *Coffee and Coffeehouses: The Origins of a Social Beverage in the Medieval Near East*. Seattle: University of Washington Press, 1988.

Haugen, Arne. *The Establishment of National Republics in Soviet Central Asia*. Basingstoke, Hampshire: Palgrave Macmillan, 2003.

Hellbeck, Jochen. *Revolution on My Mind: Writing a Diary under Stalin*. Cambridge, MA: Harvard University Press, 2006.

Hirsch, Francine. *Empire of Nations: Ethnographic Knowledge and the Making of the Soviet Union*, Culture and Society after Socialism. Ithaca, NY: Cornell University Press, 2005.

Hodgkin, Samuel. *Persianate Verse and the Poetics of Eastern Internationalism*. Cambridge, UK: Cambridge University Press, 2024.

Hodgkin, Samuel. "Revolutionary Springtimes: Reading Soviet Persian Poetry, from Ghazal to Lyric." In *Iranian Languages and Literatures of Central Asia: From the Eighteenth Century to the Present*. Edited by M. De Chiara. Paris: Peeters, 2015.

Hodgkin, Samuel. "Soviet Persian Anthologies: Transnational, Multinational, International." *Iranian Studies* 55, no. 3 (2022): 631–51.

Hoffmann, David L. *Cultivating the Masses: Modern State Practices and Soviet Socialism, 1914–1939*. Ithaca, NY: Cornell University Press, 2011.

Hölscher, Lucian. "Publichnost'/ glasnost'/ publichnaia sfera/ obshchestvennost' (Öffentlichkeit)." In *Slovar' osnovnykh istoricheskikh poniatii: Izbrannye stat'i*. Edited by D. Sdvizhkov and I. Shirle, Vol. 1. Moscow: Novoe literaturnoe obozrenie, 2014.

Holt, Katharine. "Performing as Soviet Central Asia's Source Texts: Lahuti and Džambul in Moscow, 1935–1936." *Cahiers d'Asie Centrale* 24 (2015): 213–38.

Iakubov, N. *Publitsisticheskaia deiatel'nost' Abdully Kakhkhara: avtoreferat dissertatsii*. Tashkent: TashGU, 1970.

Iashin, Komil. *Istoriia uzbekskoi sovetskoi literatury v piati tomakh, 1917–1985*. Tashkent: Fan, 1987.

İğmen, Ali F. *Speaking Soviet with an Accent: Culture and Power in Kyrgyzstan*. Central Eurasia in Context. Pittsburgh, PA: University of Pittsburgh Press, 2012.

Il'ina, I. N. *Obshchestvennye organizatsii Rossii v 1920-e gody*. Moscow: Institut rossiiskoi istorii RAN, 2000.

Inglis, Fred. *A Short History of Celebrity*. Princeton, NJ: Princeton University Press, 2010.

Ishankhodzhaeva, Zamira Raiimovna. "Repressivnaia politika sovetskoi vlasti i ee vozdeistvie na kul'turnuiu zhizn' uzbekistana (1925–1950 gg)." Dissertation. Republic of Uzbekistan Academy of Sciences, Institute of History, 2012.

Jabbari, Alexander. *The Making of Persianate Modernity: Language and Literary History between Iran and India*. Cambridge, UK: Cambridge University Press, 2023.

Jameson, Fredric. "Third-World Literature in the Era of Multinational Capitalism," *Social Text* Autumn, no. 15 (1986): 65–88.

Kaganovsky, Lilya. *How the Soviet Man Was Unmade: Cultural Fantasy and Male Subjectivity under Stalin*. Pittsburgh, PA: University of Pittsburgh Press, 2008.

Kamp, Marianne. *Collectivization Generation: Oral Histories of a Social Revolution in Uzbekistan*. Ithaca, NY: Cornell University Press, 2024.

Kamp, Marianne. "Debating Sharia: The 1917 Muslim Women's Congress in Russia." *Journal of Women's History* 27, no. 4 (2015): 13–37.

Kamp, Marianne. "Femicide as Terrorism: The Case of Uzbekistan's Unveiling Murders," in *Belief and Bloodshed: Religion and Violence across Time and Tradition*, edited by James K. Wellman. Lanham, Md.: Rowman & Littlefield, 2007.

Kamp, Marianne. "Hunger and Potatoes: The 1933 Famine in Uzbekistan and Changing Foodways," *Kritika: Explorations in Russian & Eurasian History*, 20, no. 2 (2019): 237–67.

Kamp, Marianne. *The New Woman in Uzbekistan: Islam, Modernity, and Unveiling under Communism*. Jackson School Publications in International Studies. Seattle: University of Washington Press, 2006.

Kamp, Marianne. "Pilgrimage and Performance: Uzbek Women and the Imagining of Uzbekistan in the 1920s," *International Journal of Middle East Studies*, 34, no. ii (2002): 263–78.

Kamp, Marianne R. "Three Lives of Saodat: Communist, Uzbek, Survivor," *The Oral History Review*, 28, no. 2 (2001): 21–58.

Kaplan, Isabelle R. "Comrades in Arts: The Soviet Dekada of National Art and the Friendship of Peoples." *RUDN Journal of Russian History* 19, no. 1 (2020): 78–94.

Kaplan, Vera. *Historians and Historical Societies in the Public Life of Imperial Russia*. Bloomington, IN: Indiana University Press, 2017.

Kari-Iakubova, E. *Mukhitdin Kari-Iakubov: Ocherk zhizni i tvorchestva*. Izdatel'stvo khudozhestvennoi literatury im. Gafura Guliama, 1968.

Karimov, Naim. *XX asr adabiyoti manzaralari*. Toshkent: O'zbekiston, 2008.

Karimov, Naim. *Adabiyot va tarixiy jarayon*. Tashkent: Mumtoz So'z, 2013.

Karomatov, Faizulla. *O'zbek musiqasi sovet davrida*. Tashkent: O'zbekiston KP MKning nashriyoti, 1967.

Kary-Niiazov, Tashmukhamed Niiazovich. *Ocherki istorii kul'tury Sovetskogo Uzbekistana*. Moskva: Akademiia nauk SSSR, 1955.

Kassymbekova, Botakoz. *Despite Cultures: Early Soviet Rule in Tajikistan*. Pittsburgh, PA: University of Pittsburgh Press, 2016.

Kassymbekova, Botakoz, and Aminat Chokobaeva. "On Writing Soviet History of Central Asia: Frameworks, Challenges, Prospects." *Central Asian Survey* 40, no. 4 (2021): 483–503.

Kedrina, Z. S., and S. Kasymov. *Istoriia uzbekskoi sovetskoi literatury*. Moscow: Nauka, 1967.

Keller, Shoshana. *To Moscow, Not Mecca: The Soviet Campaign against Islam in Central Asia, 1917–1941*. Westport, CT.: Praeger, 2001.

Kelly, Catriona, and David Shepherd. *Constructing Russian Culture in the Age of Revolution, 1881–1940*. Oxford: Oxford University Press, 1998.

Khalid, Adeeb. *Central Asia: A New History from the Imperial Conquests to the Present*. Princeton, NJ: Princeton University Press, 2021.

Khalid, Adeeb. "The Historiography of Modern Central Asia Today." *Kritika: Explorations in Russian and Eurasian History* 26, no. 1 (2025): 91–108.

Khalid, Adeeb. *Making Uzbekistan: Nation, Empire, and Revolution in the Early USSR*. Ithaca, NY: Cornell University Press, 2015.

Khalid, Adeeb. *The Politics of Muslim Cultural Reform: Jadidism in Central Asia*. Berkeley: University of California Press, 1999.

Khalid, Adeeb. "Printing, Publishing, and Reform in Tsarist Central Asia," *International Journal of Middle East Studies*, 26, no. 2 (1994): 187–200.

Kharkhordin, Oleg. *The Collective and the Individual in Russia: A Study of Practices*. Berkeley, CA: University of California Press, 1999.

Khazanov, Anatoly M. *Nomads and the Outside World*. Madison: University of Wisconsin Press, 1994.

Khushbekov, A. *Iz istorii kul'turnogo stroitel'stva v Uzbekistane v gody pervoi piatiletki*. Samarkand: Sredneaziatskii gosudarstvennyi universitet imeni Lenina, 1959.

Kia, Mana. *Persianate Selves: Memories of Place and Origin before Nationalism*. Stanford, CA: Stanford University Press, 2020.

Kiaer, Christina. *Collective Body: Aleksandr Deineka at the Limit of Socialist Realism*. Chicago: The University of Chicago Press, 2024.

Kılıç-Schubel, Nurten. "Writing Women: Women's Poetry and Literary Networks in Nineteenth-Century Central Asia." In *Horizons of the World: Festschrift for Isenbike Togan*. Edited by Nurten Kılıç-Schubel and Evrim Bimbaş. Istanbul: İthakı, 2011, 405–42.

Kirasirova, Masha. "The 'East' as a Category of Bolshevik Ideology and Comintern Administration: The Arab Section of the Communist University of the Toilers of the East," *Kritika: Explorations in Russian and Eurasian History*, 18, no. 1 (2017): 7–34.

Kivelson, Valerie A., and Ronald Grigor Suny. *Russia's Empires*. Oxford: Oxford University Press, 2016.

Kligman, Gail, and Katherine Verdery. *Peasants under Siege : The Collectivization of Romanian Agriculture, 1949–1962*. Princeton University Press, 2011.

Kluge, Alexander, and Oskar Negt. *Public Sphere and Experience: Analysis of the Bourgeois and Proletarian Public Sphere*. New York: Verso Books, 2016.

Kondrat'eva, Tamara. *Kormit' i pravit': o vlasti v Rossii XVI-XX vv*. Moscow: ROSSPEN, 2006.

Koshchanov, Matiakub. "Pisatel' dvukh literatur," in *Shchedrost' talanta: stat'i ob uzbekskoi literature*. Moscow: Sovetskii Pisatel', 1980.

Kotkin, Stephen. *Magnetic Mountain: Stalinism as a Civilization*. Berkeley: University of California Press, 1995.

Kotkin, Stephen. "Modern Times: The Soviet Union and the Interwar Conjuncture," *Kritika: Explorations in Russian and Eurasian History* 2, no. 1 (2001): 111–64.

Krylova, Anna. "The Tenacious Liberal Subject in Soviet Studies." *Kritika: Explorations in Russian and Eurasian History* 1, no. 1 (2000): 119–46.

Krylova, Anna. "Soviet Modernity: Stephen Kotkin and the Bolshevik Predicament." *Contemporary European History* 23, no. 2 (2014): 167.

Krylova, Anna. "Imagining Socialism in the Soviet Century." *Social History* 42, no. 3 (2017): 315–41.

Kunakhovich, Kyrill. *Communism's Public Sphere: Culture as Politics in Cold War Poland and East Germany*. Ithaca, NY: Cornell University Press, 2023.

Lahusen, Thomas. *How Life Writes the Book: Real Socialism and Socialist Realism in Stalin's Russia*. Ithaca, NY: Cornell University Press, 1997.

Latour, Bruno. *Reassembling the Social: An Introduction to Actor-Network-Theory*. Oxford: Oxford University Press, 2005.

Latypov, Alisher. "The Opium War at the 'Root of the World': The 'Elimination' of Addiction in Soviet Badakhshan." *Central Asian Survey* 32, no. 1 (2013): 19–36.

Latypov, Alisher. "Choikhonai Surkh: The Replacement of 'Opium Dens' with Red Teahouses and the Limits of the Soviet Enlightenment Project in Tajikistan." *Central Asian Affairs* 7, no. 3 (September 2020): 236–66.

Lenoe, Matthew E. *Closer to the Masses: Stalinist Culture, Social Revolution, and Soviet Newspapers*. Cambridge, MA.: Harvard University Press, 2004.

Levi, Scott C. *The Rise and Fall of Khoqand, 1709–1876: Central Asia in the Global Age*. Pittsburgh, PA: University of Pittsburgh Press, 2017.

Levi, Scott Cameron. *The Indian Diaspora in Central Asia and Its Trade, 1550–1900*. Leiden: Brill, 2002.

Levin, Theodore. *The Hundred Thousand Fools of God: Musical Travels in Central Asia (and Queens, New York)*. Bloomington, IN: Indiana University Press, 1996.

Levin, Theodore Craig, Saida Daukeeva, and Elmira Köchümkülova, eds. *The Music of Central Asia*. Bloomington: Indiana University Press, 2016.

Levin, Zeev. *Collectivization and Social Engineering: Soviet Administration and the Jews of Uzbekistan, 1917-1939*. Leiden: Brill, 2015.

Lewin, Moshe. *Russian Peasants and Soviet Power: A Study of Collectivization*. Evanston, IL: Northwestern University Press, 1968.

Loy, Thomas. "Rise and Fall: Bukharan Jewish Literature of the 1920s and 1930s." In *Iranian Languages and Literatures of Central Asia: From the Eighteenth Century to the Present*. Edited by M. De Chiara. Paris: Peeters, 2015.

Mahmood, Saba. *Politics of Piety: The Islamic Revival and the Feminist Subject*. Princeton University Press, 2012.
Mahmudov, Madirim. *Barhayot siymolar: qatag'on qurbonlari haqida lavhalar*. Tashkent: O'zbekiston, 1991.
Malikov, A. M. "The Russian Conquest of the Bukharan Emirate: Military and Diplomatic Aspects." *Central Asian Survey* 33, no. 2 (2014): 180–98.
Mansurbekova, Feruza. "Unisondan polifoniya sari: O'zbek xor san'ati tarixi." *Guliston*, no. 4 (2014): 38–9.
Martin, Terry. *The Affirmative Action Empire: Nations and Nationalism in the Soviet Union, 1923–1939*. Ithaca, NY: Cornell University Press, 2001.
Massell, Gregory J. *The Surrogate Proletariat: Moslem Women and Revolutionary Strategies in Soviet Central Asia, 1919–1929*. Princeton, NJ: Princeton University Press, 1974.
Matsui, Yasuhiro, ed. *Obshchestvennost' and Civic Agency in Late Imperial and Soviet Russia: Interface between State and Society*. Houndmills, Basingstoke, Hampshire: Palgrave Macmillan, 2015.
Matthee, Rudi. "From Coffee to Tea: Shifting Patterns of Consumption in Qajar Iran." *Journal of World History* 7, no. 2 (1996): 199–230.
Matthee, Rudolph P. *The Pursuit of Pleasure: Drugs and Stimulants in Iranian History, 1500–1900*. Princeton, NJ: Princeton University Press, 2005.
Matyakubov, Otanazar. "Nineteenth Century Khorezmian Tanbur Notation: Fixing Music in an Oral Tradition." Translated by Harold Powers. *Yearbook for Traditional Music* 22 (1990): 29–35.
Mazzarella, William. *Censorium: Cinema and the Open Edge of Mass Publicity*. Durham, NC: Duke University Press, 2013.
Mazzarella, William. "A Torn Performative Dispensation: The Affective Politics of British Second World War Propaganda in India and the Problem of Legitimation in an Age of Mass Publics," *South Asian History and Culture*, 1, no. 1 (2009): 1–24.
McChesney, Robert Duncan. "'Barrier of Heterodoxy'? Rethinking the Ties between Iran and Central Asia in the 17th Century." In *Safavid Persia: The History and Politics of an Islamic Society*. Edited by C. Melville. London: I. B. Tauris, 1996.
Meeker, Michael. "Civil Society: Coffeehouses and Cooperatives." In *A Nation of Empire: The Ottoman Legacy of Turkish Modernity*. Berkeley: University of California Press, 2002.
Merchant, Tanya. *Women Musicians of Uzbekistan from Courtyard to Conservatory*. Urbana, IL: University of Illinois Press, 2015.
Michaels, Paula A. *Curative Powers: Medicine and Empire in Stalin's Central Asia*. Pittsburgh, PA: University of Pittsburgh Press, 2003.
Miller, Frank J. *Folklore for Stalin: Russian Folklore and Pseudofolklore of the Stalin Era*. Armonk, N.Y.: M.E. Sharpe, 1990.
Millward, James A. *Eurasian Crossroads: A History of Xinjiang*. New York: Columbia University Press, 2007.
Mirzaev, I. *Puti razvitiia uzbekskoi realisticheskoi prozy*. Tashkent: Fan, 1984.
Mirzaev, Saidulla. *Oydin: adabiy portret*. Tashkent: "Tashkent" Badiiy adabiyot nashriyoti, 1965.
Morrison, Alexander. "After the War: Central Asia without Russia," *SICE Blog* (blog), October 24, 2022. http://www.oeaw.ac.at/sice/sice-blog/after-the-war-central-asia-without-russia (accessed May 9, 2025).
Morrison, Alexander. *The Russian Conquest of Central Asia: A Study in Imperial Expansion, 1814–1914*. Cambridge: Cambridge University Press, 2021.
Morrison, Alexander. *Russian Rule in Samarkand, 1868–1910: A Comparison with British India*. Oxford: Oxford University Press, 2008.
Morrison, Alexander, Cloé Drieu, and Aminat Chokobaeva, eds. *The Central Asian Revolt of 1916: A Collapsing Empire in the Age of War and Revolution*. Manchester: Manchester University Press, 2019.
Naiman, Eric. *Sex in Public: The Incarnation of Early Soviet Ideology*. Princeton, NJ: Princeton University Press, 1999.

Nalivkin, Vladimir Petrovich, and Mariia Vladimirovna Nalivkina. *Muslim Women of the Fergana Valley: A 19th-Century Ethnography from Central Asia*. Translated by Marianne Kamp and Mariana Markova. Bloomington, IN: Indiana University Press, 2016.

Nazarova, Saodat. "XX asrning 20–30 yillaridagi O'zbek sahna san'ati rivojida Muhiddin Qori Yoqubovning o'rni." *O'zMU Xabarlari*, special issue (2013).

Northrop, Douglas. *Veiled Empire: Gender & Power in Stalinist Central Asia*. Ithaca, NY: Cornell University Press, 2004.

Nuritov, A. N. "Rabota politotdelov MTS uzbekistana sredi sel'skoi molodezhi (1933–1934 gody)." *Nauchnye trudy (TashGU)*, no. 281 (1966): 97–103.

Obertreis, Julia. *Imperial Desert Dreams: Cotton Growing and Irrigation in Central Asia 1860–1991*. Göttingen: V&R, 2017.

O'Keeffe, Brigid. *New Soviet Gypsies : Nationality, Performance, and Selfhood in the Early Soviet Union*. Toronto: University of Toronto Press, 2013.

Osokina, Elena A. *Ierarkhiia potrebleniia: o zhizni liudei v usloviiakh stalinskogo snabzheniia, 1928–1935 gg*. Moscow: Izdatel'stvo MGOU, 1993.

Öztürk, Serdar. "The Struggle over Turkish Village Coffeehouses (1923–45)." *Middle Eastern Studies* 44, no. 3 (2008): 435–54.

Penati, Beatrice. "Notes on the Birth of Russian Turkestan's Fiscal System: A View from the Fergana Oblast'." *Journal of the Economic & Social History of the Orient* 53, no. 5 (2010): 739–69.

Penati, Beatrice. *Rural History of Soviet Central Asia: Land Reform and Agricultural Change in Early Soviet Uzbekistan*. Leiden: Brill, 2025.

Peterson, Maya K. *Pipe Dreams: Water and Empire in Central Asia's Aral Sea Basin*. Cambridge: Cambridge University Press, 2019.

Platt, Kevin M. F. *Border Conditions: Russian-Speaking Latvians between World Orders*. Ithaca, NY: Cornell University Press, 2024.

Platt, Kevin M. F., and David Brandenberger, eds. *Epic Revisionism: Russian History and Literature as Stalinist Propaganda*. Madison: University of Wisconsin Press, 2006.

Pulatov, Kh. *Kul'turno-vospitatel'naia deiatel'nost' sovetskogo gosudarstva v uzbekistane*. Tashkent: Gosudarstvennoe izdatel'stvo uzbekskoi SSR, 1959.

Qo'chqorov, Rahmon. "Uch 'Sarob.'" in *Iste'dod qadri*. Tashkent: G'ofur G'ulom nomidagi Adabiyot va san'at nashriyoti, 1989.

Qoriyev, Bois. "Adabiy taxalluslar haqida." *O'zbek tili va adabiyoti*, no. 1 (1967): 51–8.

Qo'shjonov, Matyoqub. *Abdulla Qahhor mahorati*. Tashkent: G'ofur G'ulom nomidagi adabiyot va san'at nashriyoti, 1988.

Qo'shjonov, Matyoqub. *Ayniy badiiyatining evolyutsiyasi*. Tashkent: Fan, 1988.

Qurbonova, Habiba. *Husayn Shams arxivi katalogi*. O'zbekiston SSR davlat fanlar akademiyasi: H. S. Sulaymonov nomidagi qo'lyozmalar instituti, 1987.

Rafael, Vicente L. *Contracting Colonialism Translation and Christian Conversion in Tagalog Society under Early Spanish Rule*. Ithaca, NY: Cornell University Press, 1988.

Rakhmatullaev, A. *Proza Aini*. Dushanbe: Irfon, 1970.

Ramsay, Rebekah. "Nomadic Hearths of Soviet Culture: 'Women's Red Yurt' Campaigns in Kazakhstan, 1925–1935." *Europe-Asia Studies* 73, no. 10 (2021): 1937–61.

Roberts, Flora. "A Time for Feasting? Autarky in the Tajik Ferghana Valley at War, 1941–45." *Central Asian Survey* 36, no. 1 (2017): 37–54.

Roberts, Flora J. "Old Elites Under Communism: Soviet Rule in Leninobod." Ph.D. Diss., Chicago, University of Chicago, 2016.

Rolf, Malte. *Soviet Mass Festivals, 1917–1991*. Pittsburgh: University of Pittsburgh Press, 2013.

Roosien, Claire. "Not by Archives Alone: The 'Revolution' in Soviet Central Asian Literary Studies." *Iranian Studies* 55, no. 3 (2022): 777–85.

Sahadeo, Jeff. *Russian Colonial Society in Tashkent, 1865–1923*. Bloomington, IN: Indiana University Press, 2007.

Sartori, Paolo. *Visions of Justice: Sharia and Cultural Change in Russian Central Asia*. Leiden: Brill, 2016.

Schild, Kathryn Douglas. "Between Moscow and Baku: National Literatures at the 1934 Congress of Soviet Writers." Ph.D. Diss. University of California, Berkeley, 2010.

Scott, Joan W. "Gender: A Useful Category of Historical Analysis." *The American Historical Review* 91, no. 5 (1986): 1053–75.

Shao, Qin. "Tempest over Teapots: The Vilification of Teahouse Culture in Early Republican China." *The Journal of Asian Studies* 57, no. 4 (1998): 1009–41.

Sharafiddinov, Ozod. *Abdulla Qahhor*. Tashkent: Yosh Gvardiia, 1988.

Shaw, Claire L. *Deaf in the USSR: Marginality, Community, and Soviet Identity, 1917–1991*. Ithaca, NY: Cornell University Press, 2017.

Shaw, Charles D. "The Many Nationalities of Tamara Khanum: Friendship of the Peoples at Home, Abroad, and Within." *The Russian Review* 82, no. 3 (2023): 433–52.

Shelekpayev, Nari. "Govorit' so stisnutymi zubami: styd, vlast' i zhenskoe telo v sovremennom Kazakhstane." *Novoe literaturnoe obozrenie*, no. 161 (1/ 2020): 157–74.

Shelekpayev, Nari. "Thinking beyond Soviet Teleologies: Perspectives for the Study of Central Asia." *Kritika: Explorations in Russian and Eurasian History* 26, no. 1 (2025): 133–59.

Shigabdinov, Renat. "Shefskoe dvizhenie v Uzbekistane v literature 20-x godov," *Obshchestvennye nauki v uzbekistane*, vol. 1, no. 12 (1990): 44–5.

Shin, Boram. "National Form and Socialist Content: Soviet Modernization and Making of Uzbek National Opera between the 1920s and 1930s." *Interventions* 19, no. 3 (2017): 416–33.

Shissler, Ada Holland. "Beauty Is Nothing to Be Ashamed Of: Beauty Contests As Tools of Women's Liberation in Early Republican Turkey." *Comparative Studies of South Asia, Africa and the Middle East* 24, no. 1 (2004): 107–22.

Shissler, Ada Holland. "'If You Ask Me': Sabiha Sertel's Advice Column, Gender Equity, and Social Engineering in the Early Turkish Republic." *Journal of Middle East Women's Studies* 3, no. 2 (2007): 1.

Shissler, Ada Holland. "Womanhood Is Not for Sale: Sabiha Zekeriya Sertel Against Prostitution and for Women's Employment." *Journal of Middle East Women's Studies* 4, no. 3 (2008): 12.

Siegelbaum, Lewis H. *Stakhanovism and the Politics of Productivity in the USSR, 1935–1941*. Cambridge: Cambridge University Press, 1988.

Şimşek, Sefa. *Bir ideolojik seferberlik deneyimi: Halkevleri 1932–1951*. İstanbul: Boğaziçi Üniversitesi Yayınevi, 2002.

Şimşek, Sefa. "'People's Houses' as a Nationwide Project for Ideological Mobilization in Early Republican Turkey." *Turkish Studies* 6, no. 1 (2005): 71–91.

Skakov, Nariman. "Eisenstein in Fergana: From Avant-Garde to National Form," *Studies in Russian and Soviet Cinema*, 15, no. 1 (2021): 23–38.

Skakov, Nariman. *Reorientalism: From Avant-Garde to Soviet National Form*. New York: Columbia University Press, 2025.

Smirnova, V. "Abdulla Kakhkhar iz ferganskoi doliny," *Druzhba narodov*, no. 7 (1963): 258–68.

Stites, Richard. *Russian Popular Culture: Entertainment and Society since 1900*. Cambridge: Cambridge University Press, 1992.

Sukhareva, Ol'ga. *Istoriia sredneaziatskogo kostiuma (2-ia polovina XIX-nachalo XX v.)*. Moscow: Nauka, 1982.

Sultonova, Mashhura. *O'zbek sovet adibalari*. Tashkent: "Qizil O'zbekiston," "Pravda Vostoka," and "O'zbekistoni Surkh" birlashgan nashriyoti va bosmaxonasi, 1963.

Suyarkulova, Mohira. "Fashioning the Nation: Gender and Politics of Dress in Contemporary Kyrgyzstan," *Nationalities Papers*, 44, no. 2 (2016): 247–65.

Thompson, E. P. "Time, Work-Discipline, and Industrial Capitalism," *Past & Present*, no. 38 (1967): 56–97.

Tlostanova, Madina. *Dekolonial'nost' bytiia, znaniia i oshchushcheniia: sbornik statei*. Almaty: Tselinnyi, 2020.

Tursunova, Husniya. *Tadqiqi muqoisavii frazeologizmhoi paralleli zabonhoi tojiki va uzbeki (dar asosi asari S. Ainii Ghulomon/Qullar)*. Dushanbe: Donish, 1979.

Valdivieso, Erika. "Searching for Dido in the Latin Epics of Colonial Mexico." *TAPA*, 154, no. 2 (2024): 537–76.

Vatlin, Alexander. *Agents of Terror Ordinary Men and Extraordinary Violence in Stalin's Secret Police*. Translated and edited by Seth Bernstein. Madison, WI: The University of Wisconsin Press, 2016.

Vejdani, Farzin. *Making History in Iran: Education, Nationalism, and Print Culture*. Stanford, CA: Stanford University Press, 2015.

Viola, Lynne. *Peasant Rebels under Stalin Collectivization and the Culture of Peasant Resistance*. New York: Oxford University Press, 1996.

Volkov, Vadim. "Obshchestvennost': Russia's Lost Concept of Civil Society." In *Civil Society in the Baltic Sea Region*. Edited by Norbert Götz and Jörg Hackmann. Aldershot, Hants, England: Ashgate, 2003.

La Vopa, Anthony J. "Conceiving a Public: Ideas and Society in Eighteenth-Century Europe." In *Enlightenment Past and Present: Essays in a Social History of Ideas*. Liverpool: Liverpool University Press, 2022.

Vyzgo, T. S., I. N. Karelova, and F. M. Karomatov, eds. *Istoriia Uzbekskoi Sovetskoi Muzyki*. Vol. 1. 2 vols. Tashkent: G'ofur G'ulom nomidagi Adabiyot va san'at nashriyoti, 1972.

Wang, Di. *The Teahouse: Small Business, Everyday Culture, and Public Politics in Chengdu, 1900–1950*. Stanford, CA.: Stanford University Press, 2008.

Wang, Di. *The Teahouse under Socialism: The Decline and Renewal of Public Life in Chengdu, 1950–2000*. Ithaca, NY: Cornell University Press, 2018.

Warner, Michael. *Publics and Counterpublics*. New York: Zone Books, 2002.

Welsford, Thomas. "Becoming Behbudiy." *Journal of Central Asian History* 1 (2022): 37–99.

Widdis, Emma. *Socialist Senses : Film, Feeling, and the Soviet Subject, 1917–1940*. Bloomington, IN: Indiana University Press, 2017.

Wilde, Andreas. *What Is beyond the River?: Power, Authority, and Social Order in Transoxania 18th-19th Centuries*. Vienna: Verlag der Österreichischen Akademie der Wissenschaften, 2016.

Wilson, Jennifer. "Queer Harlem, Queer Tashkent: Langston Hughes's 'Boy Dancers of Uzbekistan,'" *Slavic Review*, 76, no. 3 (2017): 637–46.

Yılmaz, Hale. *Becoming Turkish: Nationalist Reforms and Cultural Negotiations in Early Republican Turkey, 1923–1945*. Syracuse, NY: Syracuse University Press, 2013.

Yunusov, Ravshan. "Qo'shiqmi yo ashula?" *Guliston*, no. 2 (1997): 26–8.

Yurchak, Alexei. *Everything Was Forever until It Was No More: The Last Soviet Generation*. Princeton: Princeton University Press, 2013.

Zahra, Tara. "Imagined Noncommunities: National Indifference as a Category of Analysis." *Slavic Review* 69, no. 1 (2010): 93–119.

Zekhni, Malika. "Invisible Bodies: Civilising Mission, Sexuality, and Prostitution in Fin de Siècle Russian Turkestan." *Cultural and Social History* 19, no. 2 (2022): 141–59.

Ziad, Waleed. *Hidden Caliphate: Sufi Saints beyond the Oxus and Indus*. Cambridge, MA: Harvard University Press, 2021.

Index

For the benefit of digital users, indexed terms that span two pages (e.g., 52–53) may, on occasion, appear on only one of those pages.